The History of Cancer

Recent Titles in
Bibliographies and Indexes in Medical Studies

Federal Information Sources in Health and Medicine: A Selected
Annotated Bibliography
Mary Glen Chitty, compiler, with the assistance of Natalie Schatz

Viruses and Reproduction: A Bibliography
Ernest L. Abel, compiler

The History of Cancer

AN ANNOTATED BIBLIOGRAPHY

COMPILED BY
James S. Olson

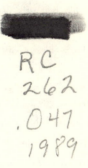

BIBLIOGRAPHIES AND INDEXES IN MEDICAL STUDIES,
NUMBER 3

Greenwood Press
New York • Westport, Connecticut • London

Library of Congress Cataloging-in-Publication Data

Olson, James Stuart, 1946-
   The history of cancer : an annotated bibliography / compiled by
James S. Olson.
      p   cm.—(Bibliographies and indexes in medical studies,
   ISSN 0896-6591 ; no. 3)
   Includes index.
   ISBN 0-313-25889-9 (lib. bdg. : alk. paper)
   1. Cancer—History—Abstracts. 2. Cancer—History—Bibliography.
   I. Title. II. Series.
   [DNLM: 1. Neoplasms—history—abstracts.   ZQZ 200 052h]
   RC262.O47   1989
   616.99'4'009—dc20
   DNLM/DLC
   for Library of Congress   89-2174

British Library Cataloguing in Publication Data is available.

Library of Congress Catalog Card Number: 89-2174
ISBN: 0-313-25889-9
ISSN: 0896-6591

First published in 1989

Greenwood Press, Inc.
88 Post Road West, Westport, Connecticut 06881

Printed in the United States of America

∞

The paper used in this book complies with the
Permanent Paper Standard issued by the National
Information Standards Organization (Z39.48-1984).

10 9 8 7 6 5 4 3 2 1

1-26-90

Contents

Preface

This project began inauspiciously eight years ago while I was getting a 100–rad dose of electrons from a megavoltage external beam radiation machine at the M. D. Anderson Hospital and Tumor Institute in Houston, Texas. Physicians had removed a lump from my left hand and diagnosed it as an epithelioid sarcoma, a rare and dangerous cancer of the soft tissues. Over the next seven years, I had three surgeries on the hand and 70 radiation treatments—nearly 13,000 rads, all to no avail. The tumor kept recurring and last year surgeons at the hospital performed what they called "radical surgery"—amputation of my left arm and a lymph node dissection in the axilla under my arm.

What does a historian think about while all this is happening? What were they doing to me? What did all the terms mean: "lymph node dissection," "en bloc resection," "biopsy," "wide excision," "bone scan," "liver scan," "blood count," "rads," "cobalt," "electrons," "neutrons," "linear accelerators," and "chemotherapy"? So I decided to read and research, partly because my curiousity was stimulated and partly just to make some sense out of what was going on. My focus became the history of cancer, actually of the more than 100 diseases which are considered cancer. The book is an annotated bibliography of that topic—the history of cancer.

At the outset, I had no idea about the vastness of the literature. Although the underdeveloped world's preoccupation with cancer still lags, primarily because infectious diseases are still their main killers, cancer has become a major health concern of the developed world, where it is the second leading cause of death. In more than 400 pages, I have described the contents of nearly 3,000 articles, most of which were written since 1945.

To locate articles in the literature, I used a variety of research devices, but especially the National Library of Medicine's annual "Bibliography of the History of Medicine." Its section on "Neoplastic Disease" lists articles from scientists and scholars all over the world. Although most of the articles included in The History of Cancer: An Annotated Bibliography were published in American, British, French, German, Italian, and Soviet journals, there are also annotated citations from Polish, Spanish, Mexican, Portuguese, Romanian, Swedish, German, Belgian, Japanese, Chinese, Indian, Australian, New Zealand, Argentinian, Canadian, Irish, Dutch, Hungarian, and Czechoslovakian journals.

There are a few points the reader should know about the book. I tried to divide the book into sections and chapters based on the way physicians and oncologists actually approach the disease. Discrepancies in dates and the spelling of names appear in several places throughout The History of Cancer. For the most part, I accepted the dates and spellings which the authors of the books and articles used. I made no attempt to reconcile or correct them. When one article covered essentially the same ground as another, I simply cross-referenced it to the description of a very similar article. That I described in full the contents of one article and only cross-referenced another does not mean that the one article was better than the other; I just encountered the cross-referenced articles at a later point in my own research.

As you can imagine, I am indebted to a number of people for their assistance in the project. Judy Olson, Susan Olson, Edgar Wolferts, Witold Lukaszewski, and Barry Hayes all helped me translate materials from languages I cannot read. A grant from the Research Council of Sam Houston State University provided me with released time and computer time to develop the project. Librarians at the Newton Gresham Library of Sam Houston State University, particularly Shirley Parotti, did yeoman service in locating and borrowing materials from some very obscure journals. Finally, Cindy Neal and Lynda Harp went beyond the call of duty in preparing the final manuscript for printing.

James S. Olson
Huntsville, Texas

I HISTORICAL BACKGROUND

1 General Histories

Abram, Harry S. "The Psychology of Terminal Illness as Portrayed in Solzhenitsyn's 'The Cancer Ward'." *Archives of Internal Medicine*, 124 (December 1969), 758-60.

Although Alexander Solzhenitsyn's work is marvelous social and political commentary, it is also an accurate portrayal of the psychology of terminal illness. The patients described in the novel at first express denial that they are suffering from cancer, often lose their identity in dehumanized hospital settings, frequently fear surgical mutilations and their sexual implications, and worry if there will ever be an end to the treatments, if they ever will be cured of cancer.

Ackernecht, E. H. "Zur Geschichte der Krebsbehandlung." *Gesnerus*, 37 (1980), 189-97.

(See Chapter 1: Gallucci and Chapter 1: Kardinal and Yarbro).

Almast, S. C. "Historical and Evolutionary Notes on Cancer." *Punjab Medical Journal*, 11 (1962), 475-78.

(See Chapter 1: Aslam, Bano, and Vohora).

"An Historical Map of Central Europe, 1850-1900." *Cancer Bulletin*, 2 (September-October 1950), 107-09.

The map shows in portrait form the lives of Rudolf Virchow, Adolph Hannover, Ernst Wagner, Karl Thiersch, Wilhelm Waldeyer, Theodor Billroth, Alexander von Winiwarter, Richard von Volkmann, Julius Cohnheim, Wilhelm Freund, Ludwig Turck, and Johann Czermak, and briefly describes their contributions to oncology.

"An Historical Map of England and France, Featuring Persons of Importance in the Evolution of Knowledge of Cancer, 1850-1900." *Cancer Bulletin*, 2 (May-June 1950), 54-55.

The map displays in portrait form the lives of John Hughes Bennett, John Adams, Charles Moore, James Paget, Hermann Lebert, Charles Philippe Robin, Henry Thompson, Victor Horsley, Byron Bramwell, and R. H. Harrison, and briefly describes their contributions to oncology.

Aslam, M., Hassina Bano, and S. B. Bohora. "Sartan (Cancer) and Its Treatment in Unani Medicine." *The American Journal of Chinese Medicine*, 9 (1981), 95-107.

Knowledge of cancer in Unani (Greco-Arabian) systems of medicine goes back to the ancient theories of people like Hippocrates and Galen. They attributed the etiology of the disease to the combustion and imbalances of the basic humors in the body, especially an excess of "black bile." To treat the disease Unani medicine advocated a variety of natural drugs derived from mineral and vegetable products; an easily digested diet with high energy value; frequent enemas to remove the excess "humors" in the body; hot baths to remove impurities from the body; surgical excision when possible; and cauterization.

Asselin, H. G. "Cancers et cancérologues au XVIIIe siècle." *L'hopital et l'aide sociale a Paris*, 5 (1964), 629-44.

In Europe during the eighteenth century a number of individuals made important contributions to scientific understanding of cancer. Claude Gendron, the physician to the royal family in France, viewed cancer as a local, not systemic disease, amenable to surgical excision if treated early in its course. French surgeons Henri Le Dran and Jean Louis Petit advocated wide surgical excision as well as removal of regional lymph nodes, and argued that the variety of caustic pastes commonly used to treat cancer were of no use. In Lyon, Bernard Peyrilhe argued that cancer was a local disease which spread throughout the body in the lymphatic system.

Barthelme, E. "Histoire de la notion du cancer." *Histoire de science et medicine*, 15 (1981), 167-72.

(See Chapter 1: Kardinal and Yarbro).

Beliaev, I. I. "K istorii izucheniia étiologii raka Kozhi Trubochistov." *Gigiena i Sanitaria*, 6 (June 1976), 43-44.

(See Chapter 1: Kardinal and Yarbro).

Berlin, Nathaniel I. "The Conquest of Cancer." *Perspectives in Biology and Medicine*, 22 (Summer 1979), 500-18.

In recent years there have been several major eras in the history of clinical oncology and treatment. The chemotherapy era began during World War II when Leon Jacobsen at the University of Chicago noted the effect of nitrogen mustard on lymphomas, and a few years later when Sidney Farber began treating childhood leukemia with folic acid antagonists. The greatest chemotherapy success came in the 1950s when the drug methotrexate began to achieve high cure rates in treating choriocarcinoma. By the 1970s combination chemotherapy was curing or providing long-term survival for 50 percent of children with acute lymphocytic leukemia. Closely related to the chemotherapy era was the endocrine era. It began in 1895 when George Beatson reported tumor regressions in premenopausal women undergoing oophorectomy for breast cancer. In 1966 Charles Huggins received a Nobel Prize for his earlier work demonstrating the effect of hormonal manipulation (castration and adrenalectomy) in prostate cancer. The 1960s was characterized by an extensive search for steroid compounds effective in breast cancer. In the 1970s Elwood Jensen identified an estrogen receptor in some breast cancers making it possible to determine the effectiveness of hormonal manipulation in individual patients. Progestational compounds are also effective in treating women with endometrial cancer. The viral era began in 1908 when Ellerman and Bang identified the fowl leukosis virus and 1911 when Peyton Rous discovered the virus that produces sarcoma in chickens. Viral research made little progress until the 1950s when Sarah Stewart identified the polyoma virus and in the 1960s when Albert Dalton found particles in the blood of children with acute leukemia which resembled animal leukemia viral particles. The era of the environment emerged as migrant studies showed that cancer incidence among migrants resembled those of the people of their new residence. Studies in the 1960s of Japanese migrants moving from Japan to California showed that their rates of stomach cancer dropped substantially while the incidence of colorectal cancer rose, a fact consistent with the general California population. The importance of diet also came to be recognized with the work of Albert Tannebaum in the 1930s and 1940s showing that a calorically restricted diet in experimental animals resulted in a lower cancer incidence. Consumption of animal fat seemed connected to high rates of colorectal and breast cancer. The chemical carcinogenesis era began in 1775 with Percivall Pott's discovery of the relationships between exposure to soot and development of squamous cell carcinomas of the skin. Subsequent research has shown that perhaps 80 to 90 percent of cancers have an environmental origin through exposure to various chemicals and tobacco use.

Bernasconi, M., C. Carminati, and C. Tamburini. "Panaroma storico sulla patalogia del cancro. Lotta tra due vite." *Krankenpflege*, 76 (November 1983), 70-71.

(See Chapter 6: Fisher and Hermann).

Blokhin, N. N. "50 let sovetskoi onkologii." *Khirurgiia,* 43 (October 1967), 3-9.

(See Chapter 1: Blokhin and Napalkov).

Blokhin, N. N. "50 let sovetskoi onkologii." *Vestnik Meditsinskaia Nauk SSR,* 22 (1967), 3-8.

(See Chapter 1: Blokhin and Napalkov).

Blokhin, N. N. "60 let sovetskoi onkologii." *Vestnik Akademii Nauk SSR,* 12 (1977), 3-7.

(See Chapter 1: Blokhin and Napalkov).

Blokhin, N. N., and N. P. Napalkov. "Razvitie onkologii v SSSR." *Voprosy Onkologii,* 28 (1982), 3-9.

The article provides a brief survey of the history of oncology in the Soviet Union, going from the experimental research of M. A. Novinsky in the late nineteenth century to the contributions of P. A. Gertsen, N. N. Petrov, and contemporary cancer specialists.

Braun, Armin C. "History of the Tumor Problem." In *The Story of Cancer. On its Nature, Causes, and Control.* New York: 1977.

The earliest references to what later became known as cancer are found in the Ebers Papyrus, which was written in Egypt around 1500 B.C. By the time of Hippocrates (c. 400 B.C.) Greek physicians were familiar with cancers of the breast, stomach, and uterus. The Roman physician Galen (c. 160 A.D.) developed his humoral theory to explain the etiology of cancer, and his views dominated western medicine for the next 1,500 years. In 1775 Percivall Pott attributed cancer of the scrotum in chimney sweeps to the accumulation of soot on their skin. The development of microscopes in the early nineteenth century greatly accelerated scientific understanding of cancer. In 1831 Robert Brown of England discovered the cell nucleus, and in 1838 Johannes Müller proposed his theory on the cellular composition of all living tissues. In 1877 J. F. Cohnheim proposed that cancer arises from "embryonic rests" which had been misplaced during the early development of an organism. The last great scientific advances of the nineteenth century concerning cancer were the pioneering experiments on the transplantability of tumors.

Breslow, Lester. *A History of Cancer Control in the United States, 1946-1971.* Bethesda: 1977.

The major efforts at cancer control in the United States during the 25 years following World War II included the public health campaigns of the National Cancer Institute and the American Cancer Society in educating the public about the seven warning signs of cancer and the need for early diagnosis; the increasing use of the Pap smear for the early diagnosis of cervical cancer; the Surgeon General's campaign against smoking; the rise of chemotherapy as a new cancer treatment; and the development of megavoltage radiotherapy machines.

Brunner, F. G. *Pathologie und Therapie der Geschwülste in der Antiken Medizin bei Celsus and Galen.* Zürich: 1977.

Aulus Cornelius Celsus was a Roman physician who lived in the first century after Christ. He is best remembered for his extraordinary compilation of the major ideas of Greek and Alexandrian medical science. Celsus understood the notion of carcinoma, which he had learned from Greek medical writings, and he urged the use of caustic pastes and surgical excision if the lesion was at an early, superficial stage. If the lump or swelling had ulcerated, Celsus argued that treatment only irritated the tumor and hastened the onset of advanced disease and death. Clarissimus Galen lived in second century Rome, and he established the theory for the etiology of cancer which survived for more than thirteen centuries. Galen attributed cancer to an excess of black bile, one of the basic humoral fluids in human beings. For Galen there was little which could be done for cancer victims. Consistent with the medical advice of Hippocrates, Galen argued that no treatment was better than any treatment for advanced, ulcerated tumors.

Bruno, Anthony. "National Cancer Institute: An Overview With Historic Footnotes: A Report on the U.S.-U.S.S.R. Health Agreement." *National Cancer Institute Monographs*, 40 (February 1974), 7-20.

In January 1956 a Soviet delegation of medical researchers visited the United States seeking assistance on a widespread polio outbreak. It was the first cooperative medical enterprise between the United States and the Soviet Union since the Bolshevik Revolution. The Lacy-Zarubin Agreement of 1958 specifically targeted cooperative work against cancer. Various conferences were held for physicians from both countries during the 1960s, and they led to the U.S.-U.S.S.R. Bilateral Health Agreement of 1972, in which both countries agreed to share information on chemotherapy, virology, cellular genetics, and cancer epidemiology.

Bryan, Cyril P. *The Papyrus Ebers.* 1930.

The Ebers Papyrus was written in Egypt around 1,600 B. C. and is a medical treatise. The manuscript recommended cauterization or surgical excision for what we would today consider benign lesions, but it was pessimistic about treatment of ulcerated, fungating lesions.

Butler, Francella. "Cancer in Colonial Days." *Daughters of the American Revolution Magazine*, 87 (1953), 1231 and 1254.

In 1748 the House of Burgesses in Virginia awarded 100 pounds to Mary Johnson for developing a cancer cure. The medicine she developed was a mixture of garden sorrel, celandine, bark from a persimmon tree, and water, to be applied topically to the wound. The article also suggests that George Washington had a malignant tumor removed in 1794, and that his mother died of breast cancer in 1789.

Butler, Francella. *Cancer Through the Ages: The Evolution of Hope.* Fairfax, Virginia: 1955.

Although people have known about cancer for thousands of years, successful treatment of the disease has primarily been a twentieth century phenomenon. Surgeons were able to cure superficial lesions centuries ago if wide excision was used, but not until post-World War II physicians began combining early diagnosis with *en bloc* surgical resection, megavoltage radiotherapy, and chemotherapy did hopes for a cure of cancer become realistic.

Cabanne, F., R. Gerard-Marchant, and F. Destaing. "Geschichte der Krebses." In J.C. Sournia, M. Martiny, and J. Poulet, eds. *Illustrierte Geschichte der Medizin.* Salsburg, Austria: 1980. Volume 8. Pp. 2849-79.

(See Chapter 1: Gallucci and Chapter 1: Kardinal and Yarbro).

Cassileth, Barrie R. "The Evolution of Oncology." *Perspectives in Biology and Medicine*, 26 (Spring 1983), 362-74.

Cancer has been recognized as a disease entity ever since the ancient Egyptians first distinguished betweeen different types of external lumps on the body. The scientific discipline of oncology, however, has emerged only very recently as efforts to conquer cancer have acquired an extraordinary intensity. Hippocrates delineated several types of cancer and coined the term "karkinos" to describe the lesion. Arsenic pastes were often applied and surgical excision was recommended when possible. By the sixteenth century the notion of metastasis was first understood, and in the late eighteenth century physicians made the first connections between certain occupations and malignant lesions. In the eighteenth century two other developments occurred. First, Zacutus Lusitanus and Daniel Sennert concluded that cancer was contagious and helped initiate the sense of shame, horror, and stigma with which cancer has become associated ever since. Second, the humoral theory, total-body-invasion view of cancer which had dominated medicine since Galen's time gave way to the modern, localistic understanding of the disease. By the end of the nineteenth century a complex disease with numerous manifestations had been recognized and the notion that cancer could be treated surgically was gaining momentum. The first trends toward medical specialization were also appearing in the nineteenth century, and a number of professional medical societies were established. Pathologists made great strides in distinguishing between benign and malignant lesions. In surgery the understanding of asepsis and antisepsis greatly reduced surgical mortality rates and improved surgical treatment of cancer. At the end of the nineteenth century the first medical journals devoted to cancer began to publish on a regular basis, and cancer hospitals began to appear. Early in the 1900s the first public and medical societies to study and control cancer were organized. Radiation was used to treat breast cancer within one year of Roentgen's discovery of x-rays in 1895, and radiotherapy soon joined surgery as a treatment modality for cancer victims. Chemotherapy first appeared in the 1940s when experiments with nitrogen mustard proved effective against lymphomas, and in the 1950s experimental trials with the antifolic acids were successful against acute childhood leukemia. By the late 1950s chemotherapy had joined radiotherapy and surgery as a major treatment for cancer. Finally, oncology evolved into a recognized, distinct medical discipline in the 1960s.

"Le cancer dans le monde. Quelques donees sur l'histoire du cancer dans l'état du Texas." *Lutte cancer*, 42 (January-February 1965), 36-39.

The major development in the history of oncology in the state of Texas was the founding of the M. D. Anderson Hospital and Tumor Institute in Houston and its evolution into one of the premier cancer centers in the world, especially in its commitment to radiotherapy.

Crile, George. "The Cancer Problem: A Speculative Review of the Etiology, Natural History, and Treatment of Cancer." *Perspectives in Biology and Medicine*, 3 (Spring 1960), 358-81.

In the last 50 years the death rate from cancer has remained essentially the same, although cure rates for some cancers, like cervical and uterine lesions, have improved, probably because of earlier diagnosis of those diseases. Recently surgeons have learned that the widest surgical excision of a tumor is not always the best treatment and that for some tumors delays in treatment are less important than formerly supposed because of improved cytological techniques and staging mechanisms, which offer better predictability of outcomes. Also, the discovery that cancer cells enter the bloodstream has changed treatment thought. The real challenge is to remove the primary tumor completely and at the same time prevent the circulating cancer cells from implanting themselves and growing. Some research indicates that traumatic surgery may actually enhance the process of metastasis and accelerate the death of the patient, perhaps because the trauma compromises the patient's immunological system and his ability to fight the disease. Some animal research indicates that radiation therapy may have the same results by destroying lymphocytes at the site of the tumor. The clinical approach to cancer has not changed much in recent years. Surgical excision performed as early as possible still seems to afford the best possibility of a cure, while radiation applied to localized, radiosensitive lesions is often equally successful. Except for the success with choriocarcinoma, chemotherapy is still largely for palliative purposes. Genuine advances have been made in treatment of endocrine-dependent cancers, particularly those of the breast, prostate, and endometrium. The future of cancer research lies in molecular biology and the understanding of cellular differentiation, mutation, and division.

Deeley, Thomas J. "A Brief History of Cancer." *Clinical Radiology*, 34 (1983), 597-608.

Cancer is a disease of modern society for several reasons: 1) the increase in life expectancy; 2) better clinical diagnosis; and 3) increased exposure to causative carcinogens. Signs of malignancy have been found in fossil remains, skeletal remains of prehistoric people, and in soft tissues of Egyptian mummies. The Greeks were the first to attempt systematic explanations of cancer. The Roman physician Galen likened cancer to a crab and gave it the name "karkinos," which in Latin is cancer. He concentrated on breast cancer and believed in surgery to excise the entire lesion. Few gains were made in the Middle Ages in understanding cancer. During the Renaissance the Greek ideas were resurrected. In the eighteenth century cancer was clearly differentiated from other lesions, such as infections, cysts, and hyperplasia. Also, the first suspicions that cancer spread through the blood and lymphatic system were expressed in the eighteenth century. In the nineteenth century there were many advances in pathology and histology as well as great advances in surgery. Cancer treatment has been very complicated and diverse over the centuries. It was delivered in several varieties. First there were the topical applications to deal with ulcerated malignancies. These included astringent or stryptic substances (lead, lime, spirits of hartshorn, hemlock, deadly nightshade, and strychnine) under the theory that poison counteracts poison. There were also soothing substances to clean away necrotic and infected tissues (massed cabbage, carrots, honey, goose dung, beeswax, plantain, celendine, poppies, roses, red onions and parsnip). Metals such as gold, lead, copper, iron, and zinc were topically applied. The recently removed internal organs of various animals were sometimes topically applied to tumors. There were also a number of internal, herbal, and metallic medications.

Dont, Hans. "Die Terminologie von Geschwür, Geschwulst und Anschwellung im Corpus Hippocraticum." Ph.D. Dissertation. University of Vienna. 1968. Pp. 105.

Hippocrates and the early Greeks were familiar with tumors of the skin, uterus, breast, and stomach, and they knew that the prognosis for patients was dismal. He differentiated between what he called "oidemata," the soft-swellings associated with cysts and inflammations, and "karkinos," or hard swellings which were tumors. Hippocrates selected the word "karkinos," which meant crabs, because of the tenacity of cancerous lesions, their ability to recur locally and spread to distant sites. From that terminology came the modern words "cancer" and "carcinoma."

Dorzhgotov, B. K. "Razvitie onkologicheskoi sluzbhy v Mongol'skoi Narodnoi Respublike." *Voprosy Onkologii*, 23 (1977), 27-29.

The article provides a brief survey of the development of clinical oncology in the Mongolian Soviet Socialist Republic. Because of the remoteness of the territory significant gains in cancer treatment did not emerge there until the 1960s. By the end of the decade patients had access to major surgical facilities, megavoltage radiotherapy equipment, and a variety of chemotherapy protocols.

Ebbell, B. *Die Alt-Agypttsche Chirurgie.* Oslo: 1939.

(See Chapter 1: Bryan).

Ebbell, B. *The Papyrus Ebers: The Greatest Egyptian Medical Document.* 1937.

(See Chapter 1: Bryan).

Fisher, Edwin R., and Cecelia M. Hermann. "Historic Milestones in Cancer Pathology." *Seminars in Oncology*, 6 (1979), 428-32.

(See Chapter 6: Fisher and Hermann).

Gallucci, Betty B. "Selected Concepts of Cancer as a Disease: From the Greeks to 1900." *Oncology Nursing Forum*, 12 (July-August 1985), 67-71.

In the Greek era growths were divided into "phymata" (growths), "oidemata" (soft swellings), and "karkinos" (hard lumps), which were probably malignant. Galen argued that cancer arose from the flux of black bile into an area that was injured or overexercised. They were especially familiar with breast cancer, which they associated with the suppression of menses. They described the course of the disease quite accurately: the breast becomes hard, pain ensues, the body becomes wasted, and death is inevitable. For the Greeks cancer was a systemic disease. Gradually the Greek theory of the humors was replaced. The theory of circulation by Harvey, the growth of modern chemistry, and the discovery of the lymphatic system led to erosion of the humoral theories. This new view incorporated a more chemical orientation where corrosive acids or ferments of the lymph were responsible for creating cancer. Lymphatic fluid was viewed as a substance responsible for maintenance of the solid parts of the body and replaced the humors in the theories of the etiology of the disease. By the early 1800s the tissue theory had replaced the lymphatic fluid theory. Physicians began to describe different kinds of tissue, although metastases were still explained as an amorphous fluid or seed that travelled to distant parts of the body. Researchers also began to liken tumors to embryonic development. The development of the microscope in the 1820s gave rise to the cellular theories. In 1855 Rudolf Virchow popularized the concept that every cell arises from a pre-existing cell, and he coined the term cellular pathology. It was easier to understand metastasis, especially after Wilhelm Waldeyer in 1869 argued that cancers arise from normal epithelium and spread by direct extension in the local region and via the lymphatic system or bloodstream to distant sites.

Gallucci, Betty B. "Selected Concepts of Cancer as a Disease: From 1900 to Oncogenes." *Oncology Nursing Forum*, 12 (September-October 1985), 69-78.

Boveri, a German professor of zoology (1862-1915), was the first to propose the somatic mutation theory. He argued that abnormalities of the chromosomes were responsible for the development of cancer. Today we know that tumor cells are genetically unstable. Mutations appear resulting in cells that have different properties and characteristics from the original line. The new cell lines may be able to metastasize, have different antigenic properties, and may be more or less resistant to chemotherapy. Also during Boveri's time, the viral theory of cancer had its beginnings. Peyton Rous led the way in showing that tumors could be induced in other animals of the same species by the injection of cell-free filtrates of tumors. Not until the 1940s and the development of the electron microscope could viruses be seen. Some tumors—Burkitt's lymphoma, nasopharyngeal carcinoma, and primary liver cancer—have a definite viral etiology, and we know now that hepatocellular carcinoma can be prevented by a vaccine. The realization of chemical carcinogenesis began with Pott's (1775) epidemiological studies of squamous cell carcinoma in chimney sweeps. Fourteen years earlier Hill had postulated a connection between the use of snuff and the development of polyps and cancers. In 1795 Soemmering reported a link between pipe smoking and oral cancer. Yamagiwa and Ichikawa reported the carcinogenic results of painting coal tar on the ears of rabbits in 1915. Research in cell biology and biochemistry accelerated after Warburg proposed in the 1920s and 1930s that the mitochondrion was the site in the cell where carcinogenesis occurred. He felt that a carcinogen damaged the cellular respiratory system which is centered in the mitochondrion. Since then, the structure of the cell has been minutely studied, and virtually every component part has been accused of playing a role in the carcinogenic process. The first immunologic experiments were conducted at the end of the nineteenth century, when Novinsky reported on transplantation of tumors in dogs. Experiments early in the 1900s demonstrated that tumors could be transplanted into other animals and even across specie lines. Because these early experiments were conducted without inbred animal strains, however, the scientists confused tumor rejection with general graft rejection. Once inbred animal strains were available, it became clear that tumor cells do have molecules on their surfaces that could distinguish them by the immune system from normal cells. Between 1975 and 1985 the use of monoclonal antibodies went from the experimental to the clinical stage. Recombinant DNA techniques have also allowed for the manufacturing and clinical trial of interferon. The newest development in the current understanding of tumor biology involves the mystery of oncogenes. Oncogenes appear in every cell of every species, scientists believe, and malfunctions in the oncogenes give rise to malignant tumors. The discovery of the function of cellular oncogenes may lead to the development of new drug therapies.

Giroux, T. E. "La medicine indienne et le traitement du cancer." *Laval medical,* 38 (December 1967), 953-62.

Beginning in the eighteenth century Roman Catholic missionaries in Québec collected information about the folk medical practices of the various Native American tribes, and in the early twentieth century, anthropologists compared the missionary information with current Indian practices. Most of the tribes recognized the danger of hard tumors and ulcerated skin lesions, and they recommended a variety of herbal pastes and potions to deal with them.

Gottlieb, Johan. "Contribución al tratamiento de los enfermos cancerosos en el siglo XVIII." *Folia Clínica Internacional,* 25 (November 1975), 613-17.

In the eighteenth century the major developments in the treatment of cancer included more systematic surgical techniques based on anatomical studies, the shift from viewing cancer as a systemic illness to one of local origin, and the recognition that such environmental factors as tobacco and soot were carcinogenic.

Haddow, Alexander. "A Perspective in Time." *Perspectives in Biology and Medicine,* 18 (Summer 1975), 433-55.

In the 1920s there was an extraordinary optimism among physicians and scientists about the prospects for conquering cancer, but the years since have shown the tenacity and complexity of the disease. More realistic expectations, and perhaps some skepticism, have replaced the optimism of the 1920s. Today much more is understood about the molecular structure of cancer cells, but improvements in cure rates have been painfully slow.

Hayward, Oliver S. "The History of Oncology. I. Early Oncology and the Literature of Discovery." *Surgery,* 58 (August 1965), 460-68.

From the time of the Greeks and the Romans cancer was viewed as a systemic disease related to an excess of black bile (atrabilis) and therefore beyond any cure by surgical excision of a local swelling. Compounding confusion, local swellings, whether due to cancer, infection, or aneurysm, were all classified together. But in the eighteenth century, because of philosophical change and the rise of medical schools and dissection rooms in London, Edinburgh, Vienna, and Paris, empirical approaches overwhelmed the older ideas of Galen. Percivall Pott (1714-1788) discovered the cause of scrotal cancer, developed a cure through wide surgical excision, and eliminated the disease in a generation through social legislation. One of Potts's students was the renowned surgeon John Hunter (1728-1793), who then trained a generation of British, American, and European surgeons.

Huard, Paul, and M. J. Imbault-Huard. "Les étapes du traitement des tumeurs par ischemie, priorite de Harvey." *Histoire de science et medicine*, 14 (1980), 171-75.

(See Chapter 1: Kardinal and Yarbro).

Imbault-Huart, H. J. "Histoire du cancer." *Histoire*, 74 (1984), 74-77.

(See Chapter 1: Gallucci).

Jackson, Robert. "St. Peregrine, O.S.M.—Patron Saint of Cancer Patients." *Canadian Medical Association Journal*, 111 (19 October 1971), 824, 827.

Peregrine Laziosi was born in 1265 in Forli, northern Italy. He joined the Order of the Servants of Mary. During his life he was allegedly cured miraculously of cancer, although historians now believe he was suffering from varicose veins. He died in 1345 and was canonized in 1726.

Kardinal, Carl G. "An Outline of the History of Cancer." Part I. *Missouri Medicine*, 74 (December 1977), 662-66; Part II: 75 (January 1978), 10-14; Part III: 75 (February 1978), 74-78.

(See Chapter 1: Kardinal and Yarbro).

Kardinal, Carl G., and John W. Yarbro. "A Conceptual History of Cancer." *Seminars in Oncology*, 6 (December 1979), 396-408.

Tumors were first described in ancient Egyptian writings, although they were not differentiated from inflammatory swellings or chronic ulcerations. They recommended poultices and surgical excision. Under the Greeks, Hippocrates was the first to use the term carcinoma (karkinoma), and he likened cancer to a crab because of its tenacious ability to spread. Hippocrates also argued for the humoral theories—that cancer was caused by an excess of "black bile." That humoral theory, expanded upon by Galen, dominated western oncology for the next 1,500 years. Galen was also the first to use the term sarcoma, which he applied to fleshy tumors. In the sixteenth and seventeenth centuries, the Renaissance brought about a dramatic shift from the Aristotelian-Galenic rationalism with its metaphysical base to a Baconian-Newtonian empiricism with an experimental base. Doubts about the black bile theory began to emerge because physicians could not see it during dissections. The fall of Galenic authority was followed by chaos, since no new theories filled the vaccuum. Not until the middle of the sixteenth century did the new lymph theory appear. People like John Hunter and Frederick Hoffman believed that cancer was composed of fermenting and degenerating lymph varying in density, acidity, and alkalinity. Not until the nineteenth century did the lymph theory decline as pathologists like Johannes Müller, Julius Vogel, and Rudolf Virchow noted the cellular composition of tumors. Virchow believed that cancers spread through a liquid process. James Paget proposed the constitutional theory—there was a hereditary or constitutional predisposition towards the reception of the neoplastic impetus, and there was an exciting cause that was a specific morbid material disseminated throughout the vascular system. Julius Cohnheim argued that tumors arose from masses of residual cells misplaced during embryonal development. These cells were distributed throughout the viscera or gathered in certain places such as the mucocutaneous junctions. They changed from embryonal cells to neoplasms because of changes in the blood supply. Another prominent theory was the trauma idea of Hugo Ribbert in the early twentieth century. He argued that cancer cells have no unusual powers of proliferation; they have merely been freed from the restraints of "tissue tension" by mechanical isolation. Trauma exposes and then isolates predisposed epithelial cells by newly formed connective tissue. The isolated cells have altered growth tendencies that have been increased by irritation. Late in the nineteenth century the parasitic theory of cancer gained credence. Johannes Fibiger received the Nobel Prize in 1926 for his theory that cancer arose from a nematode worm. Subsequent research has discredited his theories. The parasitic theory then disappeared.

Keil, Harry. "The Historical Relationship Between the Concept of Tumor and the Ending -Oma." *Bulletin of the History of Medicine*, 24 (1950), 352-77.

The ending "oma" has been customarily used for identifying neoplastic growths, both benign and malignant. Hippocrates first used the word "carcinoma," meaning crab, to describe malignant lesions. He also used the word "oedema" as a general term for tumors or swellings. Celsus used "carcinoma" only for malignant lesions and the word "steatoma" for fatty tumors. Galen used "sarcoma" to describe malignant lesions and "blastoma" for a wart or polyp. The term "apostema" was a general term for tumors until the Renaissance, when the phrase "tumores praeter naturam" (tumors against nature) came into general use. Only gradually did more specific terms become popular among physicians. Severinus used "myxosarcoma" in 1632 to describe elephantitis of the scrotum. In 1709 Littre employed the word "lipoma" for fatty tumors. Frank used "haemtoma" for bloody cysts in 1791, and Odier coined the term "neuroma" for nerve tissue tumors in 1803. The term "'melanoma" was first used by Hooper in 1828, and he suggested developing other terms ending in "oma" for all other cancerous lesions. In 1843 Hannover used epithelioma for benign skin lesions. By the middle of the nineteenth century pathologists were using the terms "papilloma," "adenoma," "fibroma," "rhabdomyoma," "angioma," "cylindroma," "chloroma," and "lymphoma."

Kiselev, A. K. "Iz istorii sovetsko-amerikanskich nauchnykh sviazei oblasti onkologii." *Voprosy Onkologii*, 21 (1975), 94-101.

(See Chapter 1: Bruno).

Kolodziejska, H. "Onkologia polska w XXX-lecie Polskiej Rzeczypospoliteudowej." *Nowotwory*, 24 (October-December 1974), 225-27.

The article provides a brief summary of the history of Polish oncology on the 30th anniversary of the Polish People's Republic.

Korbler, Johannes. "Die Krebslehre des Parcelus und die Gegenwart." *Centaurus*, 12 (1967), 182-91.

(See Chapter 1: Pagel).

Korbler, Johannes. "Die Krebslehre und die Krebsbehandlung an der Wende des 17. zum 18. Jahrhundert." *Forschung Praxis Fortbilding. Organ fur die Fesamte Praktische und Theoretische Medizin*, 18 (10 March 1967), 129-30.

By the end of the eighteenth century the traditional ideas of Galen and Hippocrates about disease, which had dominated scientific thought for nearly 2,000 years, were finally rejected under the impact of empirical observation. The humoral explanation of disease gave way to the iatrochemical school, which saw diseases in general, and cancer in particular, coming from abnormalities in lymphatic fluids. Physicians were beginning to see cancer as a localized entity which could be treated by surgical excision when possible. In the case of breast cancer, mastectomies with removal of the involved axilla were becoming more and more common.

Korbler, Johannes. "Die Spagirische Krebsbehandlung zu Beginn des 17. Jahrunderts. Ein Kapital Medizingeschichte." *Hippokrates*, 38 (30 September 1967), 732-36.

By the end of the sixteenth century Europe had passed through the Renaissance and Reformation periods, leaving behind the medieval world and its static intellectual preoccupations. But although Copernicus was revolutionizing prevailing notions about the solar system, medical thought was for the most part still mired in the past. Paracelsus (1493-1551) had rejected the humoral theory of disease in favor of his own view of disease as an external entity which took root as a seed in the body, but his views did not gain a wide following. People like the French surgeon Ambroise Paré advocated wide excision of external cancers, but his ideas too found few adherents. The humoral theories of Hippocrates and Galen still dominated scientific thought. The great age of medical advancement waited until the seventeenth and eighteenth centuries, when empirical observations altered the theoretical opinions on the origins of cancer.

Korbler, Johannes. "Eine Krebsbehandlung zu Beginn des XIX. Jahrhunderts." *Centaurus*, 10 (1964), 40-47.

The nineteenth century was a time of great discovery in oncology, even though at the beginning of the century, because adequate microscopes had not been produced yet, the field of cellular pathology and histology had not emerged. Nevertheless, physicians were convinced that both the humoral theories of the Middle Ages and the iatrochemical and iatrophysical views of the sixteenth and seventeenth centuries were inadequate explanations for the etiology of cancer. Instead of seeing the disease as a systemic problem, they viewed it as a local lesion which tended to spread and kill the patient. Proper treatment therefore involved early diagnosis and wide surgical excision of the lesion. They also realized that some cancers were environmentally induced, like scrotal cancers in chimney sweeps, and therefore controllable through public health programs.

Korbler, Johannes. "Einige Beitrage zur Geschichte der Krebskrankheit in Byzanz (die Aerzte-der Kaiser-die Prinzessin)." *Janus*, 58 (1971), 101-11.

Byzantine concepts of cancer in the Middle Ages were drawn directly from Greek and Roman notions—that cancer arose from imbalances in the body's humoral fluids, particularly an excess of "black bile." The recommended treatments involved surgery and cauterization for surface lesions, like those of the skin and breast, as well as a variety of lotions and pastes. Also, Byzantine physicians, like their Greek scientific forebears, advocated doing nothing rather than risking a surgical procedure when it was already obvious that the tumor was out of control.

Korbler, Johannes. *Geschichte der Krebskrankeit. Schicksale der Kranken, der Aerzte und der Forscher. Der Werdegang Einer Wissenschaft.* Vienna: 1973.

(See Chapter 1: Richards and Chapter 1: Rather).

Koszarowski, T. "Rozwoj onkologii w Polsce w latach 1932-1944 i 1948-1973; szkic historyczny z okazji rocznicy 25-lecia Instytutu Onkologii im. Marii Skłodowskiej-Curie w Polskiej Rzecypospolitej Ludowej." *Nowotwory*, 21 (January-June 1973), 1-5.

The article provides a brief history of the major developments in Polish oncology since the 1940s.

Krooks, James. "Man's Early Challenge to Neoplasms." *Minnesota Medicine*, 52 (July 1969), 1159-64.

(See Chapter 1: Gallucci and Chapter 1: Kardinal and Yarbro).

Kudimova, E. G. "K istorii razvitii onkologicheskoi sluzbhy v SSSR." *Voprosy Onkologii*, 16 (1970), 16-23.

(See Chapter 1: Blokhin and Napalkov).

Kutorga, V. V. "Cancerology in the First Half of the 19th Century." *Eleventh International Congress of the History of Medicine*, 5 (1968), 187-88.

During the first half of the nineteenth century great strides were made in understanding the nature of malignancies. The old humoral theories had long since been discarded in favor of new ideas concerning the lymphatic system. Scientists believed in the idea of carcinogenesis; believed that surgical excision was the only way of really affecting a permanent cure in patients; and knew that cancer could metastasize, although they were only beginning to surmise the cellular nature of the disease. Pathology was emerging as a medical discipline and leukemia and lymphoma had been identified. Anesthesiology first emerged in the 1840s, permitting more extensive surgical approaches to malignant disease.

Lemon, Henry M. "My Speciality: Oncology." *Nebraska Medical Journal*, 64 (August 1979), 259.

Lemon briefly surveys the major developments in oncology since the 1930s, including the early detection of cervical cancer, chemotherapy for some solid tumors, the development of megavoltage external beam radiotherapy, and hopes of preventing breast cancer through estriol therapy.

Ljunggren, Bengt. "Ein stor man med en sjuk hjarna." *Sydsvenska Medicinhistoriskes Sallskapets Arsskrift*, 21 (1984), 77-85.

(See Chapter 1: Gallucci).

Ljunggren, Bengt. "Reflexioner kring en hjarnsvulst hos 'En fornam herre af 30 ar'." *Sydsvenska Medicinhistoriskes Sallskapets Arsskrift*, 20 (1983), 87-102.

Changes in the practice of oncology have accelerated dramatically in the past 30 years. The major changes have been the abandonment of superradical surgical procedures in favor of more conservative, tissue-saving approaches; the rise of megavoltage radiotherapy and its curative use in various head and neck tumors and certain lymphomas; and the development of chemotherapy and its remarkable success in treating choriocarcinoma, acute lymphocytic leukemia, and a variety of lymphomas.

Lytton, D. G., and L. M. Resuhr. "Galen on Abnormal Swellings." *Journal of the History of Medicine and the Allied Sciences*, 33 (October 1978), 531-49.

Clarrisimus Galen, the famous Roman physician, wrote *On Abnormal Swellings (De Tumoribus Praeter Naturam)* in 192 A. D. His description of swellings and tumors was based on clinical observation, but his views on the etiology of tumors came strictly from the humoral theories of the Greeks. He described a variety of abnormal swellings: 1) "phlegmone" was a term describing swellings associated with distension, throbbing pain, heat, and redness, probably an inflammatory lesion; 2) "polysarkia" was a non-inflammatory cyst filled with clear fluid, not blood; 3) "kolpos" was a term describing an ulcerated, inflammatory lesion which was secreting pus; 4) "gangrainai" was used to describe the condition of gangrene; 5) "karkinoi" included all hard, cancerous lesions which started out as painless lumps but which eventually ulcerated through the skin before causing death; 6) "phagedaina" referred to a malignant tumor which had ulcerated through the skin; 7) "ecchymonia" referred to extensive bruises, particularly those affecting the elderly; 8) "aneurysma" described the swelling caused by blockage in a blood vessel or the weakening of an artery; 9) "elephas" was the term Galen employed to describe leprosy; 10) "myrmekia" was the term for warts; 11) "psydrakes" was the term for pimples; 12) "epiknyktides" was synonymous with insect bite swellings; 13) "dothien" were small boils; 14) "phygethlon" described glandular swellings; and 15) "kirsoi" was the term for varicose veins.

Maria, Eva, and Imelda Schubart. "Two Historical Maps Relating to the Evolution of Knowledge of Cancer." *Cancer Bulletin*, 2 (January-February 1950), 9-11.

Here is a brief outline map indicating the leading figures in the history of cancer research from ancient times to the present. It identifies such leading ancient physicians as Hippocrates, Galen, and Celsus, and nineteenth century luminaries like Rudolf Virchow and Theodor Billroth.

Mike, Valerie. "Clinical Studies in Cancer: A Historical Perspective." In Valerie Mike and Kenneth E. Stanley, eds. *Statistics in Medical Research. Methods and Issues with Applications in Cancer Research.* New York: 1982. Pp. 111-55.

Sophisticated clinical studies about the outcome of treatment are fairly recent developments in medical history, especially concerning cancer. Not until the late nineteenth century did cancer treatment really began to develop. The four major developments in clinical oncology are: 1) the rise of the *en bloc* resection in surgery; 2) the discovery of x-rays by Wilhelm Roentgen, which provided physicians with a new treatment modality; 3) the production of inbred systems of experimental animals and the successful transplantation of tumors into these animals; and 4) the development of the randomized clinical trials, which have become the primary method of evaluating the effectiveness of new treatments for cancer.

Nannini, M. C. "Il cancro, questo sconosciuto (considerazoni e ricordi di uno studente di trenta anni fa)." *Pagine di Storia della Medicina*, 15 (July-August 1971), 15-24.

During the last 30 years of oncology advances in the treatment of cancer, if not its cellular etiology, have been particularly important. The rise of chemotherapy has provided great improvements in survival rates for patients with trophoblastic tumors, lymphomas, and leukemias. Survival rates for childhood cancers are also improving. New developments in megavoltage radiotherapy have reduced local recurrence rates after wide surgical excision, rendered some large tumors resectable, and, most importantly, have permitted less radical surgical procedures for breast carcinomas, head and neck tumors, and some soft-tissue sarcomas. Nevertheless, no "magic bullet" cure has appeared for cancer, nor is one likely to appear in the near future until scientists come to terms with the genetic code and the real nature of cancer at the cellular level.

Noriega, Limon. "La evolución de la oncología en los tres últimos decenios." *Gaceta Médica de Mexico*, 113 (October 1977), 489-99.

In the last 30 years Mexican oncologists have incorporated and sometimes helped extend the 4 major developments in modern cancer treatment: the technique of the *en bloc* surgical resection, megavoltage external beam radiotherapy, chemotherapy, and the team approach to clinical services. On the public health level, government officials have emphasized the importance of the early warning signs of cancer, the danger of smoking, and the need for women to have Pap smears to diagnose early cervical neoplasia.

Onuigbo, Wilson I. B. "False Firsts in Cancer Literature." *Oncology*, 25 (1971), 163-67.

The author describes a number of "false firsts" in cancer research. The first notation of bile pigment in a metastatic tumor was reported by Laennec in 1834, not in 1883. The first recording of blood metastasis was by Joseph de la Charriere in 1712, not by Thiersch in 1865. Moore in 1867 first argued against incising into cancerous masses during surgery, not Ryall in 1907. Budd first proposed the cell theory of cancer metastasis in 1842, not Waldeyer in 1867. The first case of a secondary lung tumor was described by Baillie in 1793, not in 1824. In 1832 Sims first reported the invasion of the pulmonary veins by lung cancer, not Wolf in 1893. In 1786 John Hunter first described the lymphatic metastasis of breast carcinoma, not Halsted in the 1890s.

"The Origin of Cancer." *Cancer Bulletin*, 5 (November-December 1953), 135-37.

The article is a brief survey of the humoral, nutritional, genetic, and environmental theories of carcinogenesis.

"Osiagniecia onkologii w okresie xv-lecia Polski ludowej." *Nowotwory*, 19 (October-December 1969), 249-50.

(See Chapter 1: Kolodziejska).

Pack, George T., and Irving M. Ariel. "A Half Century of Effort to Control Cancer. An Appraisal of the Problem and an Estimation of Accomplishments." *Surgery, Gynecology & Obstetrics*, 100 (May 1955), 425-47.

In the twentieth century there have been a number of important developments in the treatment of cancer. The major accomplishments and developments are listed below:

1. In breast cancer the Halsted mastectomy became the treatment of choice by 1900, and in recent years there have been two divergent trends. One group of surgeons advocates a simple mastectomy followed by radiotherapy, while another group calls for the superradical mastectomy involving removal of the breast, associated axilla lymph nodes, a low neck dissection, and removal of the internal mammary nodes. Future survival rates will demonstrate which approach is the best one for saving lives. The other important change in breast cancer treatment has been the development of endocrine therapies started by George Beatson late in the 1890s.

2. Treatment of lung cancer has made dramatic advances before and since Evarts Graham's successful pneumonectomy in 1933. Successful surgical resections of lung tumors were made possible by the development of intrathoracic anesthesia, effective ligature of the pulmonary artery, and routine closing of the bronchial stump. Chevalier Jackson's perfection of the bronchoscopy and development of x-rays greatly advanced diagnostic techniques for lung cancer. For inoperable lesions various radiotherapeutic approaches have proven effective.

3. The first successful surgical resection for cancer of the esophagus was performed in 1913 by Franz Torek. In the 1920s Kirschner and Ohsawa performed resections of the inferior esophagus through an abdominothoracic incision and effected an esophagogastrostomy by bringing the stomach into the thoracic cavity. In 1938 Adams and Phemister performed a partial esophagectomy and gastrectomy with primary esophagogastric anastomosis.

4. Modern treatment of gastric cancer began on January 29, 1881, when Theodor Billroth performed the first successful human gastrectomy for carcinoma of the stomach. Four years later William Welch argued that gastrectomies might prolong life but they did not bring about a cure because distant metastases had already occurred before the initial surgery. Although the initial surgery was successful, long-term survival did not occur for the vast majority of patients. Diagnosis of gastric cancer was greatly advanced by Schindler's improvements in the gastroscope in 1923.

5. Cancer of the colon and rectum were greatly advanced by invention of the anastomosis button in 1892, new understanding of lymphatic drainage patterns in the rectum and colon, and the surgical procedures developed by Paul Kraske and William Ernest Miles in the early 1900s, which greatly reduced local recurrence rates.

6. The treatment of pancreatic tumors started historically in 1935 when Whipple, Parsons, and Mullins performed a two-stage pancreaticoduodenectomy, but the understanding of hyperinsulinism came after 1922 when Banting and Best extracted and identified insulin.

7. Liver cancer was not treated with any success until 1949 when the first liver lobectomies began to be performed. The problem with hepatic resection was post-operative liver failure from insufficient hepatic tissue.

8. Carcinoma of the vulva, vagina, and cervix in the twentieth century have been greatly improved by the combination of wide cervical excision, radiotherapy, both external beam and implants, and early diagnosis through the Pap smear.

Pack, George T., and Irving M. Ariel. "The History of Cancer Therapy." In *Cancer Management: A Special Graduate Course on Cancer Sponsored by the American Cancer Society*. Philadelphia: 1968. Pp. 2-27.

(See Chapter 1: Gallucci and Chapter 1: Kardinal and Yarbro).

Pagel, Walter. "Van Helmont's Concept of Disease—To Be or Not to Be? The Influence of Paracelsus." *Bulletin of the History of Medicine*, 46 (September-October 1972), 419-54.

Theophrastus Paracelsus (1493-1541) and Jan Baptiste Van Helmont (1579-1644) are the major figures in forging a new philosophy of medicine and disease during the Renaissance and post-Renaissance years. Both of them rejected the notions of Hippocrates and Galen which had prevailed for nearly 2,000 years, that all disease was a function of imbalance in the body's four basic humors, or fluids. In their view, disease was an excess or deficiency of one or more of the fluids. But Paracelsus and Van Helmont argued that disease was a specific entity in its own right—the essence of disease is a morbid seed of some kind which becomes implanted in a body organ. Although Van Helmont did not accept Paracelsus's notion of a relationship between astrology and disease, and both men did not really understand the origins of diseases—viral, bacterial, and genetic—they were correct in the notion of disease as a separate entity from the body's constitution.

Patterson, James T. *The Dread Disease. Cancer and Modern American Culture*. Cambridge, Mass.: 1987.

Although cancer as a disease has been known for centuries among Americans, it did not really become a preoccupation until the latter half of the nineteenth century when declines in mortality rates from infectious diseases were replaced by increasing mortality rates from cancer. Ulysses S. Grant's death in 1885 from a metastatic oral cancer received widespread public attention. In the twentieth century the United States has been characterized by an extraordinary preoccupation with cancer. Although the rise of surgical oncology, megavoltage radiotherapy, and chemotherapy have improved survival rates, there has been no "magic bullet" and the disease remains tenacious and unyielding. In the 1920s physicians were quite optimistic about finding a cure for cancer, but eventually they became far more cautious. At the same time the popular press has heralded every scientific advance, raising public hopes for a cure and, of course, stimulating public skepticism when the cures did not materialize. After World War II a huge Cancer Establishment—composed of the federal government, major pharmaceutical companies, universities, and the medical community—launched a multi-billion dollar crusade against the disease. But at the same time a "cancer counterculture" appeared, led by people who were skeptical of the medical community as well as big government. Environmentalists attributed cancer to pollution while popular psychologists looked to the stress of modern society or the frustrations of introverted people for the causes of cancer.

Pazzini, A. "Il pensiero degli antichi medici sulla patogenesi e cura dei tumori." *Pagine di Storia della Medicina*, 14 (March-April 1970), 5-13.

(See Chapter 1: Gallucci and Chapter 1: Dont).

Pazzini, A. "Il pensiero degli antichi medici sulla patogenesi e cura dei tumori." *Minerva Medicine*, 62 (7 April 1971), 1463-66.

(See Chapter 1: Gallucci and Chapter 1: Dont).

Rakov, A. I., IuV Petrov, and S. A. Kholdin. "Razvitie kliniches-koi onkologii za 50 let sovetskoi vlasti." *Voprosy Onkologii*, 13 (1967), 3-11.

(See Chapter 1: Blokhin and Napalkov).

Rather, L. J. *The Genesis of Cancer. A Study in the History of Ideas.* Baltimore: 1978.

Cancer has been a recognized disease entity for thousands of years, and people for hundreds of generations have speculated on its etiology, but it was not until the Greeks and the Romans that a physiological, rather than a religious or cosmic, explanation was offered. Hippocrates, the famous Greek physician, explained all illnesses as an imbalance in the body's four basic humors, or fluids: blood, phlegm, black bile, and yellow bile. Cancer arose because of an excess of black bile. Galen, the Roman physician, also attributed cancer to an excess of black bile. He defined cancer as "tumors against nature." For nearly 1,500 years the theories of

Hippocrates and Galen on the origins of malignant neoplasms went unchallenged
by European and Middle Eastern physicians. The first major challenges to the
humoral theories of Hippocrates and Galen appeared during the sixteenth century
when the Renaissance launched new scientific assumptions based on empirical observations rather than metaphysical assumptions. Paracelsus (1493-1551) rejected
the humoral theories and argued that disease was caused by agents external to
the body, not internal. Morbid anatomists like Vesalius, Benivieni, Ingrassia, and
Fallopius made careful examinations of the body's physical structures. During the
seventeenth century William Harvey described the circulatory system; surgeons
began arguing that complete excision of tumors was the only cure; and physicians began rejecting the black bile theory of cancer in favor of the iatrophysical
and iatrochemical theories which blamed the disease on lymphatic abnormalities.
During the eighteenth century physicians began to view cancer as a local rather
than a systemic disease, which made the need for surgical excision even more
imperative as a treatment. Claude Gendron and Hermann Boerhaave were the
leading exponents of the localist approach. The notion of chemical carcinogenesis
was born in 1761 when John Hill attributed nasal carcinomas to the use of snuff.
In 1775 Percivall Pott correctly explained scrotal cancer in chimney sweeps as a
disease caused by exposure to soot. Thomas von Soemmering, a Polish physician,
claimed in 1795 that there was a strong relationship between pipe smoking and lip
carcinoma. In the nineteenth century the understanding of cancer biology grew
by leaps and bounds. Late in the 1830s Johannes Müller and his famous student
Rudolf Virchow gave birth to the field of cellular pathology and described cancer
as a disease of cellular abnormality. Joseph Récamier first described metastasis
in 1829 and Wilhelm Waldeyer in the 1880s identified carcinomas as tumors of
epithelial origins and metastases as tumor emboli transported through the bloodstream. Julius Cohnheim argued in the 1870s that cancer arose from embryonic
cells which had failed to mature but which still existed in all tissues.

Regoly-Merel, G. "A daganat fogalma az O-Egyiptomi gyogyaszatban es hatasa
     a Gorog-Romai orvostanra." *Orvosi Hetilap*, 115 (8 September 1974), 2141-
     42.

(See Chapter 1: Bryan).

Rettig, R. A. *Cancer Crusade: The Story of the National Cancer Act of 1971.*
     Princeton: 1971.

The federal government first became involved in cancer research in 1937 when
Congress created the National Cancer Institute and provided it with an annual
appropriation of $700,000. Federal funds remained quite limited until after World
War II. In 1947 funding of the National Cancer Institute increased to $1.8 mil-
lion and to $14.5 million in 1948. By 1957 that research budget had increased
to $30 million. The increase in the volume of federal funds was commensurate
with the increase in the incidence of the disease. During the 1950s and 1960s
Americans increasingly became preoccupied with cancer as a disease, and political support for federally-backed cancer research grew geometrically. In 1968 the

National Cancer Institute budget exceeded $185 million. Success in the field of chemotherapy in the 1960s raised hopes that a cure for cancer was possible, and the successful federal program to send an exploration party to the moon reached fruition in 1969, fueling hopes that a similar crusade could be launched against cancer. President Richard M. Nixon became a visible and powerful proponent of such a federal crusade, and it reached fruition in 1971 when Congress passed the National Cancer Act, increasing the National Cancer Institute budget to more than $1 billion a year.

Richards, Victor. *Cancer: The Wayward Cell.* Berkeley: 1972. Pp. 81-92.

(See Chapter 1: Kardinal and Yarbro).

Rosso, F. and G. P. Bausani. "La terapía del cancro fino al secolo XVII." *Scientia Veterum*, 132 (1969), 141-52.

In the seventeenth century the humoral views of cancer began to give way to new iatrochemical theories of the disease. Physicians began to see cancer as a byproduct of lymphatic abnormalities. The idea of removing regional lymph nodes in surgical resections of cancer gained momentum.

Rous, Peyton. "The Challenge to Man of the Neoplastic Cell." *Science*, 157 (July 1967), 24-28.

Tumors are made up of cells that have been so singularly changed that they no longer obey the fundamental laws whereby the cellular constituents of an organism exist in harmony and act together to maintain it. Despite advances in understanding the viral origins of some animal tumors and the discovery of environmental carcinogens, we still know next to nothing about what happens when a cell becomes malignant nor how it passes that power on when it divides.

Said, H. M., and H. M. Barakati. "Cancer: The Last Two and a Half Millenia of Aetiology and Cure." *Hamdard*, 21 (July-September 1978), 28-47.

(See Chapter 1: Kardinal and Yarbro).

Senn, H. J. "Die Medizinische Onkologie—Eine Fachliche und Menschliche Herausforderung." *Wien Klinische Wochenschrift*, 131 (1981), 541-50.

The major developments in clinical oncology in the past two decades have involved the team approach to treatment—combining the skills of the surgeon, the radiotherapist, and the chemotherapist; the more conservative approach to radical surgery, with an emphasis on saving tissue and function whenever possible, primarily through the use of adjuvant radiotherapy; and the notion of rehabilitation and reconstruction of cancer patients after treatment so that their lives may return to normal.

Serebrov, A. I. "K 50-letiiu sovetskoi onkologii." *Voprosy Onkologii*, 13 (1967), 3-21.

The article surveys the history of Soviet oncology, focusing on the advances made since the Bolshevik Revolution. Included in the survey are assessments of the work of N. G. Khlopin, P. A. Gertsen, M. A. Novinsky, N. N. Petrov, and R. E. Karetskii.

Schretzenmayr, A. "Zur Geschichte der Onkogenese." *Bayerisches Aerzteblatt*, 27 (February 1972), 99-109.

(See Chapter 1: Rather).

Shimada, N., and M. Baba. "History of Cancer Therapy." *Journal of the Japanese Medical Association*, 57 (1 June 1967), 1753-57.

(See Chapter 1: Gallucci and Chapter 1: Kardinal and Yarbro).

Shimkin, Michael B. "An Historical Note on Tumor Transplantation in Man." *Cancer*, 35 (1975), 540-41.

The first recorded attempt to transfer cancer from one person to another in order to measure the transmittability of the disease is attributed to Jean Louis Alibert (1768-1837), a French dermatologist who served as physician to Louis XVIII. In 1808 Alibert allowed himself to be injected with tumor tissue from a breast cancer patient. Several medical students underwent the experiment at the same time. After an initial inflammatory reaction at the site of the injection, there was no long-term consequence of the experiment, allowing Alibert to conclude that cancer was not contagious.

Shimkin, Michael B. *Contrary to Nature*. Washington, D.C.: 1977.

In 498 pages Shimkin traces the history of cancer treatment from the Greco-Roman period to the present. The book follows a broadly chronological approach: Greco-Roman, Medieval, 16th Century, 17th Century, 18th Century, 19th Century, and 20th Century, and within those chronological classifications Shimkin looks at the major advances in understanding the nature and causes of cancer as well as the most effective treatments. Each chapter also focuses on the individual scientist and physician most responsible for the appropriate scientific or clinical discovery.

Shimkin, Michael B. "Neoplasia." In John Z. Bowers and Elizabeth F. Purcell, eds. *Advances in American Medicine: Essays at the Bicentennial*. New York: 1976. Volume 1. Pp. 210-50.

In United States history several early physicians wrote about cancer: Benjamin Rush, Nathan Smith, and John Collins Warren. But systematic oncology waited until the last of the nineteenth century to emerge in the work of pathologists like Joseph J. Woodward and surgeons like William Stewart Halsted and Hugh Young. Halsted's major contribution, in addition to development of the radical mastectomy and asepsis in surgery, was his belief that only the *en bloc* resection for all malignant tumors offered any hope of limiting recurrences and subsequent metastases. By the end of the 1800s oncology was emerging as a clinical field. The New York Cancer Hospital opened in 1884 and in 1899 became known as the Memorial Hospital for the Treatment of Cancer and Allied Diseases. It was directed by the pathologist James Ewing, considered by many as the first American oncologist. After World War II, clinical oncology exploded in unprecedented development, with radiotherapy, chemotherapy, endocrine therapy, and immunotherapy, as well as improved diagnostic and cancer control programs, transforming the medical world. Cancer, the "dread disease," became a national scientific priority, symbolized by passage of the National Cancer Act of 1971, and the 1970s and 1980s were characterized by a research and political crusade against the disease.

Shimkin, Michael B. "Oncology at the Bicentennial of the United States." *International Journal of Cancer*, 18 (15 July 1976), 132-33.

(See Chapter 1: Shimkin).

Shimkin, Michael B. "What Do We Know About Cancer?" *Western Journal of Medicine*, 125 (December 1976), 509-12.

After more than a century of research, we know five fundamental concepts about cancer: 1) cancer is a large of group of diseases, characterized by changes in somatic cells and transmissable to daughter cells; 2) cell changes involve the DNA of the nucleus; 3) cancerous change can be triggered by a wide variety of environmental stimuli, including physical, chemical, and viral agents; 4) the cancerous process is usually manifested after long exposure to carcinogenic stimuli, and evolves through a series of changes; 5) the cancerous process is influenced by a variety of host factors, including heredity, nutrition, and immunologic status.

Sontag, Susan. *Illness as Metaphor*. New York: 1978.

A leading social and literary critic, Sontag argued that the "most truthful way of regarding illness—and the healthiest way of being ill—is one most purified of, most resistant to, metaphoric thinking..." In the twentieth century cancer has become the dread disease and has displaced tuberculosis as the most metaphorically-loaded disease. Cancer is seen as a disease which is "incurable," "degenerating," "ravaging," "invasive," "corrosive," or "ruthless," and the best medical treatments for the disease are similarly loaded: surgery is synonymous with "mutilation," radiotherapy with "burning," and chemotherapy with "poison." Sontag calls for

Americans to strive to achieve a liberation from the cancer metaphors.

Stokes, S. H. "A History of Cancer in U. S. Presidents." *Journal of the Tennessee Medical Association*, 80 (January 1987), 13-16.

Like other diseases, cancer has affected the rich and famous as well as the poor and obscure, including the occupants of the White House. In 1789 George Washington's mother died of a metastatic breast carcinoma, as did John Adams's daughter in 1813. Ulysses S. Grant died of a squamous cell carcinoma of the mouth which spread locally throughout the head and neck area. Grover Cleveland had his soft palate surgically removed while he was in the White House; the rubber prosthesis which replaced the palate allowed him to keep the surgery a secret. Some historians speculate that Franklin D. Roosevelt died of a metastatic cancer which had developed from a melanoma lesion over his left eye. In 1967 Lyndon B. Johnson had a skin tumor removed from his foot, but the surgery was a closely guarded secret. Betty Ford, the wife of President Gerald Ford, underwent a mastectomy, as did Nancy Reagan, wife of President Ronald Reagan. President Ronald Reagan underwent a colon resection for cancer as well as a number of local excisions of basal cell carcinomas on his face.

Supady, J. "Udział lekarzy polskich w krajowych i międzynarodowych zjazdach onkologicznych w latach 1918-1938." *Nowotwory*, 29 (October-December 1979), 315-20.

The article describes the visits of Polish physicians and researchers to national and international oncological conventions during the 1920s and 1930s and their integration into the larger community of oncologists.

Suraiya, J. N. "Medicine in Ancient India with Special Reference to Cancer." *Indian Journal of Cancer*, 10 (December 1973), 391-402.

Ancient texts in Ayurvedic characters indicate that as early as 2,000 to 2,500 years ago cancer was recognized as a distinct disease entity. The most frequently mentioned neoplasms were lesions of the oral cavity, nasopharynx, esophagus, penis, and rectum. Cervical, bone, and breast lesions were not mentioned by the ancient Ayurvedic writers. Oropharyngeal cancers were and remain frequent neoplasms in South and Southeast Asia, probably because of the use of tobacco smoking and chewing, as well as chewing of the betel nut.

Timofeevski, A. D. "Kul'tira tkani (istoriia razvitiia i primenenie v onkologii." *Vestnik Akademii Meditsini Nauk SSSR*, 21 (1966), 59-64.

(See Chapter 1: Kardinal and Yarbro).

Trapeznikov, N. N., Iu.I Puchkov, and L. E. Komarova. "Sovetsko-Amerikanskoe strudnichestvo v oblasti onkologii." *Voprosy Onkologii*, 20 (1974), 11-16.

(See Chapter 1: Bruno).

Triolo, Victor A. "Bichats Krebstheorie in Wolffs 'Lehre von der Krebskrankeit'." *Sudhoff Archiv*, 48 (March 1964), 82-86.

(See Chapter 1: Kardinal and Yarbro).

Triolo, V. A. "Nineteenth Century Foundations of Cancer Research. II. Advances in Tumor Pathology, Nomenclature and Theories of Oncogenesis." *Cancer Research*, 24 (1965), 75-106.

(See Chapter 1: Kardinal and Yarbro and Chapter 1: Keil).

Valladares, Y. "Quince años de investigación oncología en el Departamento de Biología y Bioquímica del Cancer." *Revista de España Oncología*, 31 (1984), 539-51.

Like other research centers throughout the world, the major focus of oncology in the 1970s and 1980s at the Department of the Biology and Biochemistry of Cancer in Madrid has been the investigation of the possible viral etiology of cancer, the potential of immunotherapy, and the development of new chemotherapeutic agents for the treatment of malignancies.

Vardanyan, S. A. "Armenian Medieval Doctors on Tumours and Their Treatment." *Istoriko-Filologicheskii Zhurnal*, 74 (1976), 133-44.

(See Chapter 1: Aslam, Bano, and Vohora).

Veronesi, U. "History of the Last 100 Years of Attempts to Control Neoplastic Disease." *European Journal of Surgical Oncology*, 11 (March 1985), 1-3.

(See Chapter 1: Kardinal and Yarbro).

Wammock, Hoke. "Historical Background of Cancer in Georgia." *Journal of the Medical Association of Georgia*, 64 (July 1975), 264-66.

In 1937 the Georgia legislature passed a law requiring the state to provide facilities for the treatment of indigent cancer patients and established a Division of Cancer Control under the governor's office. The program worked until Medicaid and Medicare in 1966 and 1967 assumed financial responsibility for indigent patients. In 1955 the Georgia Tumor Registry was established. In the 1970s, with federal assistance, Georgia established the Georgia Cancer Management Network.

Watson, T. A. "The 1974 Gordon Richards Memorial Lecture: Trends in the Organization of Cancer Services." *Journal of the Canadian Association of Radiology*, 26 (December 1975), 223-30.

Until the 1920s clinical oncology was almost exclusively the domain of surgeons, who were committed to increasingly radical procedures as a means of preventing local recurrences of tumors. By the 1920s, however, radiotherapy was emerging as a discipline, and by the 1940s radiotherapists and some surgeons were advocating less radical surgical procedures and the adjuvant use of either pre-operative radiation to reduce tumor sizes or post-operative radiotherapy to destroy clinically occult malignancies. In the 1950s chemotherapy emerged as a new treatment discipline, and by the 1960s it had become, along with surgery and radiotherapy, one of the three major treatment modalities. By the 1970s the team approach, in which surgery, radiotherapy, and chemotherapy were used to treat patients, had come to dominate the clinical services of the comprehensive cancer centers.

Wood, Francis Carter. "Improvements in the Treatment of Cancer Since 1913." *Quarterly Review of the American Society for the Control of Cancer*, 8 (1943), 42-45.

The major successes since 1913 have been in the areas of radical surgical resections and the sophistication of radiotherapeutic techniques, particularly the development of external beam therapy machines in the 200 to 400 kilovoltage ranges.

Zhardetskii, A. S. "K istorii onkologii v rossii (XIII-XVIII Vek)." *Sovetskaia Meditsina*, 8 (August 1976), 148-51.

(See Chapter 1: Blokhin and Napalkov).

2 Cancer Specialists

ABRIKOSOV, ALEKSEI INVANOVICH

(See Chapter 19: "Cancer Eponym: Abrikosov's Tumor").

ALBUCASIS

Spink, M. S., and G. L. Lewis. *Abulcasis on Surgery and Instruments*. Berkeley: 1973.

Albucasis was an Islamic physician who lived in Spain between 1013 and 1106. In his commentaries on cancer, he offered only the most pessimistic opinions about the medical treatment, arguing that any internal tumor or external tumor which had existed for an extended period was all but incurable. For tumors of the breast or skin he advocated surgical excision, bleeding to remove excess "black bile," and cauterization of the wound.

ADLER, ISAAC

"Isaac Adler, M.D. (1849-1918)." *CA-A Cancer Journal for Clinicians*, 30 (September-October 1980), 294.

At the turn of the century primary lung cancer was thought to be extremely rare. Less than eighty cases had been reported in all of the literature until 1911, when Isaac Adler wrote *Primary Malignant Growths of the Lungs and Bronchi*, presenting nearly 400 cases and proving that the disease was much more common than previously expected. He also felt that physicians too often misdiagnosed the disease, confusing it with pulmonary tuberculosis. Isaac Adler was a physician in New York City who administered chest x-rays to all of his patients. Isaac Adler died 1918 at the age of 69.

ARDERNE, JOHN OF

Millar, T. M. "John of Arderne, The Father of British Proctology." *Proceedings of the Royal Society of Medicine of England*, 47 (1954), 75-84.

John of Arderne was born around 1307 and is recognized as the first physician-surgeon of England. He practiced medicine in London and wrote profusely about his clinical observations. Medical historians consider him the father of proctology because of his early descriptions of rectal carcinomas, although John of Arderne admitted there was no cure for the disease. He died in 1390.

Swain, C. P. "A Fourteenth Century Description of Rectal Cancer." *World Journal of Surgery*, 7 (March 1983), 304-07.

(See Chapter 2: ARDERNE, JOHN OF: Millar).

ARETAEUS

Leopold, E. J. "Aretaeus the Cappadocian." *Annals of the History of Medicine*, 2 (1930), 424-35.

Aretaeus the Cappadocian was a second century physician who practiced medicine in Alexandria and Rome. A follower of the theories of Hippocrates, Aretaeus attributed cancer to an excess of black bile. In his writings, which were not discovered by Europeans until the sixteenth century, Aretaeus offered clinical descriptions of a number of malignant lesions. He is also credited with naming diabetes. Among Renaissance physicians Aretaeus was considered second only to Hippocrates in his wisdom and scientific acumen.

AVICENNA

Eltorai, Ivan. "Avicenna's View on Cancer from His Canon." *American Journal of Chinese Medicine*, 7 (Autumn 1979), 276-84.

Avicenna was born in Bagdad in 980 and died there in 1037. Avicenna practiced medicine in Isfahan but travelled widely throughout Persia. He was the author of more than 200 books on science, medicine, and philosophy. Avicenna was a great physician whose work *Canon of Medicine* was the classical medical text of the Middle Ages. In the *Canon*, Avicenna clearly recognized cancer as a lesion which progressively grows larger and "spreads roots which insinuate themselves amongst the tissue-elements." He strongly advised surgical removal of cancerous lesions whenever possible. Otherwise, local recurrence was virtually guaranteed.

Musaev, T. M. "Vzgliady Abu Ali Ibn Siny (Avitsenny) na opukholevye zabole-vaniia." *Voprosy Onkologii*, 26 (1980), 72-74.

(See Chapter 2: AVICENNA: Eltorai).

Wicken, G. M. *Avicenna. Scientist and Philosopher.* London: 1952.

(See Chapter 2: AVICENNA: Eltorai).

BABES, AUREL

Douglass, L. E. "A Further Comment on the Contributions of Aurel A. Babes to Cytology and Pathology." *Acta Cytologica*, 11 (1967), 217-24.

(See Chapter 13: Douglass).

BAILLIE, MATTHEW

Crainz, Franco. "The Editions and Translations of Dr. Matthew Baillie's 'Morbid Anatomy'." *Medical History*, 26 (1982), 443-52.

(See Chapter 2: BAILLIE, MATTHEW: "Matthew Baillie").

Grossman, I. W. "The Diagnosis of Neoplasm in Matthew Baillie's Atlas of Anatomy (1812)." *Bulletin of the New York Academy of Medicine*, 47 (December 1971), 1504-08.

(See Chapter 2: BAILLIE, MATTHEW: "Matthew Baillie").

"Matthew Baillie (1761-1823)." *CA-A Cancer Journal for Clinicians*, 24 (January-February 1974), 47-48.

Matthew Baillie was born in Scotland in 1761. He studied at Glasgow University and at Oxford University in England. A member of the Royal College of Physicians, Baillie is best remembered for his 1793 text *The Morbid Anatomy in Some of the Most Important Parts of the Human Body.* Although Baillie was not really concerned with the etiology or the process of disease, his work was the first systematic, codified pathology study. It was also the first systematic description of malignant lesions, clearly distinguishing them from inflammatory or cystic tumors. Matthew Baillie died in 1823.

Rodin, Alvin. *The Influence of Matthew Baillie's Morbid Anatomy: Biography, Evaluation, and Reprint.* Springfield, Ill.: 1973.

(See Chapter 2: BAILLIE, MATTHEW: "Matthew Baillie").

BEATSON, GEORGE

Gilbertsen, V. A. "Beatson's Contribution to Cancer Research." *Surgo*, 32 (1964), 17-19.

(See Chapter 11: Goldenberg).

Paul, James. "Sir George Thomas Beatson and the Royal Beatson Memorial Hospital." *Medical History*, 25 (1981), 200-01.

(See Chapter 11: Goldenberg).

Stockwell, Serena. "Classics in Oncology: George Thomas Beatson, M. D. (1848-1933)." *CA-A Cancer Journal for Clinicians*, 33 (March-April 1983), 105-21.

George Thomas Beatson was born in Ceylon in 1848 and received his undergraduate degree from the University of Edinburgh in 1874 and his medical degree from Cambridge University in 1878. After teaching at the University of Edinburgh, Beatson went to the Glasgow Cancer Hospital. In 1896 he published his monumental paper "On the Treatment of Inoperable Cases of Carcinoma of the Mamma: Suggestions for a New Method of Treatment, with Illustrative Cases," where he recommended bilateral oophorectomy for advanced breast cancer. Eventually surgical castration became the primary form of therapy for premenopausal women with advanced breast cancer. George Beatson died in 1933, by which time the practice of oophorectomy had largely been abandoned with the development of synthetic hormones.

BENNETT, ALEXANDER HUGHES

"Alexander Hughes Bennett (1848-1901) and Rickman John Godlee (1849-1925)." *CA-A Cancer Journal for Clinicians*, 24 (May-June 1974), 169-70.

Alexander Hughes Bennett was born in Scotland in 1848. His father, John Hughes Bennett, was a prominent physician at Edinburgh University. When his father died of a benign brain tumor, Bennett became interested in neurosurgery and practiced at the Westminister Hospital in London. In 1885, along with Rickman John Godlee, Bennett performed the first successful surgical removal of a brain tumor. All previously recorded intracranial operations had been performed only upon external evidence of brain injury, not upon clinical evidence of neuromuscular dysfunction. Bennett died in 1901.

BERENBLUM, ISAAC

Berenblum, Isaac. "Cancer Research in Historical Perspective: An Autobiographical Essay." *Cancer Research*, 37 (January 1977), 1-7.

(See Chapter 2: BERENBLUM, ISAAC: Stockwell).

Stockwell, Serena. "Isaac Berenblum, M. D." *CA-A Cancer Journal for Clinicians,* 31 (July/August 1981), 239-40.

Isaac Berenblum was born in Bialystock, Poland, in 1903. His family emigrated to Belgium in 1906 and then to England in 1914, when World War I broke out. Educated at Leeds University, Berenblum spent his career as a cancer specialist at Leeds University, Oxford University, and the Weizmann Institute of Science. He is credited with being the first person to explain the basic mechanism of carcinogenesis. In 1941 Berenblum conducted experiments which showed that carcinogenesis involves three separate, independent stages: initiation, promotion, and latency. He applied benzpyrene to mouse skin and found that the chemical induced a few, very small tumors. But when he applied croton resin with benzpyrene, there was a dramatic increase in the size and number of tumors. The benzpyrene (initiator) caused a mutation in stem cells that became apparent only when the croton resin (the promoter) was applied. The mutation caused by the initiation process can remain dormant (the latency period). The promoter alters or inhibits cell differentiation without stopping growth.

BERNHARD, WILHELM

Marbach, J. U. "Wilhelm Bernhard, 1920-1978." *Gesnerus,* 36 (1979), 303-11.

Wilhelm Bernhard was born in 1920 and spent his career as a pathologist and cellular biologist. He did his postgraduate training at the Medical School of the University of Paris and eventually became the assistant to Charles Oberling at the Institute for Cancer Research at the University of Paris. Bernhard died in 1978.

BILLROTH, CHRISTIAN ALBERT THEODOR

Mann, Ruth J. "Theodor Billroth, 1829-1894." *Mayo Clinic Proceedings,* 49 (1974), 132-35.

Theodor Billroth was born on the island of Rugen, Germany, in 1829. He received his medical degree from the University of Berlin in 1852. After studying surgery at Gottingen between 1852 and 1860, Billroth began teaching in Zürich, where he remained until 1867. He then became a professor of surgery at the University of Vienna. Billroth spent the rest of his career there. Billroth is credited with being the father of modern surgery. Billroth was an early user of the principles of antisepsis, and because of that he made extraordinary contributions to modern surgery. He was the first to perform a resection of the esophagus (1871), total excision of the larynx (1873), partial gastrectomy (1881), and a gastrojejunostomy (1885). Theodor Billroth died in 1894.

BOERHAAVE, HERMANN

Lindeboom, G. A. *Boerhaave and His Times.* Leyden: 1970.

(See Chapter 2: BOERHAAVE, HERMANN: Lindeboom).

Lindeboom, G. A. *Hermann Boerhaave. The Man and His Work.* London: 1968.

Hermann Boerhaave was born in Leiden, Holland, in 1668, where he practiced medicine and wrote scientific expositions throughout his life. From 1708 until his death, Boerhaave was a professor of medicine at the University of Leiden. Medical historians look to him as the father of contemporary methods of clinical instruction, having students accompany a senior physician on hospital rounds on a daily basis. Because he wrote so prodigiously, Boerhaave became an influential figure in early eighteenth century medicine. He believed that cancer developed out of "scirrhus" lesions, which themselves came from fluid blockages in the body. Boerhaave died in 1738.

Underwood, E. Ashworth. *Boerhaave's Men at Leyden and After.* Edinburgh: 1977.

(See Chapter 2: BOERHAAVE, HERMANN: Lindeboom).

BOGOMOLETS, ALEKSANDR ALEKSANDROVICH

Neiman, I. M. "Onkologicheskie vozzreniia A. A. Bogomol'tsa v svete sovremennykh dannykh." *Patologicheskaia Fiziologiia i Eksperimental'naia Terapiia,* 4 (July-August 1976), 3-7.

(See Chapter 2: BOGOMOLETS, ALEKSANDR ALEKSANDROVICH: Pinchuk).

Pinchuk, V. G. "Razvitie idei A. A. Bogomolets v oblasti izucheniia reaktivnosti pri poukholevom protsesse." *Fiziologii Zhournal,* 27 (May-June 1981), 327-31.

A. A. Bogomolets was born in Kiev on May 12, 1881. He graduated from Novorossiia University at Odessa in 1906, specializing in medicine, particularly pathophysiology. Between 1911 and 1925 he was a professor at the University of Saratov, and then he moved to the Second Moscow University. From 1931 to his death in 1946, Bogomolets was director of the Institute of Experimental Biology and Pathology and of the Institute of Clinical Physiology at Kiev.

BORDET, JULES

Beumer, J. "Jules Bordet, 1870-1961." *Journal of General Microbiology*, 29 (1962), 1-13.

Jules Bordet was born in Belgium in 1870 and trained as a bacteriologist at the Free University of Brussels. Bordet became a world renowned bacteriologist and immunologist, and from 1907 to 1940 he served as director of the Pasteur Institute of Brussels. In 1917 Bordet won the Nobel Prize for his research. He died in 1961.

BORREL, AMÉDÉE

Le Guyon, Rene. "Borrel et le theorie virusale des cancers." *Bulletin de le Academie National de Medecine*, 151 (21 November 1967), 585-93.

(See Chapter 4: Le Guyon).

BORST, MAX

Steffen, Charles. "Max Borst (1869-1946)." *American Journal of Dermatopathology*, 7 (February 1985), 25-27.

Max Borst was born in 1869 and raised in Würzburg, Germany. He received his medical training at the university there, graduating in 1892, and he then spent 6 years studying at the Pathologic Institute at Würzburg. During his academic career Borst taught at the universities of Bonn, Cologne, Gottingen, Würzburg, and Munich. A famed cellular anatomist, Borst specialized in neoplastic disease and was the first to classify lesions according to their histogenesis and to attempt to describe the natural history of the lesions from their pathological appearance. Max Borst died in 1946.

BOVERI, THEODOR

Baltzer, Fritz, *Theodor Boveri. Life and Work of a Great Biologist 1862-1915.* Berkeley: 1967.

Theodor Boveri was born in Germany in 1862 and eventually became a professor of zoology at the University of Wurzberg. In his studies of mitosis in sea urchins, Boveri observed anatomically irregular cell divisions, and he compared them with mitoses in tumor cells. In 1902 Boveri proposed his somatic mutation theory of oncogenesis, in which he argued that the etiology of cancer could be found in abnormal chromosomes. His ideas did the not find a wide audience at the time, because Amédée Borrel's infectious theories held sway, but in recent years medical historians have realized that Boveri's proposals were ahead of their time. Theodor Boveri died in 1915.

BOWEN, JOHN TEMPLETON

White, C. J. "John Templeton Bowen, M. D." *Archives of Dermatology*, 43
(February 1941), 386.

(See Chapter 18: "Cancer Eponyms: Bowen's Disease").

BRUNSCHWIG, ALEXANDER

"Alexander Brunschwig (1901-1969)." *CA-A Cancer Journal for Clinicians*, 24
(November-December 1974), 361-62.

Alexander Brunschwig was born on September 11, 1901, in El Paso, Texas.
He received bachelor's and master's degrees from the University of Chicago in
1923 and 1924, and he earned a medical degree at the Rush Medical College in
Chicago in 1927. During his career Brunschwig taught pathology and surgery at
the Boston City Hospital, the University of Strasbourg, the University of Chicago,
and the Memorial Hospital for the Treatment of Cancer and Allied Diseases. In
1937 Brunschwig performed the first successful resection of the entire head of the
pancreas and most of the duodenum for cancer. By the late 1940s Brunschwig was
developing the surgical procedure which became known as the "Brunschwig Pelvic
Exenteration." Theorizing that cervical and endometrial cancer were often confined to the lower pelvis, he called for ultraradical dissection of the organs in the
pelvic area. Although controversial, his pelvic exenteration is considered by many
to be a major breakthrough in gynecologic oncology during the mid-twentieth
century. He is remembered as one of the medical world's primary advocates of
superradical surgical procedures. In addition to the massive pelvic exenteration,
Brunschwig had also performed superradical mastectomies, hempelvectomies, and
hemicorporectomies. Alexander Brunschwig died on August 7, 1969.

BURKITT, DENIS PARSONS

"Denis Parsons Burkitt (1911-)." *CA-A Cancer Journal for Clinicians*, 22
(November-December 1972), 345-47.

(See Chapter 2: BURKITT, DENIS PARSONS: Glemser).

Ellis, H. "Eponyms in Oncology: Denis Burkitt." *European Journal of Surgical
Oncology*, 13 (April 1987), 167.

(See Chapter 2: BURKITT, DENIS PARSONS: Glemser).

Glemser, Bernard. *Mr. Burkitt and Africa*. New York: 1970.

Denis Burkitt was born in Northern Ireland in 1911 and received his medical degree from Dublin University in 1935. Between 1941 and 1964 Burkitt
served as a military and later British government physician in Uganda, and in
1958 he described the lesion which now bears his name—Burkitt's lymphoma, a

rapidly growing neoplasm which most frequently appeared in the jaws of young children. Along with Dr. Joseph Burchenal of the Sloan-Kettering Institute for Cancer Research in New York City, Burkitt developed a highly successful antifolate chemotherapy treatment for the disease. Subsequent research has indicated a strong suspicion that the Epstein-Barr virus is central to the etiology of Burkitt's lymphoma.

BURNET, FRANK MACFARLANE

"Sir Frank MacFarlane Burnet (1899-)." *CA-A Cancer Journal for Clinicians*, 26 (March-April 1976), 116-17.

Frank MacFarlane Burnet was born on September 3, 1899, in Traragon, Australia. He earned his medical degree at the University of Melbourne and then went into pathology. Burnet earned a Ph.D. from the Lister Institute in 1928 and then returned to Australia where he spent the rest of his career at the Hall Institute, a center for virology research. While there he changed his own research focus from virology to immunology, demonstrating, after injecting blood from an adult chicken into a chick embryo, that the "adult" cells recognized the embryo cells as "non-self." Burnet was awarded the Nobel Prize in 1960. After receiving the Nobel Prize, Burnet spent the remaining years of his career focusing on autoimmune diseases.

CELSUS, AULUS CORNELIUS

Castiglioni, Arturo. "Aulus Cornelius Celsus as a Historian of Medicine." *Bulletin of the History of Medicine*, 8 (1940), 857-73.

(See Chapter 1: Brunner).

CHEEK, J. HAROLD

Stockwell, Serena. "J. Harold Cheek, M. D." *CA-A Cancer Journal for Clinicians*, 33 (July-August 1983), 242-43.

J. Harold Cheek was born in Eldorado, Oklahoma, and earned his medical degree in 1944 from the University of Texas, Southwestern Medical School, in Dallas, Texas. Specializing in surgery, Cheek eventually confined his practice exclusively to breast cancer patients. In 1953 Cheek surveyed 55 prominent surgeons on the question of breast cancer, pregnancy, and lactation. At the time conventional wisdom insisted that breast cancer associated with pregnancy or lactation was categorically inoperable. The survey posed five questions about breast cancer and pregnancy—incidence, operability, recurrence, therapeutic abortion, and sterilization. Most of the physicians responded, but none of the responding physicians believed that pregnancy alone should be considered a factor that ruled out radical mastectomy. Because of Cheek's article, standard surgical practice changed. Pregnant women with breast cancer presenting themselves to an oncologist were considered candidates for radical surgery.

CHURG, JACOB

Grishman, Edith. "The Man Behind the Eponym: Dr. Jacob Churg." *American Journal of Dermatopathology*, 8 (August 1986), 358-59.

Jacob Churg was born in Poland in 1910 and received his medical training there. He moved to the United States and worked as a pathologist at Mt. Sinai Hospital in New York City. Churg specialized in histology and made a major contribution in discovering the relationship between asbestos exposure and the development of mesothelioma.

CLARK, JOHN

Harvey, A. McGehee. "Early Contributions to the Surgery of Cancer: William S. Halsted, Hugh H. Young, and John G. Clark." *The Johns Hopkins Medical Journal*, 135 (December 1974), 399-417.

(See Chapter 23: Harvey).

CLARK, R. LEE

Macon, N. D. *Clark and the Anderson. A Personal Profile.* Houston: 1976.

R. Lee Clark was born in Texas and specialized in surgical oncology. The M. D. Anderson Hospital and Tumor Institute in Houston, Texas, was established in 1942, with Ernest W. Bertner as its first director. Four years later Clark succeeded him as director, and in the next three decades he built the hospital into one of the premier cancer research and clinical facilities in the world. M. D. Anderson was especially noted for its aggressive and finely-tuned approach to the radiotherapy of tumors.

CLAUDE, ALBERT

Florkin, M. "Pour Saluer Albert Claude." *Archives International des Physiologie et Biochimistrie*, 80 (October 1972), 632-47.

Albert Claude was born in Belgium in 1899 and is widely considered the father of modern molecular biology. He spent his career as director of the Jules Bordet Institute for Cancer Research in Brussels, after working nearly twenty years with the Rockefeller Institute in New York City. Claude perfected the technique of fractionating cells through differential centrifugation and then explaining the function of cellular constituents. In 1974 Claude received the Nobel Prize.

COHNHEIM, JULIUS

Grundmann, E. "Die Vorstellungen von Julius Cohnheim zur Geschwülstentstehung und Metastasierung im Blickwinkel neuer Forschungsergebnisse." *Zentralblatt für Allgemeine Pathologie und Pathologische Anatomie*, 130 (1985), 323-31.

(See Chapter 8: Grundmann).

COOPER, ASTLEY

Brock, Russell. *The Life and Work of Astley Cooper.* London: 1952.

(See Chapter 2: COOPER, ASTLEY: Keynes).

Keynes, Geoffrey. "The Life and Works of Astley Cooper." *St. Bartholomew's Hospital Reports*, 15 (1922), 9-36.

Astley Cooper, the gifted anatomist and surgeon, was born in England in 1768. He studied medicine and surgery under John Hunter and practiced medicine in London at Guy's Hospital. Committed to the notion of empirical research, Cooper was an active dissectionist and writer and concentrated particularly on diseases of the breast in women and testicles in men. In Europe he was widely considered the successor to John Hunter as the dean of surgery. His writing included an accurate description of the anatomy of the breast and associated lymphatic tissues, as well as tumors of the testicle. In surgery Cooper was the first to tie off the aorta to treat an aneurysm. Cooper was aware of the metastatic routes of testicular carcinomas, and he advocated orchiectomy as the only curative treatment. Astley Cooper died in 1841.

CURIE, MARIE SKLODOWSKA

Curie, Eva. *Madame Curie.* Garden City, N. Y.: 1937.

Marie Sklodowska was born in Warsaw, Poland, in 1867 and studied physics at the Sorbonne in Paris, where she met her husband, Pierre Curie. They were married in 1895. Curie earned her Ph.D. at the Sorbonne in 1904. In their experiments with uranium, they discovered that pitchblende mineral showed an unusually high radioactivity. Eventually they separated out polonium and radium in their experiments. She coined the term "radioactivity" in 1898. Shortly after their discovery in the late 1890s, radium was being used to treat malignant neoplasms, giving birth to the new discipline of radiotherapy. The Curies received the Nobel Prize in 1903 for their work in physics, and in 1911 Marie Curie won the Nobel Prize in chemistry for isolating polonium and radium. Madame Curie died in 1934 of a radiation-induced leukemia.

CUSHING, HARVEY WILLIAMS

Fulton, John F. *Harvey Cushing: A Biography.* New York: 1946.

Harvey Cushing was born in Cleveland, Ohio, in 1869. A gifted surgeon, he served as chief of surgery at Peter Bent Brigham Hospital in Boston and as professor of surgery at Harvard University, between 1912 and 1932, and then he was associated with Yale University between 1932 and 1937. Cushing specialized in neurosurgery and was the author of *The Pituitary Body and its Disorders* (1912) and *Intracranial Tumors* (1932). During his career Cushing removed more than two thousand brain tumors and is widely considered the father of brain surgery. Harvey Cushing died in 1939.

German, William J., and Stevenson Flanigan. "Pituitary Adenomas: A Follow-Up on the Cushing Series." *Clinical Neurosurgery*, 10 (1964), 72-81.

(See Chapter 10: German and Flanigan).

Thomson, Elizabeth H. *Harvey Cushing: Surgeon, Author, Artist.* New York: 1981.

(See Chapter 10: CUSHING, HARVEY: Fulton).

CZERNY, VINCENZ

Wyklicky, H. "Vincenz Czerny. Pionier der Interdisziplinaren Krebsbekamp-fung." *Rheuma*, 6 (1986), 1-4.

Vincenz Czerny was born in Germany in 1842. A surgeon at the University of Heidelberg, Czerny founded the Institute for Experimental Cancer Research in 1906. Czerny was the leader of the idea of the team approach to clinical cancer, fully supporting the idea of radiotherapy working hand-in-hand with surgery to treat cancer patients. In doing so Vincent Czerny set the stage for the development of modern clinical oncology. The Institute was a pioneer in the early development of radiotherapy as a scientific discipline. Czerny died in 1916.

DONNE, ALFRED FRANÇOIS

Thorburn, A. Lennox. "Alfred François Donne 1801-1878, Discoverer of Tri-chomonas Vaginalis and Leukemia." *British Journal of Venereal Diseases*, 50 (October 1974), 377-80.

(See Chapter 16: Thorburn).

DORN, HAROLD FRED

Henson, Pamela. "Harold Fred Dorn." *Dictionary of American Biography.* Suppl. 7. 1981. Pp. 191-99.

Harold Dorn was born in Ithaca, New York, on July 30, 1906. He graduated from Cornell University with a degree in rural sociology and then went on to the University of Wisconsin for a Ph.D. in sociology and statistics. Dorn spent his career with the United States Public Health Service and concentrated on developing the statistical methodology for large-scale epidemiological studies of cardiovascular and neoplastic diseases. His work was important in the establishment of the epidemiological branch of the National Cancer Institute and the discipline of cancer epidemiology.

DUKES, CUTHBERT ESQUIRE

"Cuthbert Esquire Dukes (1890-1977)." *European Journal of Surgical Oncology,* 13 (February 1987), 77.

Cuthbert Dukes was born in 1890 and received his medical degree in 1914. After World War I he joined the staff of St. Mark's Hospital in London where he worked as a pathologist. He joined St. Peter's Hospital in 1929 and there developed his famous staging system for rectal carcinoma. Cuthbert Dukes died in 1977.

Fitzgerald, R. H. "What is the Dukes' System for Carcinoma of the Rectum?" *Diseases of the Colon and Rectum,* 25 (July-August 1982), 474-77.

In the 1930s C. Dukes and H. Westhues demonstrated clinically and statistically that downward lymphatic and tissue spread of rectal carcinomas was unusual. At the time surgical resection of rectal tumors usually required removal of the sphincter muscle, leaving patients incontinent and necessitating colostomies. Because of the work of Dukes and Westhues, surgical removal of the sphincter became unusual.

EHRLICH, PAUL

Gutt, R. W. "Pawel Ehrlich i obecna nauka o limfocytach." *Przeglad Lekarski,* 35 (1978), 707-10.

Paul Ehrlich was born in Germany in 1854 and became a world-renowned bacteriologist and chemist. He is widely considered the scientific father of modern chemotherapy because of his animal experiments with various chemical agents. Ehrlich also made important contributions to the understanding of leukemia. Using panoptic staining, he first elaborated cellular details of different types of leukemia, and he also traced the origins of granular cells to a precursor cell—the myelocyte. In 1887 Paul Ehrlich concluded that leukemia was a primary disease of the hemapoietic system—that more and more cells are produced and released into the bloodstream. Paul Ehrlich won the Nobel Prize in physiology and medicine in 1909. Ehrlich is also considered the father of modern chemotherapy because of his theory that administered drugs went through a molecular bonding process in a patient which either killed the malignant cells or rendered them vulnerable to normal immunological processes. Paul Ehrlich died in 1915.

Parascandola, John. "The Theoretical Basis of Paul Ehrlich's Chemotherapy." *Journal of the History of Medicine and the Allied Sciences,* 36 (January 1981), 19-43.

(See Chapter 25: Swann).

Swann, John Patrick. "Paul Ehrlich and the Introduction of Salvarsan." *Medical Heritage,* 1 (March-April 1985), 137-38.

(See Chapter 25: Swann).

EWING, JAMES

"Cancer Eponyms: Ewing's Sarcoma." *Cancer Bulletin*, 6 (September-October 1954), 105, 114.

(See Chapter 9: "Cancer Eponyms: Ewing's Sarcoma").

"James Ewing (1866-1943)." *CA-A Cancer Journal for Clinicians*, 22 (March-April 1972), 93-94.

(See Chapter 2: EWING, JAMES: Stewart).

Regato, J. A. "James Ewing." *International Journal of Radiation Oncology, Biology, and Physics*, 2 (January-February 1977), 185-98.

(See Chapter 2: EWING, JAMES: Stewart).

Stewart, F. W. "James Ewing, M. D." *Archives of Pathology*, 36 (September 1954), 325-40.

James Ewing was born December 25, 1866, in Pittsburgh, Pennsylvania. He received his undergraduate degree from Amherst and his medical degree from Columbia University. In 1899 Ewing became head of the pathology department of the Cornell University Medical School, and in 1919 he wrote his pathbreaking book *Neoplastic Diseases*. There Ewing argued that cancer was actually a collection of dozens of different disease entities, and that treatment should be geared to the tumor type and the stage of the disease. Ewing served as the first president of the American Association for Cancer Research (1907-09). In 1913 Ewing joined the staff of the Memorial Hospital for the Treatment of Cancer and Allied Diseases in New York City, and he became director of the hospital in 1931. Ewing is best remembered for his initial description of endotheliomas— non-osteogenic tumors of the bone, the tumor which now bears his name. James Ewing died of cancer on May 16, 1943.

Stewart, F. W. "Retirement in New York: Prognosis and Reminiscences of a Non-Optimist." *Bulletin of the New York Academy of Medicine*, 47 (1971), 1342-49.

(See Chapter 2: EWING, JAMES: Stewart).

FARBER, SIDNEY

Foley, George E. "Obituary of Sidney Farber, M. D." *Cancer Research*, 34 (1974), 658-61.

(See Chapter 2: FARBER, SIDNEY: "Sidney Farber 1903-1973").

"Sidney Farber (1903-1973)." *CA-A Cancer Journal for Clinicians*, 24 (September-October 1974), 294-96.

Sidney Farber was born in Buffalo, New York, on September 30, 1903. He graduated from the University of Buffalo in 1923, studied at the Universities of Freiburg and Heidelberg, and then received a medical degree from Harvard in 1927. He spent two years in pathology residencies at Harvard and the University of Munich, and in 1929 Farber returned to Harvard, where he remained for the rest of his distinguished career. Late in the 1940s and early in the 1950s, Farber pioneered the field of chemotherapy after discovering that folic acid deprivation actually retarded the growth of leukemia cells. In the winter of 1947, Farber administered aminopterin, an antifolic drug, to a child critically ill with acute leukemia and induced a temporary remission. In 1954 Farber demonstrated that actinomycin D was effective against metastatic Wilms' tumor in children. In addition to being one of the founders of modern chemotherapy, Farber is also recognized as the father of pediatric oncology, through his founding of the Children's Cancer Research Foundation in Boston. Sidney Farber died in 1973.

FELL, JESSE WELDON

Farrow, Ruth T. "Odyssey of an American Cancer Specialist of a Hundred Years Ago." *Bulletin of the History of Medicine*, 23 (1949), 236-52.

Jesse Weldon Fell was an American physician of the mid-nineteenth century practicing in London. He specialized in cancer treatment. Fell treated cancer with a herbal potion taken from Indian tribes near Lake Superior. The plant was known as sanguinaria canadensis. He mixed the fluid from the plant with zinc chloride and applied it topically to tumors. Fell was eventually invited to join the staff of the Middlesex Hospital in 1857. Clinical trials proved his "Fell's Paste" to be useless and he was ridiculed by the London medical establishment.

Montagu, M. F. Ashley and W. J. Musick. "A Yankee Doctor in England in 1859." *Bulletin of the History of Medicine*, 13 (1943), 217-28.

(See Chapter 2: FELL, JESSE WELDON: Farrow).

FERGUSON, ALEXANDER ROBERT

Mustacchi, P., and L. Jassey. "Alexander Robert Ferguson, M. D. "On 'The Irritation Cancer of Egypt'." *Cancer*, 15 (1962), 215-16.

Alexander Robert Ferguson was born in Scotland in 1870 and spent much of his medical career as a pathologist at the School of Medicine in Cairo, Egypt. In 1911 Ferguson made the connection between the disease bilharziasis, a parasitical bladder infection common in Africa, and bladder carcinoma. He made the connection after extensive autopsy studies. Widespread parasitical presence in the bladder induced epithelial lesions which evolved into carcinoma. Ferguson died in 1920.

FURTH, JACOB

Furth, Jacob. "The Making and Missing of Discoveries: An Autobiographical Essay." *Cancer Research*, 36 (March 1976), 871-80.

An experimental oncologist trained at the University of Budapest and the Charles University of Prague, Jacob Furth immigrated to the United States early in the 1920s and taught and worked successively at the University of Pennsylvania, the Rockefeller Institute, the Cornell-New York Hospital, the Southwestern Medical College in Dallas, the Oak Ridge National Laboratory, Harvard University, the Roswell Park Institute, and Columbia University. Furth specialized in the chemical, viral, and radiation etiology of animal leukemias.

GALEN, CLARISSIMUS

Lytton, D. G., and L. M. Resuhr. "Galen on Abnormal Swellings." *Journal of the History of Medicine and the Allied Sciences*, 33 (October 1978), 531-49.

(See Chapter 1: Lytton and Resuhr).

Rather, L. J. "Disturbance of Function (Functio Laesa): The Legendary Fifth Sign of Inflammation, Added by Galen to the Four Cardinal Signs of Celsus." *Bulletin of the New York Academy of Medicine*, 47 (1971), 303-322.

(See Chapter 2: GALEN, CLARISSIMUS: Temkin).

Reedy, James. "Galen on Cancer and Related Diseases." *Clio Medica*, 10 (September 1975), 227-38.

(See Chapter 2: GALEN, CLARISSIMUS: Temkin).

Sarton, George. *Galen of Pergamon*. Lawrence, Kansas: 1954.

(See Chapter 2: GALEN, CLARISSIMUS: Temkin).

Siegel, Rudolf. *Galen's System of Physiology and Medicine*. Basel: 1968.

(See Chapter 2: GALEN, CLARRISIMUS: Temkin).

Temkin, Owsei. *Galenism. Rise and Decline of a Medical Philosophy*. New York: 1973.

Clarissimus Galen was born in 139 A. D. in Pergamon, Asia Minor. He studied medicine at Alexandria and became the most renowned physician in the Roman world. In 157 he was appointed physician to the gladiators at Rome; after service there he became physician to the Emperors Marcus Aurelius and Commodus.

Galen followed the lead of Hippocrates in describing cancers as growths arising from an excess of black bile. Because of injury or overexercise, some part of the body would attract the black bile, giving rise to a tumor. Galen believed in the humoral theory, which argued that the body possesses four fundamental humors: blood, phlegm, yellow bile, and black bile, and that individual health requires that they all be in balance. Illness develops when one of the humors increases or decreases in amount. For cancer the culprit was black bile. Galen recommended no treatment for cancer, unless they were lesions of the skin, which he believed should be surgically excised. Galen returned to Pergamon in 190, and he died in 201, but his theories about health, illness, and physiology dominated medical thinking for the next thirteen centuries. The humoral theories remained the prevailing approach to medicine and disease throughout the Middle Ages and into the Renaissance.

Toledo-Pereryva, Luis H. "Galen's Contribution to Surgery." *The Journal of the History of Medicine and the Allied Sciences*, 28 (October 1973), 357-75.

(See Chapter 2: GALEN, CLARISSIMUS: Temkin).

GENDRON, CLAUDE DESHAIS

Mustacchi, P. and Michael B. Shimkin. "Gendron's Enquiries into the Nature, Knowledge and Cure of Cancers." *Cancer*, 9 (1956), 645-47.

Claude Deshais Gendron was born in France in 1663 and received his medical training at the Montpellier school. Gendron spent most of his career as a physician to the royal family at Versailles, France, following in the footsteps of his uncle, Abbott Gendron. Gendron believed in empirical observations and regularly performed dissections to study cancer. In 1700 his book *Recherches sur la nature et la guerison des cancer* was published, and in it he rejected the humoral theory of cancer etiology as well as the iatrochemical school. Instead, Gendron claimed that tumors originated locally in tissues and could not be cured without wide surgical excision. Although he did not understand the real etiology of cancer, his rejection of the humoral theories was ahead of his time. Claude Gendron died in 1750.

GERTSEN, PETR ALEKSANDROVICH

Kozhevnikov, A. I. "Petr Aleksandrovich Gertsen (K 75-letiiu Moskovskogo nauch-noissledovatel'skogo Onkologicheskogo Instituta im. P. A. Gertsena). *Vestnik Khirurgiia*, 121 (December 1978), 104-07.

Petr Aleksandrovich Gertsen was born April 26, 1871, in Florence. He was one of the founders of oncology in the Soviet Union. Gertsen received his medical education at the Lausanne in Switzerland. He was a founder of what became known as the P. A. Gertsen Central Oncological Institute in Moscow. Gertsen was a surgeon who pioneered a number of techniques, including the creation of an artificial prethoracic esophagus from the small intestine, colon and gallbladder resections, and head and neck tumors. Gertsen died on January 2, 1947.

GODLEE, RICKMAN JOHN

"Alexander Hughes Bennett (1848-1901) and Rickman John Godlee (1849-1925)." *CA-A Cancer Journal for Clinicians*, 24 (May-June 1974), 169-70.

Rickman John Godlee was born in London in 1849 and studied medicine at Edinburgh University where his uncle, John Lister (the father of modern surgery), taught medicine. Godlee returned to London in 1877 to practice surgery at the University College Hospital. In 1885, along with Alexander Hughes Bennett, Godlee performed the first successful surgical removal of a brain tumor. In 1914 Godlee was elected president of the Royal College of Surgeons. He died in 1925.

GRAHAM, EVARTS

"Evarts A. Graham (1883-1957)." *CA-A Cancer Journal for Clinicians*, 24 (July-August 1974), 236-37.

Evarts A. Graham was born in Chicago, Illinois, on March 19, 1883. He graduated from Princeton University in 1903 and the Rush Medical College in Chicago in 1907. After leaving the army medical corps in 1919, Graham secured a position as professor of surgery at Washington University in St. Louis. On April 5, 1933, Evarts won his place in medical history by performing the first successful one-stage pneumonectomy for lung cancer with individual ligation of the hilar structures. By the 1950s that surgery had become the preferred treatment for lung carcinoma. Evarts A. Graham died of lung cancer on March 4, 1957.

Olch, Peter D. "Evarts A. Graham, The American College of Surgeons, and the American Board of Surgery," *Journal of the History of Medicine and Allied Sciences*, 27 (July 1972), 247-62.

(See Chapter 2: GRAHAM, EVARTS: "Evarts A. Graham").

GRAWITZ, PAUL ALBERT

"Cancer Eponyms: Grawitz's Tumor." *Cancer Bulletin*, 9 (March-April 1957), 30.

Paul Albert Grawitz was born October 1, 1850, in Butow, Germany. He studied medicine in Berlin and at the Pathology Institute there. Grawitz served as professor of pathology at the University of Griefswald. In 1883 he proposed the theory that epithelial tumors of the kidney were derived from aberrant adrenal tissue. By 1920 the so-called "Grawitz's Tumor" was refuted and identified as renal adenocarcinoma.

GREEN, HARRY NORMAN

Bonser, G. M., and H. B. Stoner. "Harry Norman Green. 21 September 1902-16 May 1967." *Journal of Pathology and Bacteriology*, 96 (July 1968), 243-52.

Harry Green was born in Sheffield, England, on September 21, 1902. He received his undergraduate and medical degrees from Sheffield University and then specialized in pathology. Green taught at Sheffield University (1926-1933 and 1935-1953), Cambridge University (1933-1935), and the University of Leeds (1953-1967). Green's research interests involved the immune process in cancer induction and growth. Carcinogenic activity is essentially the result of an individual immune reaction, the carcinogen combining with certain "identity proteins" within the cells of the tissue to which it is applied. These proteins are rendered foreign to the animal and elicit an antibody response as would any other foreign protein, leading to the death of most of the affected cells. The survivors lose the carcinogen-affected protein and become no longer foreign. Green called it the "protein-depletion theory." Harry Green died on May 16, 1967.

GRUBBE, EMIL

Hodges, Paul C. *The Life and Times of Emil H. Grubbe*. Chicago: 1964.

(See Chapter 24: Hodges).

HADDOW, ALEXANDER

Bergel, F. "Alexander Haddow, 18 January 1907-21 January 1976." *Biographies of the Members of the Royal Society*, 23 (1977), 133-91.

Alexander Haddow was born in England on January 18, 1907, and spent his medical career as an oncologist with a special interest in carcinogenesis and the nature of clinical services. In 1946 Haddow was appointed as director of the Chester Beatty Institute, the premier cancer research facility in Great Britain. While in that position he emphasized developments in chemotherapy, tumor induction, carcinogenesis, and the team approach to treatment. Alexander Haddow died on January 21, 1976.

Haddow, Alexander. "An Autobiographical Essay." *Cancer Research*, 34 (1964), 3159-64.

(See Chapter 2: HADDOW, ALEXANDER: Haddow).

HALSTED, WILLIAM STEWART

Beckhard, A. J. and W. D. Crane. *Cancer, Cocaine and Courage: The Story of Dr. William Halsted.* New York: 1960.

William Stewart Halsted was born on September 27, 1852, in New York City. He graduated from Yale in 1872 and earned his medical degree at the College of Physicians and Surgeons of Columbia University in 1877. Halsted practiced medicine in New York City in the 1880s, and in 1889 he joined the medical faculty of Johns Hopkins University, where he remained until his death on September 7, 1922. A renowned surgeon, Halsted is primarily remembered for development of the radical mastectomy for treatment of breast carcinoma. He first performed the radical mastectomy in 1891 and delivered the famous paper justifying the procedure in 1894. Halsted is also remembered for a variety of other surgical accomplishments: introduced silver sutures in place of catgut because of the need for bacterial control; introduced the use of rubber gloves during surgery; invented the use of delicate, pointed forceps for hemostasis; developed methods for slowly constricting major blood vessels in treating aneurysms, ligating the left subclavian artery, reinfusing patients with their own blood, and providing neuroregional anesthesia; and developed surgical procedures for inguinal hernia, common bile duct disease, and bowel anastomosis. William Halsted died on September 22, 1922.

Ellis, H. "Eponyms in Oncology: William Stewart Halsted (1852-1922)." *European Journal of Surgical Oncology,* 11 (June 1985), 203.

(See Chapter 2: HALSTED, WILLIAM STEWART: Beckhard and Crane).

Harvey, A. McGehee. "Early Contributions to the Surgery of Cancer: William S. Halsted, Hugh H. Young, and John G. Clark." *The Johns Hopkins Medical Journal,* 135 (December 1974), 399-417.

(See Chapter 23: Harvey).

Heuer, G. J. "Dr. Halsted." *Bulletin of the Johns Hopkins Hospital,* 90 (1952) 1.

(See Chapter 2: HALSTED, WILLIAM STEWART: Beckhard and Crane).

"The Heritage of Halsted." *Cancer Bulletin,* 5 (September-October 1953), 110-11.

(See Chapter 2: HALSTED, WILLIAM STEWART: Beckhard and Crane).

Leriche, R. "A Tribute to Dr. Halsted." *Surgery,* 32 (September 1952), 538.

(See Chapter 2: HALSTED, WILLIAM STEWART: Beckhard and Crane).

Moorhead, J. J. "Halsted, The Surgeon's Preceptor." *Bulletin of the New York Academy of Medicine*, 28 (October 1952), 673.

(See Chapter 2: HALSTED, WILLIAM STEWART: Beckhard and Crane).

"William Stewart Halsted (1852-1922)." *CA-A Cancer Journal for Clinicians*, 23 (March-April 1973), 94-98.

(See Chapter 2: HALSTED, WILLIAM STEWART: Beckhard and Crane).

HANAU, ARTHUR

Bucher, H. W. "Zur Ersten Homologen Tumorubertragung in Zürich durch Arthur Hanau 1889." *Gesnerus*, 21 (1964), 193-200.

(See Chapter 2: HANAU, ARTHUR: Shimkin).

Shimkin, Michael B. "Arthur Nathan Hanau: A Further Note on the History of Transplantation of Tumors." *Cancer*, 13 (1960), 211.

Arthur Hanau (1858-1900) was a German pathologist who was trained at the University of Bonn and spent much of his career in Zürich. Following the lead of M. A. Novinsky in Russia, Hanau focused on the experimental transplantation of tumors. He succeeded in transplanting a carcinoma of the vulva from one rat to several other rats, confirming, in his own mind, the credibility of Novinsky's work. Arthur N. Hanau died in 1900 from a metastatic rectal carcinoma.

HARDY, JULES

Molina-Negro, Pedro. "Jules Hardy, M.D." *Surgical Neurology*, 22 (August 1984), 109-12.

Jules Hardy pioneered microsurgery in the 1960s and was the first to demonstrate the possibilities of identifying and preserving the normal gland during removal of large pituitary adenomas. He was the author of 100 papers. Hardy was born on July 16, 1932, in Sorel, Canada. He received his medical degree from the University of Montreal. In patients with hypersecreting pituitary disorders with normal-size sella turcica, he first described removal of intrapituitary microadenomas and advocated the transsphenoidal microsurgical exploration as the approach to therapeutic management of Cushing's disease and acromegaly. He first described prolactinmicroadenomas in the syndrome of amenorrhea-galactorrhea-infertility, thus clarifying a cause of hyperprolactinemia. Restoration of fertility after transsphenoidal microsurgical selective adenomectomy proved to be major medical advances and guaranteed Hardy's place in medical history.

HEIDELBERGER, CHARLES

Potter, V. R. "Years with Charles Heidelberger." *Carcinogenic Comparative Survey*, 10 (1985), 1-13.

(See Chapter 25: Potter).

HERTZ, ROY

"Roy Hertz (1909-)." *CA-A Cancer Journal for Clinicians*, 23 (July-August 1977), 242-43.

Roy Hertz was born on June 19, 1909, in Cleveland, Ohio. He was educated at the University of Wisconsin, receiving the B.A. in 1930, Ph.D. in physiology in 1933, and M.D. in 1939. An endocrinologist, Hertz demonstrated in 1934 that ovulation depends upon the sequential effects of follicle-stimulating and luteinizing hormones of the anterior pituitary on the ovary. He joined the U.S. Public Health Service in 1944 and the National Cancer Institute in 1946. In 1955, with Min Chiu Li, Hertz achieved the first remission of a solid tumor through chemotherapy. Speculating that the high folic acid demand of the female genital tract and normal embryonic development would subject trophoblastic tumors of the chorion to the action of folic acid antagonists, Hertz and Li administered methotrexate to a young woman with lung metastases from a choriocarcinoma. Within four months she was, and remained, disease free. He kept working with the disease, and by 1961 had added vincaleukoblastine to methotrexate therapy. By the 1960s methotrexate therapy had replaced hysterectomy as the treatment of choice for choriocarcinoma. Later Hertz succeeded in achieving tumor regression in patients with metastatic adrenocortical carcinoma by the use of ortho-para-prime DDD.

HIPPOCRATES

Barrow, Mark V. "Portraits of Hippocrates." *Medical History*, 16 (1972), 85-88.

Hippocrates was born on the island of Cos, Greece, in 460 B.C. Widely considered the father of medicine, Hippocrates was familiar with cancer and knew the difference between malignant and cystic or inflammatory lumps. Hippocrates coined the term "karkino" to describe cancer. The word in Greek meant "crab," which seemed appropriate to Hippocrates because of the tenacity of the disease. He attributed cancer to an excess of "black bile" in the body, and for nearly 2,000 years that idea prevailed. Hippocrates died in 370 B.C.

Glaser, S. "Hippocrates and Proctology." *Proceedings of the Royal Society of Medicine*, 62 (1969), 380-81.

Hippocrates was familiar with the problem of anal and rectal carcinomas, and he used digital proctology techniques to examine the tumors. His familiarity with the disease, however, did not lead to any treatments. Most of the time the lesions were not amenable to surgical excision, and Hippocrates preferred no treatment when the outlook was overwhelmingly negative. One of his primary rules for physicians was not to make the patient worse off.

HODGKIN, THOMAS

Onuigbo, Wilson I. B. "Thomas Hodgkin (1798-1866) on Cancer Cell Carriage." *Medical History*, 11 (October 1967), 406-11.

(See Chapter 8: Onuigbo).

Rose, Michael. *Curator of the Dead: Thomas Hodgkin (1798-1866)*. Atlantic Highlands, N. J.: 1982.

(See Chapter 2: HODGKIN, THOMAS: "Thomas Hodgkin").

"Thomas Hodgkin (1798-1866)." *CA-A Cancer Journal for Clinicians*, 23 (January- February 1973), 52-53.

Thomas Hodgkin was born in Tottenham, England, on January 16, 1798. Early in the 1820s he studied medicine under Laènnec in Paris, and in 1823 he received a doctorate in medicine from Edinburgh University. Hodgkin became a member of the Royal College of Physicians of London and curator of the Museum of Pathological Anatomy at Guy's Hospital in London in 1825. He presented his famous paper "On Some Morbid Appearances of the Absorbent Glands and Spleen" in 1832, where he described a malignant disease characterized by enlargement of the lymph nodes, liver, and spleen and diffuse nonsupportive adenopathy. Today the disease is known as Hodgkin's disease, a malignant lymphoma. Thomas Hodgkin died on April 4, 1866.

HOUDRY, EUGENE JULES

Stine, J. K. "Eugene Jules Houdry." *Dictionary of American Biography*, Suppl.7, 1981. Pp. 367-69.

Eugene Houdry was born in Domont, France, on April 18, 1892. He studied mechanical engineering and went into the automobile industry, specializing in refining crude petroleum into gasoline. Houdry came to the United States in 1930 and established the Houdry Process Corporation. After World War II Houdry became convinced that the increase in lung cancer rates was due to carcinogenic hydrocarbons emitted into the atmosphere by automobiles. Houdry patented the catalytic converter in 1962 and eliminated carbon monoxide and unburned hydrocarbons from exhaust fumes. He then spent the rest of his life in a political campaign to require installation of the catalytic converter on all new automobiles. Houdry died on July 18, 1962.

HUGGINS, CHARLES BRENTON

"Charles Brenton Huggins (1901-)." *CA-A Cancer Journal for Clinicians*, 22 (July-August 1972), 230-31.

Charles Huggins was born in Halifax, Nova Scotia, Canada, on September 22, 1901. He graduated from Acadia University, received a medical degree from Harvard University, and then trained in surgery at the University of Michigan. Specializing in urology, Huggins spent his career at the University of Chicago. In 1941 Huggins established a definite relationship between hormones and prostatic cancer. Prostatic cancer was dramatically affected by castration or administration of estrogens, treatment which reduced the levels of acid phosphatase in the tumor cells. Huggins's observation that the synthetic estrogen diethylstilbestrol caused regression in disseminated prostatic cancer helped launch the modern era of chemotherapy. The antiandrogenic therapy Huggins proposed was widely adopted in treating prostatic carcinoma. In 1966 Charles Huggins was awarded the Nobel Prize.

HUNTER, JOHN

Dobson, Jessie. "John Hunter's Views on Cancer." *Annals of the Royal College of Surgeons of England*, 25 (1959), 167-81.

John Hunter was born in Scotland in 1728. He practiced medicine at St. George's Hospital in London. Historians widely recognize Hunter as the father of modern surgery. He published widely on surgical anatomy. As far as cancer was concerned, Hunter believed the disease had local origins in some cases, as well as humoral or systemic beginnings, realized it was usually a disease of older people, suspected that there was a hereditary connection in the occurrence of the disease, and advocated wide surgical excision unless there was obvious lymphatic involvement, in which he viewed the disease as incurable and surgery as unjustifiable. John Hunter died in 1793.

Gloyne, S. Roodhouse. *John Hunter*. Edinburgh: 1950.

(See Chapter 2: HUNTER, JOHN: Dobson).

Oppenheimer, Jane M. *New Aspects of John and William Hunter*. New York: 1946.

(See Chapter: HUNTER, JOHN: Dobson).

JONES, HENRY BENCE

"Henry Bence Jones (1813-1873)." *CA-A Cancer Journal for Clinicians*, 28 (January-February 1978), 47-48.

Henry Bence Jones was born in Thorington Hall, England, on December 31, 1813. He attended Trinity College, Cambridge, receiving undergraduate, master's and medical degrees in 1836, 1842, and 1849. Jones practiced medicine at St. George's Hospital in London. He is best remembered for his work with multiple myeloma. In 1845 he analyzed a urine sample from a dying patient. Upon boiling, the urine sample exhibited a strange opacity, which Jones identified as albumen. An autopsy on the patient indicated a softening of the major bones, which Jones identified as a malignancy. Today the disease is known as multiple myeloma, and the urine substance so frequently associated with the disease as the "Bence Jones Protein." Multiple myeloma today is recognized as a plasma cell neoplasm. Henry Bence Jones died in 1873.

KAPLAN, HENRY SEYMOUR

Fuks, Z., and M. Feldman. "Henry S. Kaplan 1918-1984: A Physician, A Scientist, A Friend." *Cancer Survey*, 4 (1985), 294-311.

Henry S. Kaplan was born in Chicago, Illinois, in 1918 and received his medical training at the Rush Medical College there, graduating in 1940. Kaplan completed a residency in radiology at the University of Minnesota. He joined the faculty of the medical school at Stanford University, and from 1948 to 1972 he served as chairman of the radiology department. In addition to his experimental work in radiobiology and with the viral etiology of rat leukemia, Kaplan pioneered in the radical radiotherapy of Hodgkin's disease. He was a central figure in the rise of radiotherapy to the status of a new discipline in oncology. Henry S. Kaplan died in 1984.

Ginzton, Edward L., and Craig S. Nunan. "History of Microwave Electron Linear Accelerators for Radiotherapy." *International Journal of Radiation Oncology, Biology, and Physics*, 11 (February 1985), 205-16.

(See Chapter 2: KAPLAN, HENRY: Fuks and Feldman).

KAPOSI, MORITZ

Bluefarb, S. M. *Kaposi's Sarcoma*. Springfield, Ill.: 1957.

Moritz Kaposi was born in Kaposvar, Hungary, on October 23, 1837, and received a medical degree from the University of Vienna in 1861. Kaposi spent the rest of his life practicing dermatology and teaching at the University of Vienna. He is best remembered in the history of medicine for his description of "Idiopathic Multiple Pigment Sarcoma of the Skin." The malignant lesion occurs most often in the extremities of adult men and is characterized by spindle cell tumors and appearing as blue, hemorrhaged nodules on the skin. Today the disease is known as "Kaposi's sarcoma." Moritz Kaposi died in 1903.

Braun, Michael. "Moritz Kaposi, M.D." *CA-A Cancer Journal for Clinicians*, 32 (November-December 1982), 340-41.

(See Chapter 2: KAPOSI, MORITZ: Bluefarb).

"Cancer Eponyms: Kaposi's Sarcoma." *Cancer Bulletin*, 9 (January-February 1957), 5.

(See Chapter 2: KAPOSI, MORITZ: Bluefarb, S. M.).

"Eponyms in Oncology: Moritz Kaposi (1837-1902)." *European Journal of Surgical Oncology*, 12 (June 1986), 199.

(See Chapter 2: KAPOSI, MORITZ: Bluefarb).

KENNAWAY, ERNEST

Haddow, Alexander. "Sir Ernest Lawrence Kennaway FRS, 1881-1958: Chemical Causation of Cancer Then and Today." *Perspectives in Biology and Medicine*, 17 (Summer 1974), 543-88.

(See Chapter 2: KENNAWAY, ERNEST: "Sir Ernest Kennaway").

"Sir Ernest Kennaway." *Cancer Bulletin*, 11 (January-February 1959), 18.

Ernest Kennaway was born on May 23, 1881, and graduated from New College, Oxford, and the Middlesex Hospital. In 1921 he joined the Royal Cancer Hospital and eventually became director of research. Kennaway was also a professor of pathology at the University of London. Between 1925 and 1955 he worked on identifying the carcinogenic hydrocarbons from coal tar. He found the five-ring hydrocarbon known as 3:4-benzpyrene. Kennaway was also active in the study of cancer epidemiology, and in the late 1950s he was among the first to describe the connection between smoking and lung cancer. Kennaway died on January 1, 1958.

KHLOPIN, NIKOLAI GRIGOR'EVICH

Shcherbakova, M. G., Puchkov, IuG. "Znachenie nauchnogo naslediia N. G. Khlopina dlia onkologii." *Voprosy Onkologii*, 23 (1977), 99-107.

Nikolai Khlopin was born July 16, 1897, in the city of Iur'ev. He graduated from the Petrograd Military Medical Academy in 1921 and the University of Petrograd in 1922. Khlopin specialized in histology and embryology. Khlopin spent his career teaching at the Medical Military Academy and the Oncological Institute in Leningrad. Between 1932 and 1954 he was head of histology and pathology at the Institute of Experimental Medicine in Leningrad, and from 1955 to his death on June 21, 1961, Khlopin was head of the Laboratory of Experimental Morphology at the Institute of Oncology of the Academy of Medical Sciences in Leningrad. Khlopin was a world renowned figure in evolutionary histology.

KRUKENBERG, FRIEDRICH ERNST

"Cancer Eponyms: Krukenberg Tumor." *Cancer Bulletin*, 7 (January-February 1955), 5.

(See Chapter 13: "Cancer Eponyms: Krukenberg Tumor").

LACASSAGNE, ANTOINE

Latarjet, R. *Notice sur la vie et les travaux de Antoine Lacassagne, 1884-1971.* Paris: 1973.

Antoine-Marcellin-Bernard Lacassagne was born in Paris in 1884 and spent his professional life studying the relationship between carcinogenesis and hormones. In 1932 Lacassagne described his experimental success in inducing breast cancer in mice which had been repeatedly injected with female sex hormones. By studying several generations of mice, Lacassagne also argued that certain strains were more genetically susceptible to tumor formation. Antoine Lacassagne died in 1971.

del Regato, J. A. "Antoine Lacassagne." *International Journal of Radiation Oncology, Biology, and Physics*, 12 (December 1986), 165-73.

(See Chapter 2: LACASSAGNE, ANTOINE: Latarjet).

LITTLE, CLARENCE COOK

Heston, W. E. "Obituary of Clarence Cook Little." *Cancer Research*, 32 (1972), 1354-56.

Clarence Cook Little was born in 1888 and received his scientific training at Harvard University. He specialized in genetics and became president of the University of Michigan in 1924. In 1929 Little founded the Roscoe B. Jackson Memorial Laboratory in Bar Harbor, Maine. The Jackson Laboratory quickly became one of the premier institutions in the world for the study of cancer genetics. Clarence Little died in 1971.

Snell, G. D. "Clarence Cook Little." *Biographies of the Members of the National Academy of Science*, 46 (1975), 241-63.

(See Chapter 2: LITTLE, CLARENCE COOK: Heston).

LOBSTEIN, JOHN GEORG
(See Chapter 19: "Primary Retroperitoneal Sarcoma—Lobstein's Tumor").

LOEB, LEO

Hartroff, W. Stanley. "Leo Loeb, 1869-1959." *Archives of Pathology*, 70 (1960), 269-74.

Leo Loeb was born on September 21, 1869, in Mayen, Germany. He received his medical degree in Zürich in 1897 and then emigrated to the United States. Loeb taught pathology at Rush Medical College (1902-1903), McGill University (1903-1910), the University of Pennsylvania (1910-1915), and Washington University (1915-1941). Loeb is considered one of the founders of experimental cancer research. Along with A. E. C. Lathrop, he established the influence of genetic factors in the incidence of tumors in mice and the influence of estrogen on the origin of such tumors. Loeb also demonstrated the susceptibility of cancerous mice to implanted tumors and the tendency of malignant cells treated with colloidal copper to give rise to resistant strains, which led to new approaches to cancer therapy. Leo Loeb died in 1959.

"Leo Loeb (1869-1959)." *CA-A Cancer Journal for Clinicians*, 28 (November-December 1978), 367-68.

(See Chapter 2: LOEB, LEO: Hartroff).

Loeb, Leo. "Autobiographical Notes." *Perspectives in Biology and Medicine*, 2 (1958), 21-23.

(See Chapter 2: LOEB, LEO: Hartroff).

Shaffer, P. A. "Biographical Notes on Dr. Leo Loeb." *Archives of Pathology*, 50 (1950), 661-75.

(See Chapter 2: LOEB, LEO: Hartroff).

Witkowski, Jan A. "Experimental Pathology and the Origins of Tissue Culture: Leo Loeb's Contribution." *Medical History*, 27 (December 1983), 269-88.

(See Chapter 7: Witkowski).

MARJOLIN, JEAN-NICOLAS

Cruickshank, L. H. and Gaskell, E. "Jean Nicolas Marjolin: Destined to be
   Forgotten?" *Medical History*, 7 (1984), 383-84.

(See Chapter 18: Cruikshank and Gaskell).

Steffen, Charles. "Jean-Nicolas Marjolin." *The American Journal of Dermatopathology*, 6 (April 1984), 163-65.

Jean-Nicolas Marjolin, discoverer of the lesion known as Marjolin's ulcer, was
a physician at L'Hotel Dieu in Paris during the late eighteenth and early nineteenth centuries. He was born on December 6, 1780, in Ray-sur-Saone, France,
and studied medicine at the University of Paris. In 1828 he described the cancer
arising in the scars of burn victims. These are primarily squamous cell carcinomas. Marjolin died in 1850. Squamous cell carcinomas appearing in burn scars
are now known as "Marjolin's Ulcers."

Steffen, Charles. "Marjolin's Ulcer: Report of Two Cases and Evidence that
   Marjolin Did Not Describe Cancer Arising in Scars of Burns." *The American
   Journal of Dermatopathology*, 6 (April 1984), 187-93.

(See Chapter 18: Cruikshank and Gaskell).

MARTLAND, HARRISON STANFORD

"Harrison Stanford Martland (1883-1954)." *CA-A Cancer Journal for Clinicians*,
   23 (November-December 1973), 367.

Harrison Martland was born in Newark, New Jersey, in 1883. He graduated from Western Maryland College and in 1904 earned his medical degree from
Columbia University. As the city pathologist for Newark, Harrison Martland specialized in radiation-induced diseases, including malignant neoplasms. Martland
died on May 1, 1954.

MEIGS, JOE VINCENT

"Joe Vincent Meigs (1892-1963)." *CA-A Cancer Journal for Clinicians*, 25
   (January-February 1975), 31-32.

Joe Vincent Meigs was born in Lowell, Massachusetts, on October 24, 1892. He
graduated from Princeton in 1915 and received his medical degree from Harvard
in 1919. Meigs specialized in surgical gynecology and in 1927 helped found the
state-supported Pondville Hospital for Cancer. He served as its chief gynecologist
until 1960. Meigs was simultaneously a professor of gynecology for the Harvard
Medical School. Meigs is especially remembered for his revival of the Wertheim
surgical procedure—an abdominal hysterectomy—for uterine and cervical cancer.

The radical Wertheim procedure, which involved removal of the uterus, tubes, ovaries, parametria, much of the vagina, and the paravaginal tissues, had been largely abandoned in favor of radiotherapy early in the 1900s because surgical mortality rates were about 20 percent. In 1939, however, Meigs was convinced that new surgical advances, blood replacement techniques, and infection-fighting sulpha drugs would reduce those mortality rates while eliminating the high rates of localized recurrence after radiotherapy. His ideas proved correct, so he revived the Wertheim procedure and added bilateral pelvic lymph node dissection. Joe Meigs died on October 24, 1953.

MEYER, ROBERT

Fischer, H. "Die Wissenschaftliche Leistung Robert Meyer im Spiegel Seiner Arbeiten über das Verhalten des Epithels am Collum Uteri." *Wissenschaftliche Zeitschrift der Humboldt-Universitaet zu Berlin Mathematisol-Natur-Wissenschaftliche Reihe*, 13 (1964), 547-51.

Robert Meyer was born in Germany in 1870 and became a prominent pathologist and embryologist, specializing in ovarian tumors and their classification. Fleeing the Nazis, he came to the United States in 1940 and remained there until his death in 1947.

MILES, WILLIAM ERNEST

Gilbertsen, V. A. "Contributions of William Ernest Miles to Surgery of the Rectum for Cancer." *Diseases of the Colon and Rectum*, 7 (September-October 1964), 375-80.

(See Chapter 23: Gilbertsen).

"William Ernest Miles (1869-1947)." *CA-A Cancer Journal for Clinicians*, 21 (November-December 1971), 360.

William Ernest Miles was born in Trinidad in 1869 and trained at Queen's Royal College there. He studied medicine and then surgery at St. Bartholomew's in London, and there he also focused on the study of rectal cancer metastases. Miles is best remembered for developing the abdominal-perineal surgery for rectal carcinoma, which permitted dissection of the upward lymphatic spread of the disease. By dramatically improving surgical mortality rates, Miles's procedure replaced the perineal approach, which had not been effective in arresting lymphatic metastasis. William Ernest Miles died on September 24, 1947.

MONDEVILLE, HENRI DE

Clarke, Clement C. "Henri de Mondeville." *Yale Journal of Biology and Medicine*, 3 (1931), 459-81.

Henri de Mondeville was a prominent surgeon born in France in 1260. He spent most of his career as the court physician to King Philip the Fair. Mondeville believed in the humoral theory for the origin of cancer, although he viewed the etiology of the disease in terms of complex interactions between the various bodily humors. He died in 1320.

MORGAGNI, GIOVANNI BATTISTA

Jarcho, Saul. *The Clinical Consultations of Giambattista Morgagni.* Charlottesville: 1984.

Giovanni Morgagni was born in Bologna, Italy, in 1682, and practiced medicine there and later at Padua, where he taught anatomy at the university. Morgagni's 1761 publication *De sedibus et causis morborum* is considered the beginning of modern pathology. By performing hundreds of autopsies, Morgagni tried to relate the clinical history of the patient with the disease structures of his or her body. He described a variety of gastrointestinal and lung tumors, as well as distant metastases from the primary sites. Giovanni Morgagni died in 1771.

MÜLLER, JOHANNES

Haggard, Howard W., and G. M. Smith. "Johannes Müller and the Modern Conception of Cancer." *Yale Journal of Biology and Medicine*, 10 (1938), 419-38.

Johannes Müller was born in Coblenz, Germany, in 1801. He received his medical degree at the University of Bonn, concentrated in comparative anatomy and pathology, and spent his medical career as a professor at the universities of Bonn and Berlin. Müller made a number of contributions to medical history, including the idea of the specific energy of nerves, the nature of retinal images, hermaphroditism, and embryology, but he is best remembered as the father of cellular pathology and the mentor of Rudolf Virchow. In 1836 Müller began a systematic study of normal and malignant tissues using a microscope, and he realized that cancer was a cellular disease. Malignant cells, at least compared to normal cells, were abnormal and inconsistent in size with misshapen, internal components. Johannes Müller died in 1858.

Koller, Gottfried. *Das Leben des Biologen Johannes Müller, 1801-1858.* Stuttgart: 1958.

(See Chapter 2: MÜLLER, JOHANNES: Haggard and Smith).

MURPHY, JAMES BUMGARDNER

Corner, George W. "James Bumgardner Murphy." *Dictionary of American Biography*, Suppl. 4. 1974. Pp. 615-17.

James Murphy was born in Morgantown, West Virginia, on August 4, 1884. He graduated from the University of North Carolina in 1905 and then took his medical degree at Johns Hopkins in 1909. Murphy studied under Peyton Rous at the Rockefeller Institute. A pathologist, his research helped describe the mechanism of the body's resistance to the grafting of foreign tissue and the role of the lymphatic system in immunological reactions. His later research demonstrated the role of the endocrine glands and hormones in resistance to transplanted tumors and leukemia in rats and mice. Murphy died on August 24, 1950.

Davis, A. B. "James Bumgardner Murphy." *Dictionary of Scientific Biography*, 9 (1974), 586-87.

(See Chapter 2: MURPHY, JAMES BUMGARDNER: Corner).

NELATON, AUGUSTE

"Cancer Eponyms: Nelaton's Tumor." *Cancer Bulletin*, 12 (July-August 1960), 67- 68.

(See Chapter 9: "Cancer Eponyms: Nelaton's Tumor").

NORRIS, WILLIAM

Davis, Neville C. "William Norris, M.D.: A Pioneer in the Study of Melanoma." *Medical Journal of Australia*, 1 (January 26, 1980), 52-54.

In 1812 R. T. H. Laènnec of the University of Paris first used the word "melanoses" to describe melanoma tumors. The first published description of melanoma in English came in 1820 by William Norris, a physician who practiced medicine in Stourbridge, England, between 1817 and 1877. The patient died of a disseminated malignant melanoma. Norris performed an autopsy and observed metastases in the abdomen, lungs, heart, and brain. After years of studying melanoma patients, Norris wrote in 1857 the following conclusions: 1) there is a relationship between melanoma and moles; 2) the disease is more common in industrial than in rural areas; 3) patients usually have light hair and a fair complexion; 4) there is a hereditary disposition to the disease; 5) trauma may accelerate tumor growth; and 6) the best treatment is an early, wide excision of the primary melanoma along with surrounding healthy tissue.

NOVINSKY, MISTISLAV ALEKSANDROVICH

Beliaev, I. I. "M. A. Novinskii i problema profilakiti raka (k 100-letiiu eksperimental'noi onkologii)." *Gigiena i Sanitaria*, 6 (June 1977), 47-48.

(See Chapter 7: Shabad).

Shabad, L. M. "Mistislav Novinsky, Pioneer of Tumour Transplantation." *Cancer Lett*, 2 (September, 1976), 1-3.

(See Chapter 2: NOVINSKY, MISTISLAV ALEKSANDROVICH: Shabad).

Shabad, L. M. *M. A. Novinsky, Forefather of Experimental Oncology.* New York: 1950.

Mistislav Aleksandrovich Novinsky was born in 1841 in St. Petersburg, Russia. He was a veterinary student at the Medical-Surgical Academy of St. Petersburg and his master's thesis involved the successful transplantation of a nasal carcinoma in a dog to another dog and the subsequent transplantation of the first transplant to three other dogs. Novinsky was the first to show that tumors could be transplanted in animals of the same species. The work was done in 1875 and 1876.

Shimkin, Michael B. "M. A. Novinsky: A Note on the History of Transplantation of Tumors." *Cancer*, 8 (1955), 653-55.

(See Chapter 2: NOVINSKY, MISTISLAV ALEKSANDROVICH: Shabad).

OBERLING, CHARLES

Bernard, W. "Charles Oberling, 1895-1960." *Cancer Research*, 20 (1960), 1274-76.

(See Chapter 2: OBERLING, CHARLES: Haguenau).

Haguenau, Francoise. "Charles Oberling, M.D. (1895-1960)." *Cancer*, 13 (1960), 868-70.

Before his death in 1960 Charles Oberling was an outstanding pathologist. He specialized in kidney and Bright's disease. He showed that Ewing's sarcoma was a tumor of reticular cell origin, which he called reticulosarcoma. Oberling also demonstrated the possibility of inducing reticular cell proliferation in chickens inoculated with leukemia viruses. He also showed that meningioma tumors had mesenchymal as well as neuroectodermic origin. Oberling was director of the Institute for Cancer Research at the University of Paris at the time of his death.

Rous, Peyton. "Charles Oberling, Research Worker on the Nature of Cancer." *Science*, 132 (November 25, 1960), 1534-35.

(See Chapter 2: OBERLING, CHARLES: Haguenau).

OSLER, WILLIAM

Beth, W. R. *Osler: The Man and the Legend.* London: 1951.

(See Chapter 2: OSLER, WILLIAM: Robb-Smith).

Robb-Smith, A. H. T. "Did Sir William Osler Have Carcinoma of the Lung?" *Chest*, 66 (December 1974), 712-16.

Early in the 1970s rumors began circulating in the medical-research community that Sir William Osler had died of lung cancer. Although Osler was a smoker, he did so in moderation, usually after a meal. Pathologists at the time of his death could not yet distinguish between mediastinal lymphosarcoma and oat cell carcinoma, but they were able to recognize lung neoplasms. An autopsy was performed on William Osler after his death in 1919, and it indicated bronchiectasis of the right lower lobe with unresolved pneumonia, multiple lung abscesses, and an empyema.

PAGET, JAMES

Ellis, H. "Eponyms in Oncology: Sir James Paget (1814-1899)." *European Journal of Surgical Oncology*, 12 (December 1986), 393.

(See Chapter 2: PAGET, JAMES: Schoenberg and Schoenberg).

Goldstein, Howard B. "Sir James Paget." *The American Journal of Dermatopathology*, 2 (Spring 1980), 27-31.

James Paget was born in 1814 in Yarmouth, England. He apprenticed out to a local surgeon in 1830 and in 1836, after studying medicine in London, Paget passed the examinations of the Royal College of Surgeons. Paget joined the teaching and clinical staff at St. Bartholomew's Hospital in London. He is best remembered today for his descriptions of the diseases which became known as Paget's disease of the breast, extramammary Paget's disease, and Paget's disease of the bone. James Paget died in 1899.

Schoenberg, D. G., and Bruce S. Schoenberg. "Eponym: Paget's Disease of the Bone and Breast." *Southern Medical Journal*, 72 (1979), 997-98.

(See Chapter 2: Goldstein).

PAPANICOLAOU, GEORGES

Bedrossian, C. W. "Philatelic Honors (Georges Papanicolaou)." *Diagnostic Cytopathology*, 1 (January-March 1985), 77-78.

(See Chapter 2: PAPANICOLAOU, GEORGES: Carmichael).

Carmichael, Erskine. "Dr. Papanicolaou and the Pap Smear." *The Alabama Journal of Medical Science*, 21 (January 1984), 101-04.

(See Chapter 2: PAPANICOLAOU, GEORGES: Carmichael).

Carmichael, Erskine. *The Pap Smear: The Life of Georges N. Papanicolaou.* New York: 1973.

Georges N. Papanicolaou was the founder of cytology. He was born in Euboea, Greece, in 1883. In 1904 he received a medical degree from the University of Athens. Papanicolaou studied further at the University of Jena in Germany. He did not want to practice medicine but preferred research, so he joined the Hertwig Institute in Munich. In 1910 Papanicolaou received the Ph.D. He left for New York City in 1913, where he joined the staff of the Cornell Medical College. Papanicolaou worked on cytological smears in guinea pigs. In 1928 he wrote a paper claiming that pre-cancerous cells appeared in the cytologic smears of the the human female's vagina and uterus. In 1933 Papanicolaou published *The Sexual Cycle in the Human Female as Revealed by Vaginal Smears.* The first formal monograph on the detection of cancer by vaginal smears appeared in 1943, when Papanicolaou and his colleague, Herbert F. Traut, wrote *Diagnosis of Uterine Cancer by the Vaginal Smear.* Georges Papanicolaou died on February 22, 1962. Since then his cytological technique has become one of the most important diagnostic tools in gynecologic oncology.

"Georges Nicholas Papanicolaou (1883-1962)." *CA-A Cancer Journal for Clinicians,* 23 (May-June 1973), 171-79.

(See Chapter 2: PAPANICOLAOU, GEORGES: Carmichael).

"Georges Nicholas Papanicolaou." *Cancer Bulletin,* 14 (July-August 1962), 72.

(See Chapter 2: PAPANICOLAOU, GEORGES: Carmichael).

Riley, H. D. "Georges Nicholas Papanicolaou." In *Dictionary of American Biography, 1961-1965.* Suppl. 7. 1981. Pp. 598-99.

(See Chapter 2: PAPANICOLAOU, GEORGES: Carmichael).

PANCOAST, HENRY KHUNRUTH

Brown, P. "Henry Khunrath Pancoast." *American Journal of Roentgenology,* 42 (August 1939), 507.

(See Chapter 2: PANCOAST, HENRY KHUNRATH: "Cancer Eponyms: Pancoast's Tumor").

"Cancer Eponyms: Pancoast's Tumor." *Cancer Bulletin,* 7 (July-August 1955), 67.

Henry Khunrath Pancoast was born on February 26, 1875, in Philadelphia, Pennsylvania. He received his medical degree from the University of Pennsylvania in 1898 and then went into radiology. In 1912 he was appointed professor of radiology at University Hospital in Philadelphia, where he worked for the next 25 years. Pancoast was the first president of the American Board of Radiology. He died in 1939.

In 1924 Pancoast described a clinical syndrome diagnostic of apical lung tumor which he called "superior pulmonary sulcus tumor." In 1932 Henry Pancoast argued that the tumor had embryonic origins. Today we know that "Pancoast's tumor" is not a distinct neoplastic entity but many types of neoplasms developing in the thoracic apex. They all produce similar symptoms: shoulder pain, Horner's syndrome, muscle atrophy in the hand, drooping eyelids, and pupil constriction. It may be either a primary carcinoma or metastatic lesions found in the apex of the lung. By extension it involves the brachial plexus, the subclavian and cartoid arteries, and sometimes the first two or three ribs.

PARACELSUS, THEOPHRASTUS

Grabman, James P. "Theophrastus Paracelsus." *The Journal of the History of Medicine and the Allied Sciences*, 29 (April 1974), 228-29.

(See Chapter 2: PARACELSUS, THEOPHRASTUS: Pagel).

Pachter, Henry M. *Paracelsus: Magic Into Science.* New York: 1951.

(See Chapter 2: PARACELSUS: THEOPHRASTUS: Pagel).

Pagel, Walter. *Das Medizinische Weltbild des Paracelsus: Seine Zusammenhänge mit Neuplatonismus und Gnosis.* Wiesbaden: 1962.

(See Chapter 2: PARACELSUS, THEOPHRASTUS: Pagel).

Pagel, Walter. *Paracelsus. An Introduction to Philosophical Medicine in the Era of the Renaissance.* Basel: 1958.

(See Chapter 2: PARACELSUS, THEOPHRASTUS: Pagel).

Pagel, Walter. "Van Helmont's Concept of Disease—To Be or Not to Be? The Influence of Paracelsus." *Bulletin of the History of Medicine*, 46 (September-October 1972), 419-54.

Theophrastus Paracelsus (1493-1541) and Jean Baptiste Van Helmont (1579-1644) are the major figures in forging a new philosophy of medicine and disease during the Renaissance and post-Renaissance years. Both of them rejected the notions of Hippocrates and Galen which had prevailed for nearly two thousand years, that all disease was a function of imbalance in the body's four basic humors, or fluids. In their view disease was an excess or deficiency of one or more of the fluids. But Paracelsus and Van Helmont argued that disease was a specific entity in its own right—the essence of disease is a morbid seed of some kind which becomes implanted in a body organ. Although Van Helmont did not accept Paracelsus's notion of a relationship between astrology and disease, and both men did not really understand the origins of diseases—viral, bacterial, and genetic—they were correct in the notion of disease as a separate entity from the body's constitution.

PARÉ, AMBROISE

Bongartz, R. R. "Die Neoplasmen bei Ambroise Paré, 1510-1590." Ph.D. Dissertation. University of Dusseldorf. 1967. Pp. 200.

Ambroise Paré was born in France in 1510 and trained as a barber and as a surgeon. He spent years as a military surgeon whose skills eventually brought him to the royal family as a personal physician. Paré is remembered for many important medical developments, including abandonment of the application of boiling oil to gunshot wounds and replacing cauterization with ligature for control of bleeding. Paré also believed in wide surgical excision of cancerous lesions. He died in 1590.

Boyd, Howard Hill, Jr. "Ambroise Paré: Sawbones or Scientist." *Journal of the History of Medicine and Allied Sciences*, 15 (January 1960), 268-81.

(See Chapter 2: PARÉ, AMBROISE: Bongartz).

Hamby, Wallace B. *The Case Reports and Autopsy Records of Ambroise Paré.* Springfield: 1960.

(See Chapter 2: PARÉ, AMBROISE: Bongartz).

PETROV, NIKOLAI

Bershtein, L. M. "K 75-letiiu vykhoda v svet rukovodstva N. N. Petrova 'obshcheee uchenie ob opukholiakh'." *Voprosy Onkologii*, 31 (1985),75-78.

(See Chapter 2: PETROV, NIKOLAI: Shabad).

Demin, V. N. "N. N. Petrov–osnovopolozhnik pervoi kafedry onkologii v SSSR." *Voprosy Onkologii*, 21 (1975), 9-12.

(See Chapter 2: PETROV, NIKOLAI: Shabad).

Demin, V. N. "Razvitie idei N. N. Petrova v deiatel'nosti Kafedry Onkologii Leningradskogo Giduv." *Vestnik Khirurgiia*, 135 (October 1985), 145-48.

(See Chapter 2: PETROV NIKOLAI: Shabad).

Kavetskii, R. E. "Idei N. N. Petrova i nekotorye teoreticheskie voprosy sovremennoi onkologii." *Voprosy Onkologii*, 22 (1976), 12-15, and 23 (1977), 3-7.

(See Chapter 2: PETROV, NIKOLAI: Shabad).

Kholdin, S. A. 'Rol'N. N. Petrova v razvitii otechestvennoi klinicheskoi onkologii." *Voprosy Onkologii*, 18 (1972), 112-17.

(See Chapter 2: PETROV, NIKOLAI: Shabad).

Mel'nikov, R. A. "N. N. Petrov–osnovopolozhnik eksperimental'nogo izucheniia kantserogenezu u primatov." *Voprosy Onkologii*, 22 (1976), 34-40.

(See Chapter 2: PETROV, NIKOLAI: Shabad).

Napalkov, N. P. "Razvitie idei N. N. Petrova o profilaktike raka v eksperimental'nykh issledovaniiakh, posviashchennyk, transplatsentarnomu kantserogenezu." *Voprosy Onkologii*, 22 (1976), 23-34.

(See Chapter 2: PETROV, NIKOLAI: Shabad).

Napalkov, N. P., V. I. Mishura, and V. M. Merabishvili. "Razvitie idei N. N. Petrova v oblasti organizatsii protivorakovoi bor'by." *Voprosy Onkologii*, 28 (1982), 126-32.

(See Chapter 2: PETROV, NIKOLAI: Shabad).

Shabad, L. M. "Znachenie issledovanii N. N. Petrova v razvitii eksperimental'noi onkologii." *Voprosy Onkologii*, 18 (1972), 104-11.

Nikolai Nikolaevich Petrov (1876-1964) was one of the most important experimental oncologists in the Soviet Union. In 1926 he founded and then headed the Leningrad Institute of Oncology. Petrov's major research accomplishment was the experimental induction of gallbladder carcinoma and osteogenic sarcoma in monkeys.

POTT, PERCIVALL

Potter, Michael. "Percivall Pott's Contribution to Cancer Research." *National Cancer Institute Monograph*, 10 (1963), 1-13.

(See Chapter 2: POTT, PERCIVALL: "Sir Percivall Pott").

"Sir Percivall Pott (1714-1788)." *CA-A Cancer Journal for Clinicians*, 24 (March-April 1974), 108-09.

Percivall Pott was born in London in 1714. He was apprenticed in the late 1720s to Edward Nourse, a surgeon at St. Bartholomew's Hospital in London, and in 1736 he began to practice surgery in his own right. He spent his entire professional life there, retiring in 1787 and dying the next year. Pott is best remembered as the premier surgeon of his time and for his 1775 observation that cancer of the scrotum in chimney sweeps was caused by the accumulation of soot over a long period of time in the groin area. Pott's observation is considered to be the beginning of the modern era of chemical carcinogenesis. Percivall Pott died in 1788.

RAMAZZINI, BERNARDINO

Wright, Wilmer C. *"De Morbis Artificum" by Bernardino Ramazzini. The Latin Text of 1713.* Chicago: 1940.

Bernardino Ramazzini was an Italian physician born in 1633. In 1700 he published his book *De Morbis Artificum*, which provided one of the first systematic descriptions of various occupationally associated diseases. He was an early epidemiologist who also noted the high incidence of breast carcinomas in Roman Catholic nuns. Ramazzini believed that breast cancer hid its origins in uterine abnormalities, and that nuns, because of their commitment to celibacy, imposed abnormal stress on the uterus, which eventually led to breast cancers. Bernardino Ramazzini died in 1714.

REGAUD, CLAUDIUS

Regaud, Jean. *Claudius Regaud (1870-1940): Pionnier de la cancerologie, créateur de la Fondation Curie: Chronique de sa vie et son oeuvre.* Paris: 1982.

Claudius Regaud was born in 1870 and died in 1940. He spent his professional career as a professor of histology at the University of Lyon until 1906, when he moved to Paris as director of radiation research at the Institute of Radium. There he was a founder of the Marie Curie Foundation. In his own research Regaud showed the superiority of radiotherapeutic dosages over time through fractionated applications rather than single exposures and pioneered the discipline of radiotherapy.

RHOADS, CORNELIUS PACKARD

Burchenal, Joseph H. "Cornelius P. Rhoads, M.D. (1898-1959)." *Cancer,* 12 (1959), 1073.

(See Chapter 2: RHOADS, CORNELIUS PACKARD: Stock).

Heller, John R. "Cornelius Packard Rhoads, Leader in Cancer Research." *Science,* 131 (February 19, 1960), 486-87.

(See Chapter 2: RHOADS, CORNELIUS PACKARD: Stock).

Karnofsky, David A. "Cornelius Packard Rhoads (1898-1959)." *Transactions of the New York Academy of Sciences,* 22 (1959), 3-6.

(See Chapter 2: RHOADS, CORNELIUS PACKARD: Stock).

Stock, C. Chester. "Obituary: Cornelius Packard Rhoads, 1898-1959." *Cancer Research*, 20 (April 1960), 409-11.

Born on June 20, 1898, in Springfield, Massachusetts, Cornelius Rhoads received his bachelor's degree from Bowdin College in 1920 and his medical degree from Harvard in 1924. Cornelius Rhoads was a brilliant scientist and administrator. He spent his career as a professor of medicine at Harvard, chief pathologist for the Rockefeller Institute, and head of the Memorial Center for Cancer and Allied Diseases. During his career, he published more than 300 scientific papers on osteoblastoma, leukemia, gastrointestinal carcinoma, nitrogen mustard therapy, and various other chemotherapeutic agents. He is widely considered as the father of modern chemotherapy. Until his death on August 13, 1959, Rhoads was head of the Sloan-Kettering Institute for Cancer Research in New York City.

RICH, ARNOLD RICE

"Arnold Rice Rich (1893-1968)." *CA-A Cancer Journal for Clinicians*, 29 (March-April 1979), 112-14.

Arnold Rich was born in Birmingham, Alabama, in 1893, and educated at the University of Virginia and the Johns Hopkins University Medical School. A pathologist, Rich remained at Johns Hopkins for his entire career. He is best remembered for his work on occult prostate carcinoma. Until 1935 prostate carcinoma was considered a rare disease. In 1935, however, Rich published a landmark study indicating that in autopsy studies he found a 14 percent incidence of occult prostate carcinoma and a 28 percent incidence in men above the age of 70. It proved to be a major epidemiological study and had an immediate clinical impact when physicians made prostate examinations a routine part of physicals. Arnold Rich died in 1968.

RIGONI-STERN, DOMENICO ANTONIO

Scotto, Joseph, and John C. Bailar. "Rigoni-Stern and Medical Statistics. A Nineteenth Century Approach to Cancer Research." *Journal of the History of Medicine and Allied Sciences*, 24 (January 1969), 65-75.

(See Chapter 5: Scotto and Bailar).

ROENTGEN, WILHELM CONRAD

Glasser, Otto. *Dr. W. C. Roentgen.* Springfield, Ill.: 1945.

(See Chapter 2: ROENTGEN, WILHELM CONRAD: "Wilhelm Conrad Roentgen 1845-1923").

"Wilhelm Conrad Roentgen (1845-1923)." *CA-A Cancer Journal for Clinicians,* 22 (May-June 1972), 151-52.

Wilhelm Roentgen was born on March 27, 1845, in Lennep, a small town along the lower Rhine in Germany. He was raised in Holland and received a doctorate in physics from the University of Zürich. Roentgen taught physics at the University of Würzburg, and in 1895 he discovered x-rays, for which he received the Nobel Prize in 1901. Roentgen's discovery was almost immediately applied to cancer as a diagnostic and therapeutic tool. Wilhelm Roentgen died on November 10, 1923.

ROUS, PEYTON

Andrewes, C. H. "Francis Peyton Rous 1879-1970." *Biographical Memoirs of the Fellows of the Royal Society,* 17 (1971), 643-62.

(See Chapter 2: ROUS, PEYTON: Huggins).

Dulbecco, R. "Francis Peyton Rous." *Biographies of the Members of the National Academy of Science,* 48 (1976), 275-306.

(See Chapter 2: ROUS, PEYTON: Huggins).

Henderson, J. S. "Peyton Rous." *Archives of Pathology,* 90 (1970), 189-90.

(See Chapter 2: ROUS, PEYTON: Huggins).

Huggins, Charles B. "Peyton Rous and His Voyages of Discovery." *Journal of Experimental Medicine,* 150 (October 1, 1979), 733-34.

Peyton Rous was born in Baltimore on October 5, 1879. He took undergraduate and medical degrees at Johns Hopkins University, and he became head of the laboratory for cancer research at the University of Michigan. In 1922 he became editor of the *Journal of Experimental Medicine* and remained a contributing force to it until his death in 1970. In his research Rous demonstrated that chicken sarcoma has a viral etiology and that solid tumors were transplantable.

Koebling, H. M. "Scientific Autographs. IV. Peyton Rous (1879-1970) and His Nobel Prize." *Agents Actions,* 1 (August 1970), 211-14.

(See Chapter 2: ROUS, PEYTON: Huggins).

"Peyton Rous (1879-1970)." *CA-A Cancer Journal for Clinicians,* 22 (January-February), 21-22.

(See Chapter 2: ROUS, PEYTON: Huggins).

RUSH, BENJAMIN

Binger, Carl. *Revolutionary Doctor, Benjamin Rush, 1746-1813.* New York: 1966.

(See Chapter 2: RUSH, BENJAMIN: Shimkin).

Shimkin, Michael B. "Benjamin Rush on Cancer." *Cancer Research,* 36 (July 1976), 2117-18.

Benjamin Rush was born in Philadelphia, Pennsylvania, in 1745. He was educated at Princeton and at the University of Edinburgh and practiced medicine in Philadelphia. Rush was a professor of medicine at the University of Pennsylvania and a signer of the Declaration of Independence in 1776. During his career he treated many cancer patients, but he was quite skeptical of the curative pastes circulating at the time. He offered the opinion that little could be done for the breast cancer which eventually killed Mary Washington, mother of George Washington, in 1789, but he did urge Abigail Smith, the daughter of President John Adams, to undergo a mastectomy for her breast cancer. She did not have the operation and died of cancer in 1813. Benjamin Rush died in 1813.

RUSSELL, WILLIAM

King, D. Friday and Debra Eisenberg. "Russell's Fuchsine Body. 'The Characteristic Organism of Cancer'." *The American Journal of Dermatopathology,* 3 (Spring 1981), 55-58.

In 1890 William Russell, a pathologist at the Royal Infirmary of Edinburgh, claimed to have identified the "characteristic organism of cancer" by double staining tumor tissue with fuchsine and iodine green. He said he could identify an organism in the cells, which he believed was a fungus. So he supported the germ theory of cancer. Many others at the time also believed in an infectious etiology of cancer, but most disagreed with Russell beceause they had also isolated his "fuchsine bodies" in syphlitic and tuberculer tissues. Today we know the "Russell bodies" are accumulations of immunoglobin. Their function remains a mystery.

SCHABEL, FRANK

Freireich, Emil. "A Memorial Issue for Dr. Frank M. Schabel, Jr." *Cancer,* 54 (September 15, 1984), 1132-52.

Frank M. Schabel was a leading figure in the development of chemotherapy at the Cancer Chemotherapy National Service Center. His own research was particularly important in determining dose rates in clinical cancer chemotherapy and showing the steep dose-response relationships for both tumor and host toxicity. Schabel was also a leading figure in developing the use of chemotherapy for microscopic metastatic disease in patients where the primary tumor has been controlled by surgery and/or radiotherapy and adjuvant chemotherapy. Finally, Schabel pioneered the use of combinations of alkylating agents in chemotherapy.

SCHERESCHEWSKY, JOSEPH

Andervont, H. B. "J. W. Schereschewsky: An Appreciation." *Journal of the National Cancer Institute*, 19 (1957), 331-33.

J. W. Schereschewsky was an epidemiologist at Harvard University and later at the National Cancer Institute. He was one of the first researchers to note the declining mortality rate in the United States from infectious disease as well as the concomitant increase in the cancer mortality rate. Schereschewsky's work led to the establishment of the epidemiological unit at the National Cancer Institute in 1939. He died in 1940 at the age of 67.

SCHIMMELBUSCH, CURT

Dalton, Martin L., and Karl H. Grozinger. "Curt Schimmelbusch and Schimmelbusch's Disease." *Surgery*, 63 (May 1968), 859-61.

(See Chapter 11: Dalton and Grozinger).

SEVERINO, MARCO AURELIO

Trent, Josiah C. "Five Letters of Marcus Arelius Severinus to the Very Honourable English Physician." *Bulletin of the History of Medicine*, 15 (1944), 306-23.

Marco Aurelio Severino was born in Naples, Italy, in 1580. He practiced medicine and taught surgery at the university there. Severino published widely in comparative anatomy and is considered one of the patriarchs of surgical pathology. Because of his careful comparative observations of surface lesions and breast tumors, Severino was able generally to distinguish between malignant and benign neoplasms. He died in 1656.

SHIMKIN, MICHAEL

Shimkin, Michael B. "The Written Word and Cancer—Some Personal Involvement, 1940-1977: Autobiographical Essay." *Cancer Research*, 38 (February 1978), 241-52.

The article surveys Shimkin's career at the United States Public Health Service and the medical schools of Temple University and the University of California, San Diego, and his editorships of *The Journal of the National Cancer Institute* and *Cancer Research*.

SIMS, JAMES MARION

Baer, Joseph L. "The Life of James Marion Sims." *American Journal of Obstetrics and Gynecology*, 60 (1950), 949-66.

(See Chapter 2: SIMS, JAMES MARION: Harris and Brown).

Carmichael, E. B. "Early Alabama Physicians." *Journal of the Medical Association of Alabama*, 28 (1958), 81-84.

(See Chapter 2: SIMS, JAMES MARION: Harris and Brown).

Carmichael, Erskine. "J. Marion Sims: Inventor, Physician, Surgeon." *Journal of the International College of Surgeons*, 33 (1960), 757-62.

(See Chapter 2: SIMS, JAMES MARION: Harris and Brown).

Dabney, M. Y. "James Marion Sims, Father of Modern Gynecology." *Journal of the Medical Association of Alabama*, 9 (1940), 333-36.

(See Chapter 2: SIMS, JAMES MARION: Harris and Brown).

Harris, Seale. "Marion Sims and Other 19th Century Pioneers: The Dawn of Scientific Medicine and Surgery." *Journal of the Medical Association of Alabama*, 15 (1945), 128-34, 152-59, 185-92.

(See Chapter 2: SIMS, JAMES MARION: Harris and Brown).

Harris, Seale, and Frances Williams Brown. *Woman's Surgeon: The Life of J. Marion Sims*. New York: 1950.

J. Marion Sims, the father of gynecology, was born on January 25, 1813, in Lancaster County, South Carolina. He graduated from South Carolina College, studied at the Charleston Medical School, and received his medical degree from Jefferson Medical College in Philadelphia. Sims began his practice in Mount Meigs, Alabama, and soon earned a wide reputation as a skilled surgeon. Late in the 1840s, he developed a successful surgical procedure for treatment of vesicovaginal fistulas, and when he published an article describing the operation in 1852 his reputation became international. Sims moved to New York City in 1853, and when the Civil War broke out in 1861, he moved to Paris. His 1866 book *Clinical Notes on Uterine Surgery* became a major factor in the establishment of gynecology as a separate medical discipline. Sims returned to New York City after the Civil War and in 1884 founded the New York Cancer Hospital, which later evolved into the Memorial Sloan-Kettering Cancer Center. Sims died on November 13, 1883.

Jervey, Allen J. "James Marion Sims, A Biographical Sketch of One of South Carolina's Men of Medicine." *Bulletin of the Greenville County Medical Society*, 7 (1944), 173-79.

(See Chapter 2: SIMS, JAMES MARION: Harris and Brown).

Johnson, Wingate M. "James Marion Sims: Medical Pioneer." *Virginia Medical Monthly*, 70 (1943), 385-96.

(See Chapter 2: SIMS, JAMES MARION: Harris and Brown).

Marr, James Pratt. "Obstetrics and Gynecology in America. VIII. James Marion Sims (1813-1883)." *North Carolina Medical Journal*, 8 (1947), 447-49.

(See Chapter 2: SIMS, JAMES MARION: Harris and Brown).

Marr, James Pratt. *Pioneer Surgeons of the Woman's Hospital. The Lives of Sims, Emmett, Peaslee, and Thomas.* Philadelphia: 1957.

(See Chapter 2: SIMS, JAMES MARION: Harris and Brown).

Martin, Hayes, Harry Ehrlich, and Francella Butler. "J. Marion Sims—Pioneer Cancer Protagonist." *Cancer*, 3 (1950), 189-204.

(See Chapter 2: SIMS, JAMES MARION: Harris and Brown).

Moir, Chassar. "J. Marion Sims and the Vesico-Vaginal Fistula: Then and Now." *British Medical Journal*, 2 (1940), 773-78.

(See Chapter 2: SIMS, JAMES MARION: Harris and Brown).

Pitts, Nadine. "James Marion Sims: Pioneer Woman's Surgeon." *Journal of the Medical Association of Alabama*, 24 (1955), 236-38.

(See Chapter 2: SIMS, JAMES MARION: Harris and Brown).

Souchon, Edmond. "A Century of Gynecology." *Illinois Medical Journal*, 108 (1955), 241.

(See Chapter 2: SIMS, JAMES MARION: Harris and Brown).

SLYE, MAUD

McCoy, J. J. *The Cancer Lady: Maud Slye and Her Heredity Studies.* New York: 1977.

Maud Slye (1879-1954) was a geneticist and cancer specialist at the University of Chicago. After raising hundreds of generations of mice and testing more than 100,000 of them, Slye became convinced that neoplasms originated from a recessive gene. Her hypothesis raised a great deal of controversy in the scientific community, especially with her colleague, Clarence Little, who strongly believed that carcinogenesis was not primarily a genetic phenomenon. Subsequent research has rejected Slye's notion of recessive gene carcinogenesis.

Parascandola, John. "Maud Caroline Slye." In *Notable American Women,* 4 (1980), 651-52.

(See Chapter 2: SLYE, MAUD: McCoy).

SMITH, NATHAN

Hayward, O. S. "A Search for the Real Nathan Smith." *Journal of the History of Medicine,* 15 (1960), 268-81.

Nathan Smith was born on September 30, 1762, in Rehoboth, Massachusetts. He studied medicine at Harvard, Edinburgh, and Glasgow, practiced medicine at Cornish, New Hampshire, and served on the faculty of Dartmouth College. Between 1813 and 1828 Smith was a professor at the Yale Medical School. Smith was an early leader in recognizing gynecological cancers, and in 1821 he performed the second ovariotomy in the United States. Nathan Smith died on January 26, 1829.

Linskog, Gustaf E. "Yale's First Professor of Surgery: Nathan Smith, M. D. (1762-1829)." *Surgery,* 64 (August 1968), 524-28.

(See Chapter 2: SMITH, NATHAN: Hayward).

"Nathan Smith's Views on Cancer Therapy." *Cancer Bulletin,* 18 (January-February 1966), 7-8.

(See Chapter 2: SMITH, NATHAN: Hayward).

Oughterson, Ashley Webster. "Nathan Smith and Cancer Therapy." *Yale Journal of Biology and Medicine,* 12 (1939), 123-36.

(See Chapter 2: SMITH, NATHAN: Hayward).

STRONG, LEONELL

"Leonell C. Strong." *CA-A Cancer Journal for Clinicians,* 29 (January-February 1979), 54-56.

Leonell C. Strong was born in Renovo, Pennsylvania, in 1894. He graduated from Allegheny College in 1917 with a degree in biology and then earned a Ph.D. in genetics from Columbia University in 1922. In the 1920s Strong taught at the University of Michigan, and in 1930 he joined the Roscoe B. Jackson Laboratory in Bar Harbor, Maine. Between 1933 and 1953 he taught genetics at Yale. Between 1953 and 1964 Strong worked at the Roswell Park Institute, and then he began a five year term at the Salk Institute in La Jolla, California. Through developing genetically selected mice strains and testing them for their susceptibility to a variety of malignant lesions, Strong became one of the premier figures in cancer genetics in the twentieth century.

Strong, Leonell C. "A Baconian in Cancer Research: Autobiographical Essay." *Cancer Research*, 36 (1976), 3545-3553.

(See Chapter 2: STRONG, LEONELL: "Leonell C. Strong").

SUTHERLAND, ARTHUR

"Portrait of Arthur M. Sutherland." *CA-A Cancer Journal for Clinicians*, 31 (May-June 1981), 157-58.

Arthur Sutherland was born September 29, 1910, in White Plains, New York. He earned a B.A. from Yale in 1932 and the M.D. from Columbia in 1936. Specializing in psychiatry, Sutherland taught at the Cornell University Medical School from 1937 to 1961, serving as chief of psychiatric services at Memorial Hospital in the 1950s. Sutherland died on August 1971. He is best remembered for his research on the quality of life of cancer victims and the process of rehabilitation from mutilating surgery. His work foreshadowed the emergence of the field of health psychology.

THEODORIC

Campbell, Eldridge, and James Colton. *The Surgery of Theodoric*. New York: 1955.

Teodorico Borgognomi, or Theodoric, was born in Salerno in 1205 and became a well-known physician there. In treating malignant lesions Theodoric advocated early surgery where possible, before the tumor had invaded muscle tissue and become too vascular in nature. He wanted wide surgical excisions, with the tumor and a margin of normal tissue removed, and the entire wound cauterized after the procedure. Theodoric also called for treatment of persistent tumors with an arsenic solution. He died in 1296.

TRACY, RICHARD THOMAS

Forster, Frank M. C. "A Case of Ovariotomy Instruments Sent by Thomas Spencer Wells to Richard Thomas Tracy." *Journal of Obstetrics & Gynecology of the British Commonwealth*, 72 (1965), 810-15.

(See Chapter 13: Forster).

Forster, Frank M. C. "Richard Thomas Tracy and His Part in the History of the Ovariotomy." *The Australian New Zealand Journal of Obstetrics and Gynecology*, 4 (1964), 128-38.

(See Chapter 13: Forster).

VAN HELMONT, JAN BAPTISTE

Pagel, Walter. *Jan Baptiste Van Helmont: Reformer of Science and Medicine.* New York: 1982.

Jan Baptiste Van Helmont was a Flemish physician born in 1579. In addition to identifying the notion of gases in the air and of digestive acids breaking food down into what he called "living flesh," Van Helmont was a leading figure in the rejection of the notions of Galen and Hippocrates on the nature of disease. Instead of the humoral theory, Van Helmont insisted on a rigidly empirical approach to biology and medicine, and he argued that disease entities, including cancer, are caused by the deposition of "seeds" external to the body, making most diseases local rather than systemic phenomena. Van Helmont died in 1644.

VIRCHOW, RUDOLF

Ackerknecht, Edwin H. *Rudolf Virchow. Doctor. Statesman. Anthropologist.* Madison, Wisconsin: 1953.

(See Chapter 2: VIRCHOW, RUDOLF: Gottleib).

Andree, Christian. *Rudolf Virchow als Prahistoriken.* Cologne: 1976.

(See Chapter 2: VIRCHOW, RUDOLF: Gottleib).

Churchill, Frederick B. "Rudolf Virchow and the Pathologist's Criteria for the Inheritance of Acquired Characteristics." *The Journal of the History of Medicine and Allied Sciences*, 31 (April 1976), 117-48.

(See Chapter 6: Fisher and Hermann and Chapter 6: Krumblaar).

Clark, William D., and Francis B. Quinn. "Erroneous Reporting of Errors." *Journal of the American Medical Association*, 252 (July 13, 1984), 207-08.

(See Chapter 3: FREDERICK III: Clark and Quinn).

deR Kolisch, Paul. "Errors of the Great." *Journal of the American Medical Association*, 250 (December 2, 1983), 2926.

(See Chapter 3: FREDERICK III: Lin).

Gottleib, Johan. "La transcendencia de Rudolf Virchow para la investigacion del cancer." *Folia Clínica Internacional*, 19 (October 1969), 507-12.

Rudolf Virchow was born on October 13, 1821, in Schivelbein, Pomerania, a part of Prussia. He was educated in Berlin, Germany, where he studied under Johannes Müller and went on to become the father of cellular pathology. After several years teaching at the University of Würzburg, Virchow became head of the Pathological Institute in Berlin in 1856, where he remained for the rest of his career. Virchow is credited with identifying a number of neoplasms, including leukemia, soft-tissue sarcomas, bone sarcomas, and head and neck carcinomas. In 1847 he founded *Virchow's Archives*, which remains today the premier journal of pathology in the world. He was also fascinated with archaeology and pre-history. A liberal in politics, Virchow was also known for his opposition to Otto von Bismarck. Rudolf Virchow died on September 5, 1902.

Kettler, L. J. "Rudolf Virchow und Seine Bedetung für die Lehre von den Geschwülsten." *Archiv Geschwulstforsch*, 38 (1971), 97-108.

(See Chapter 2: VIRCHOW, RUDOLF: Gottlieb).

Lin, Jain I. "Virchow's Pathological Reports on Frederick III's Cancer." *The New England Journal of Medicine*, 311 (November 1984), 1261-64.

(See Chapter 3: FREDERICK III: Lin).

Onuigbo, Wilson I. B. "The Paradox of Virchow's Views on Cancer Metastasis." *Bulletin of the History of Medicine*, 36 (1962), 444-49.

(See Chapter 8: Onuigbo).

Rather, L. J. *Rudolf Virchow: Cellular Pathology*. New York: 1971.

(See Chapter 2: VIRCHOW, RUDOLF: Gottlieb).

"Rudolf Virchow (1821-1902)." *CA-A Cancer Journal for Clinicians*, 25 (March-April 1975), 91-92.

(See Chapter 2: VIRCHOW, RUDOLF: Gottlieb).

Wilson, J. Walter. "Virchow's Contribution to the Cell Theory." *Journal of the History of Medicine*, 2 (Spring 1947), 163-78.

(See Chapter 2: VIRCHOW, RUDOLF: Gottlieb).

VON RECKLINGHAUSEN, FRIEDRICH DANIEL

"Cancer Eponyms: von Recklinghausen's Disease." *Cancer Bulletin*, 7 (May-June 1955), 49.

(See Chapter 18: "Cancer Eponyms: von Recklinghausen's Disease").

WARBURG, OTTO HEINRICH

Krebs, Hans A. "Otto Heinrich Warburg." *Biographies of the Members of the Royal Society*, 18 (1972), 629-99.

Otto Warburg was born in Germany in 1883 and spent his career as a chemist, most of it as director of the Kaiser Wilhelm Institute for Cell Physiology at the University of Berlin. Blessed with an authoritarian personality but an eclectic mind, Warburg was the leading figure in the biochemistry of cancer until the age of molecular biology dawned. He received the Nobel Prize in 1931 for his work in the physiology of cells, both normal and malignant. Otto Warburg died in 1970.

Krebs, Hans A. and Roswitha Schmid. *Otto Warburg: Zellphysiologe-Biochemiker-Mediziner*, 1883-1970. Stuttgart: 1979.

(See Chapter 2: WARBURG, OTTO: Krebs).

WARREN, JOHN COLLINS

Truax, Rhoda. *The Doctors Warren of Boston.* Boston: 1968.

John C. Warren was born in Boston in 1778 and educated at Harvard. He studied medicine and surgery in London under Sir Astley Cooper and spent his career as a professor of medicine and surgery at Harvard. Warren is also remembered for three primary accomplishments: his founding of the Massachusetts General Hospital, establishment of the journal which evolved into the *New England Journal of Medicine*, and his use of ether to anesthetize a patient undergoing surgery in 1846 for removal of tumor in the neck. John Warren died in 1856.

WARTHIN, ALDRED SCOTT

Baugh, Reginald F. "Aldred Scott Warthin. The Man Behind the Tumor." *Archives of Otolaryngology—Head and Neck Surgery*, 113 (April 1987), 365-67.

(See Chapter 2: WARTHIN, ALDRED SCOTT: Lynch).

Lynch, Henry T. "Aldred Scott Warthin, M.D., Ph.D. (1866–1931)." *CA-A Cancer Journal for Clinicians*, 35 (November/December 1985), 345-47.

Aldred S. Warthin was born in Indiana in 1866 and earned a music degree from the Cincinnati Conservatory of Music before going into medicine. Warthin then received undergraduate and master's degrees from Indiana University, and the M.D. and Ph.D. there in 1891 and 1893. Between 1903 and 1931 Warthin was director of the Pathology Laboratory at the University of Michigan. In 1929 he described a papillary cystadenoma, a benign, encapsulated tumor of the parotid gland which today is known as "Warthin's Tumor." Warthin is also known as the "father of cancer genetics." Several years prior to the rediscovery of the genetic theories of Gregor Mendel, Warthin began his work on "Family G," the family of his seamstress, most of whom died of cancer. He developed documented pedigree charts showing both geneaology and pathology for hundreds of relatives. Warthin also identified the hereditary pattern of nonpolyphosis colorectal cancer. Aldred Warthin died in 1931.

Simpson, W. M. "Aldred Scott Warthin, 1866–1931." *American Journal of Surgery*, 14 (1931), 502-04.

(See Chapter 2: WARTHIN, ALDRED SCOTT: Lynch).

Soule, M. H. "Aldred Scott Warthin (1866-1931)." *Journal of Laboratory and Clinical Medicine*, 16 (1931), 1043-46.

(See Chapter 2: WARTHIN, ALDRED SCOTT: Lynch).

WEIR, ROBERT FULTON

Corman, Marvin L. "Classic Articles on Colonic and Rectal Surgery. Robert Fulton Weir, 1838-1927." *Diseases of the Colon and Rectum*, 25 (July-August 1982), 503-07.

Robert Weir was born in New York City on February 16, 1838. After receiving a bachelor's and master's degree from the City College of New York, Weir earned a medical degree from the New York College of Physicians and Surgeons in 1859. He spent his career as chief of surgical services at Roosevelt Hospital, the Women's Medical College, and the College of Physicians and Surgeons. Among his surgical accomplishments were the adoption of Listerian techniques of antisepsis, pioneering brain surgery, appendicostomy, and recognition of duodenal ulcers as pathologic entities. Weir's surgical procedure for high-seated carcinomas of the rectum provided great improvements in surgical survival rates. Instead of the prevailing Kraske operation, Weir favored an abdominal approach from just above the pubis. Weir developed the procedure in 1900. He died on April 6, 1927.

WILLIAMS, MICHAEL

Dodd, Charles. "Michael Williams's Contribution to Industrial Hygiene with Reference to Cancer." *Proceedings of the Royal Society of Medicine*, 57 (1964), 1165-69.

Michael Williams was born in England in 1917 and received his education and medical training at Oxford University and St. George's Hospital. He worked as an epidemiologist for many years at several prominent hospitals and at Oxford University, and then he joined the Imperial Chemical Industries as medical officer for the Dyestuffs Division. Williams played a central role in the Association of British Chemical Manufacturers' program to identify the link between bladder cancer and exposure to industrial chemicals, particularly the naphthylamines and benzidines. Michael Williams died on July 9, 1961.

WILMS, MAX

Ellis, H. "Eponyms in Oncology. Max Wilms (1867-1918)." *European Journal of Surgical Oncology*, 12 (September 1986), 311.

(See Chapter 2: WILMS, MAX: Rohl).

Rohl, Lars. "Max Wilms (1867-1918)." *Investigations in Urology*, 4 (1966), 194-96.

Max Wilms was born in Aachen, Germany, in 1867. He received his medical degree from the University of Bonn in 1890 then specialized in pathology. In 1899 Wilms wrote a famous treatise on mixed-tissue tumors. His correct decision in describing a renal tumor of embryonic mesodermal origin led to the eponym of Wilms' tumor. Wilms later trained as a surgeon at the University of Leipzig and taught at the universities of Basel and Heidelberg. He died in 1918.

WOODWARD, JOSEPH JANVIER

Edmonds, Henry W. "Woodward and the Changing Concept of Cancer, 1858-1873." *The Military Surgeon*, 109 (1951), 314-19.

Joseph J. Woodward was best known for his years as head of the Army Medical Museum and author of the medical section of *History of the War of the Rebellion*. He also specialized in cancer as a histologist, and in his writings one can see the changing concept of cancer emerging in the second half of the nineteenth century. Woodward came to accept the theories of Rudolf Virchow on the epithelial nature of carcinoma and was beginning to accept the idea of metastasis. He also observed the infiltration of wandering cells into the stroma of neoplasms. Although Woodward's early theory that cancer cells originated in leukocytes migrating through the bloodstream did not survive later empirical research, he was responsible for promoting the science of pathologic histology in the United States.

Schoenberg, Bruce S. "Joseph Janvier Woodward and an Early American View of Cancer." *Surgery, Gynecology, & Obstetrics*, 136 (March 1973), 456-62.

(See Chapter 2: WOODWARD, JOSEPH JANVIER: Edmonds).

YAMAGIWA, KATSUSABURO

Henschen, F. "Yamagiwa's Tar Cancer and Its Historical Significance." *Gann*, 59 (1968), 447-51.

(See Chapter 2: YAMAGIWA, KATSUSABURO: "Katsusaburo Yamagiwa").

"Katsusaburo Yamagiwa (1863-1930)." *CA-A Cancer Journal for Clinicians*, 27 (May-June 1977), 172-74.

Katsusaburo Yamagiwa was born in Ueda, Japan, on February 23, 1863. He studied medicine and pathology at the Tokyo Imperial University and joined the teaching staff there in 1891. Between 1891 and 1894 he studied pathology under Rudolf Virchow in Germany; he then returned and spent the rest of his career at the Tokyo Imperial University. In 1905 Yamagiwa demonstrated his belief that chronic gastric ulcers could lead to gastric carcinoma, and over the next several years he developed his own irritation theory of carcinogenesis, arguing that chronic irritation of tissues caused precancerous alterations in normal epithelium. If the irritant continued, carcinoma would develop. In 1915, with his assistant Koichi Ichikawa, Yamagiwa reported his experiments producing squamous cell carcinomas in rabbit skin by constant applications of coal tar. Yamagiwa died in 1930.

Yoshida, T. "A History of Cancer Research in Japan, With Particular Reference to Yamagiwa's Coal-Tar Carcinoma of 1915." In H. Yukawa, ed. *Profiles of Japanese Science and Scientists*. Tokyo: 1970. Pp. 44-56.

(See Chapter 2: YAMAGIWA, KATSUSABURO: "Katsusaburo Yamagiwa").

YOUNG, HUGH

"Hugh Hampton Young (1870-1945)." *CA-A Cancer Journal for Clinicians*, 27 (September-October 1977), 305-07.

Hugh H. Young was born on September 18, 1870, in San Antonio, Texas. He received all of his degrees at the University of Virginia and in 1895 interned at the Johns Hopkins University Medical School, where he specialized in urology and surgery and studied under William Halsted. Young is remembered for his consummate surgical skills as well as his 1904 performance of the first successful radical prostatectomy. Hugh Young died in 1945.

Harvey, A. McGehee. "Early Contributions to the Surgery of Cancer: William S. Halsted, Hugh H. Young, and John G. Clark." *The Johns Hopkins Medical Journal*, 135 (December 1974), 399-417.

(See Chapter 23: Harvey).

ZILBER, LEV ALEXANDEROVICH

Abelev, G. I., and I. N. Kriukova. "Rol'L'va Aleksandrovicha Zil'bera v stanovlenii sovremennoi virusologii i immunologii raka." *Molecular Biology (Moskow)*, 18 (November-December 1984), 1697-1701.

(See Chapter 4: Shevlyaghin).

Shevlyaghin, V. Y. "The Scientific Heritage of Professor Zilber and His Contribution to Virus-Genetic Theory of Malignant Tumours." *Neoplasma*, 26 (1979), 113-23.

(See Chapter 4: Shevlyaghin).

3 Historical Personalities

ADAMS, JOHN

(See Chapter 2: RUSH, BENJAMIN: Shimkin).

ANNE OF AUSTRIA

Kleinmann, Ruth. "Facing Cancer in the Seventeenth Century: The Last Illness of Anne of Austria, 1664-1666." *Advances in Thanatology*, 4 (1978), 37-55.

Anne of Austria, the mother of Louis XIV of France, first noticed a nodule in her left breast in May 1664. Worried about the implications of the lump, primarily since she had witnessed breast cancer cases in local convents, she delayed treatment. The delay, of course, was not critical since the vast majority of cancers at the time were incurable. By October 1664 she was experiencing some nausea and dizziness, and court physicians diagnosed the lesion as malignant. Anne underwent the typical treatments of bleeding and purgings, as well as topical applications of a variety of herbs and an arsenic paste, which mortified some of the diseased tissue. Surgeons progressively removed the dead tissue, hoping the entire tumor would eventually die. By October 1665 she had developed deep coughs, a sign of lung metastases, and on January 20, 1666, she died. During the course of her illness, Anne illustrated all the psychological stages of contemporary, terminally ill patients: denial, guilt, anger, and ultimately acceptance. An added dimension was the notion among the French royal family that the well-to-do ought to be immune from such personal disasters. But even their wealth and power could not halt the course of the disease.

Pasteur, L. "Les médecins et le sein d'Anne d'Autriche." *Historama*, 6 (1984), 40-45.

(See Chapter 3: ANNE OF AUSTRIA: Kleinman).

BEETHOVEN, LUDWIG VON

Bankl, H. "Beethoven's krankheit—morbus Paget? Neue quellen, neue deutun-
gen." *Pathologe*, 6 (January 1985), 46-50.

The author argues that, from the symptoms of his final illness, the great
eighteenth century composer, Ludwig Von Beethoven, suffered from and died of
Paget's disease, a type of bone cancer.

CLEVELAND, GROVER

Barber, Douglas. "Secret Operation on U.S. President." *The Probe*, 23 (May
1982), 415-16.

(See Chapter 3: CLEVELAND, GROVER: Seelig).

Brooks, J. J., H. T. Enterline, and G. E. Aponte. "The Final Diagnosis of
President Cleveland's Lesion." *Transactions and Studies of the College of
Physicians of Philadelphia*, (March 1980), 1-25.

(See Chapter 3: CLEVELAND, GROVER: Seelig).

Cooper, P. H. "President Cleveland's Palatal Tumor." *Archives of Dermatology*,
122 (July 1986), 747-48.

(See Chapter 3: CLEVELAND, GROVER: Seelig).

Cross, Wilbur, and John Moses. "My God, Sir, I Think the President is Doomed."
American History Illustrated, 17 (November 1982), 41-45.

(See Chapter 3: CLEVELAND, GROVER: Seelig).

Morreels, C. L. "New Historical Information on the Cleveland Operations."
Surgery, 62 (September 1967), 542-51.

(See Chapter 3: CLEVELAND, GROVER: Seelig).

Seelig, M. G. "Cancer and Politics. The Operation on Grover Cleveland."
Surgery, Gynecology & Obstetrics, 85 (1947), 372-76.

In June 1893 physicians examining President Grover Cleveland noticed a suspicious lesion of 1.5 centimeters in diameter on the left side of the hard palate. A
biopsy indicated a soft-tissue sarcoma. Surgeons recommended a wide excision,
but presidential advisers worried, given the depressed state of the economy, that a
cancer operation on the president might precipitate a financial panic. So on July
1, 1893, aboard a yacht on the East River in New York City, surgeons secretly
operated on the president, removing the entire left jaw from the first bicuspid
tooth to just beyond the last molar as well as part of the soft palate. On July
17 more suspicious tissue was removed and the entire wound cauterized. A New

York dentist fitted Cleveland with an artificial jaw of vulcanized rubber. With the prosthesis in place, Cleveland appeared and spoke normally. He lived another fifteen years without a recurrence of the disease and died of natural causes in 1908. Knowledge of the surgery remained confined to only a few people for many years.

DICKENS, CHARLES

Markel, H. "Charles Dickens and the Art of Medicine." *Archives of Internal Medicine*, 10 (April 1984), 408-11.

The author speculates that Paul Dombey, a character in Charles Dickens's novel *Dombey and Son*, died of acute lymphocytic leukemia, at least from the symptoms that Dickens described.

EISENHOWER, DWIGHT DAVID

Pillsbury, Donald M. "General Eisenhower's 'Melanoma'." *Journal of the American Academy of Dermatology*, 4 (May 1981), 631-32.

In September 1944 General Dwight D. Eisenhower, supreme commander of Allied forces in Europe, had a lesion surgically removed from his chest which doctors initially diagnosed as a melanoma. It caused considerable stress among the Allied military elite, since the invasion of Europe had been underway for only three months. Their worst fears were relieved, however, when pathology reports indicated it was not a melanoma but a seborrheic keratosis.

FREDERICK III

Clark, William D. and Francis B. Quinn. "Erroneous Reporting Errors." *Journal of the American Medical Association*, 252 (July 13, 1984), 207-08.

They contest the claim made by Paul deR Kolisch (Chapter 3: deR Kolisch) that famed cancer pathologist Rudolf Virchow of Berlin misdiagnosed Frederick III's laryngeal lesion as a benign tumor. Virchow correctly diagnosed it as malignant and recommended surgical excision. He was not responsible for the delay in treatment which accelerated the course of the disease and the Kaiser's death.

deR Kolisch, Paul. "Errors of the Great." *Journal of the American Medical Association*, 250 (December 2, 1983), 2926.

He argues that Rudolf Virchow, the father of cellular biology, probably misdiagnosed the laryngeal carcinoma of Frederick III of Germany as a benign tumor and indirectly contributed to his death because surgical excision of the lesion did not take place. It led to a tremendous controversy between English and German pathologists over the Kaiser's death. (See Chapter 3: FREDERICK III: Clark and Quinn).

Ellis, M. "A Letter from Sir Morell Mackenzie." *British Journal of Medicine*, 4 (December 30, 1967), 799-800.

(See Chapter 3: FREDERICK III: Lin).

Gejrot, T. "Morell Mackenzie och Fredrik III." *Lakartidningen*, 63 (20 July 1966), 2737-42.

(See Chapter 3: FREDERICK III: Lin).

Gerlings, P. G. "Enkele beschouwingen over het larynxcarcinoom naar aanleiding van de ziekte Keizer Friedrich 3d." *Neederlands Tijdschrift voor Geneeskunde*, 110 (5 November 1966), 1977-80.

(See Chapter 3: FREDERICK III: Lin).

Gerlings, P. G. "Laryngeal Carcinoma—Some Considerations with Reference to the Illness of Emperor Frederick III." *The Eye, Ear, Nose and Throat Monthly*, 47 (November 1968), 566-71.

(See Chapter 3: FREDERICK III: Lin).

Lin, Jain I. *Death of a Kaiser: A Medical Historical Narrative*. New York: 1985.

(See Chapter 3: FREDERICK III: Lin).

Lin, Jain I. "Virchow's Pathological Reports on Frederick III's Cancer." *The New England Journal of Medicine*, 311 (November 1984), 1261-64.

At the time of Frederick III's laryngeal cancer, pathologists refused to accept the concept of carcinoma *in situ*. As long as a tumor had not invaded surrounding tissue, it was not considered cancer, and Rudolf Virchow, the famed German pathologist, was functioning under that assumption. Virchow saw several tissue samples and described them as "pachydermia laryngis" or "pachydermia verrucosa." Not until nine months later, in 1888, did Virchow's associate, Dr. Waldeyer, confirm the disease as a malignant carcinoma. The German press accused the British physician treating Frederick III, Dr. Morell Mackenzie, of purposely delaying treatment by not performing a laryngectomy, but Mackenzie cited the dangers of laryngectomy as well as Virchow's pathological report in his own defense.

Massey, R. U. "The Ninety-Nine Day Kaiser." *Connecticut Medicine*, 51 (January 1987), 61.

(See Chapter 3: FREDERICK III: Lin).

McInnis, W. D., W. Egan, and J. B. Aust. "The Management of Carcinoma of the Larynx in a Prominent Patient, or Did Morell Mackenzie Really Cause World War I?" *American Journal of Surgery*, 132 (October 1976), 515-22.

(See Chapter 3: FREDERICK III: Lin).

Minnigerode, B. "The Disease of Emperor Frederick III." *Laryngoscope*, 96 (February 1986), 200-03.

(See Chapter 3: FREDERICK III: Lin).

Ober, William B. "The Case of the Kaiser's Cancer." *Pathology Annual*, 5 (1970), 207-16.

(See Chapter 3: FREDERICK III: Lin).

Oliva, H., and B. Aguilera. "Las maleficas biopsias del Kaiser Federico III." *Revista Clínica de España*, 178 (May 1986), 409-11.

(See Chapter 3: FREDERICK III: Lin).

Seiferth, L. B. "Ein Beitrag zur Krankheit Kaiser Friedrichs 3d." *HNO*, 15 (February 1967), 63.

(See Chapter 3: FREDERICK III: Lin).

Shapiro, S. L. "The Missing Biopsy." *The Eye, Ear, Nose and Throat Monthly*, 43 (September 1964), 86-88, 92.

(See Chapter 3: FREDERICK III: Lin).

Wyk, A. J. "Medisyne uit Suid-Afrika vir die Keiser." *Historia*, 24 (1979), 63-65.

(See Chapter 3: FREDERICK III: Lin).

FREUD, SIGMUND

Brown, C. T. "Freud and Cancer." *Texas Medicine*, 70 (January 1974), 62-64.

(See Chapter 3: FREUD, SIGMUND: Golub).

Golub, Sharon. "Coping With Cancer: Freud's Experiences." *Psychoanalytic Review*, 68 (Summer 1981), 191-200.

In February 1923 Sigmund Freud, the renowned father of psychoanalysis, discovered a lesion in his mouth. At the time Freud was 67 years old. His physician recognized the lesion as a malignant epithelioma but kept the truth from Freud, calling it instead a leucoplakia. It was actually a well-differentiated squamous cell carcinoma, a fairly common malignant lesion of the oral cavity. Freud underwent out-patient surgery for removal of the lesion, but the surgeon was not highly skilled and Freud suffered a large blood loss. Still thinking the lesion had been benign, Freud agreed to two x-ray treatments and local radium applications. By October 1923 the lesion had recurred, invading the hard palate, jaw, and cheek. Now informed of the nature of the illness, Freud underwent radical surgery, including the removal of the upper jaw, submaxillary glands, and part of the palate. Despite a prosthesis, eating and speaking were difficult for him for the rest of his life, and his days were spent trying to deal with constant pain and the debilities brought on by the disease. During the next sixteen years Freud underwent a number of subsequent operations to deal with local recurrences, but in 1939 a new tumor appeared which was inoperable. The tumor had invaded the orbit of his eye and ulcerated through his cheek. In tremendous pain, Freud asked his personal physician to end his misery, and on September 23, 1939, after two doses of 20 milligrams of morphine, Freud died.

Jones, Ernest. *The Life and Work of Sigmund Freud.* New York: 1953-57.

(See Chapter 3: FREUD, SIGMUND: Golub).

Luce, E. A. "The Ordeal of Sigmund Freud." In Sharon Romm, ed. *Symposium on Historical Perspectives in Plastic Surgery.* Philadelphia: 1983. Pp. 715-16.

(See Chapter 3: FREUD, SIGMUND: Golub).

Romm, Sharon. "The Oral Cancer of Sigmund Freud." In Romm, Sharon, ed. *Symposium on Historical Perspectives in Plastic Surgery.* Philadelphia: 1983. Pp. 709-14.

(See Chapter 3: FREUD, SIGMUND: Golub).

Romm, Sharon. *The Unwelcome Intruder: Freud's Struggle with Cancer.* New York: 1983.

(See Chapter 3: FREUD, SIGMUND: Golub).

Schur, Max. *Freud: Living and Dying.* New York: 1972.

(See Chapter 3: FREUD, SIGMUND: Golub).

GERSHWIN, GEORGE

Ljunggren, Bengt. "The Case of George Gershwin." *Neurosurgery,* 10 (June 1982), 733-36.

George Gershwin, the famous composer, was a gentle, friendly man and a musical genius. But he was also shy and insecure, constantly worried about his health and given to nervous disorders and frequent nausea. After 1936 close friends began to notice that he was increasingly distant and introverted, and that

periodically he suffered dizziness and unconsciousness. He also began to complain
of a loathsome and repulsive smell of burning rubber before blacking out. By
early 1937 he began to appear apathetic and dazed and he complained of persistent
headaches. He soon began to suffer from serious disabilities in motor coordination.
In July 1937 he was admitted to the Johns Hopkins Hospital in Baltimore in a
deep coma with a left-sided hemiparesis and papilledema with severe protrusion.
Examinations indicated a large brain tumor in the right temporal region. Surgery
on July 10, 1937, resulted in the partial resection of a malignant glioma, and
George Gershwin died the next morning at the age of 38.

A common symptom of temporal lobe epilepsy is a visceral aura or rising epigastric sensation from the pit of the stomach, accompanied by nausea and followed
by a brief clouding of consciousness. One may speculate that in Gershwin's case,
there was at first a low grade astrocytoma in the right temporal lobe that caused
abortive temporal lobe seizures with a rising epigastric sensation. Then, in the
final phase, the astrocytoma may have undergone rapid malignant degeneration
and turned into a fulminating glioblastoma multiforme.

GRANT, ULYSSES

Bickmore, J. T. "Grant's Cancer." *Transactions of the American Academy of
Ophthalmology and Otolaryngology*, 80 (July-August 1975), 366-74.

(See Chapter 3: GRANT, ULYSSES: Steckler and Shedd).

Bricker, E. M. "Ulysses S. Grant's Dental Dilemma." *Ticonium*, 44 (November
1985), 4-6, 16.

(See Chapter 3: GRANT, ULYSSES: Steckler and Shedd).

Nelson, Rodney B. "The Final Victory of General U. S. Grant." *Cancer*, 47
(February 1, 1981), 433-36.

(See Chapter 3: GRANT, ULYSSES: Steckler and Shedd).

Steckler, Robert M. and Donald P. Shedd. "General Grant: His Physicians and
His Cancer." *The American Journal of Surgery*, 132 (October 1976), 508-14.

Ulysses S. Grant died on July 23, 1885, a victim of a squamous cell carcinoma
with keratin pearl formation. The lesion had originated on the right tonsillar
pillar and quickly spread locally to the tongue, soft palate, and down the throat,
with lymphatic metastases in the right submandibular region. Physicians considered but abandoned an attempt at a wide surgical excision because of the extent
of the disease and Grant's weakened condition. Grant was also afraid of surgery
because of his financial condition. He wanted to finish his memoirs, which would
provide some security to his family after his death. A period of thirteen months
passed between the first symptoms and the former president's death. Physicians
administered palliative treatments of topical Iodoform, salt water and carbolic
acid gargols, and cocaine, applied topically at first and hypodermically at the end
stage.

Wold, K. C. "Ulysses S. Grant—His Last Battle." *Ticonium*, 34 (July 1975), 10-12.

(See Chapter 3: GRANT, ULYSSES: Steckler and Shedd).

JAMES, HENRY

Mercer, Caroline G., and Sarah D. Wangensteen. "Consumption, Heart Disease, or Whatever: Chlorosis, A Heroine's Illness in The Wings of the Dove." *The Journal of the History of Medicine and Allied Sciences*, 40 (July 1985), 259-86.

(See Chapter 3: JAMES, HENRY: Tintner and Janowitz).

Tintner, Adeline R., and Henry D. Janowitz. "Inoperable Cancer: An Alternate Diagnosis for Milly Theale's Illness." *The Journal of the History of Medicine and Allied Sciences*, 42 (January 1987), 73-76.

The author argues that Milly Theale, the character in Henry James's novel *The Wings of the Dove*, did not die of chlorosis, as several medical historians and literary critics have claimed, but of a metastatic carcinoma. The evidence he cites is her visit to a surgeon early on in her illness and her general malaise. Also, at the time he was writing the novel, Henry James was trying to deal with the declining health and death of his sister Alice, who suffered from a metastatic breast carcinoma.

MAXIMINUS I

Klawans, Harold L. "The Acromegaly of Maximinus I: The Possible Influence of a Pituitary Tumor on the Life and Death of a Roman Emperor." In F. Clifford Rose and W. F. Bynum. *Historical Aspects of the Neurosciences*. New York: 1982. Pp. 317-26.

The portraits of Emperor Maximinus I (173-238) indicate heavy features, a prominent suborbital ridge, and a protruding lower jaw, clinically suggestive of acromegaly. He also underwent a dramatic personality change late in life, rendering him cruel and paranoid. All these symptoms indicate the possibility of a pituitary tumor which expanded out of the sella turcica into the hypothalamus.

MERRICK, JOSEPH CAREY

Carswell, Heather. "'Elephant Man' Had More than Neurofibromatosis." *Journal of the American Medical Association*, 248 (September 3, 1982), 1032-33.

Joseph Carey Merrick suffered from neurofibromatosis and fibrous dysplasia, as well as tuberculosis, scoliosis, pyarthrosis, and Paget's disease. Neurofibromatosis patients have high rates of cancer—especially schwannoma, Wilms' tumor, rhabdomyosarcoma, leukemia, and sarcomatous degeneration of the neurofibromas.

MICHELANGELO

Rosenzweig, William. "Disease in Art: A Case for Carcinoma of the Breast in Michelangelo's 'La Notte'." *Paleopathology Newsletter*, 41 (March 1983), 8-11.

Because of the unanatomical, dimpled nature of the woman's breasts in Michelangelo's "La Notte," the author argues that the model was suffering from cancer of the breasts. Since the statue was symbolic of "night" or the end stage of life, perhaps Michelangelo intentionally chose a diseased woman as his model.

NAPOLEON

Courtney, J. F. "A History and Physical on Napoleon Bonaparte." *Medical Times*, 99 (February 1971), 142-47.

(See Chapter 3: NAPOLEON: Holmes).

Daglio, P. "Napoleone e morto d cancro?" In *Congresso Nazionale di Storia della Medicina.* Roma: 1969. Pp. 330-35.

(See Chapter 3: NAPOLEON: Holmes).

Godlewski, G. "Comment mourut Napoleon." *Semaine des hopitaux de Paris*, 47 (December 20, 1971), 3027-37.

(See Chapter 3: NAPOLEON: Holmes).

Hillemand, P. "A propos de la mort de Napoleon." *Nouvelle presse médicale*, 1 (August 26, 1972), 1972-74.

(See Chapter 3: NAPOLEON: Holmes).

Holmes, Walter R. "The Illness and Death of Napoleon." *Journal of the Medical Association of Georgia*, 72 (March 1983), 201-04.

According to the author, Napoleon Bonaparte died on May 5, 1821, of an advanced carcinoma of the stomach.

Iveson-Iveson, Joan. "Napoleon: His Final Years." *Nursing Mirror*, 155 (August 18, 1982), 22-4.

She reviews the theories of Napoleon's death: gastric cancer, amoebic dysentary, dystrophia adiposogenitalia, and Zollinger-Ellison syndrome.

Pointillart, Jean. "A Propos de corps et de la destinée de Napoleon." *Nouvelle presse médicale*, 1 (August 26, 1972), 1972.

(See Chapter 3: NAPOLEON: Holmes).

QUASIMODO

Cox, Jonathan. "Quest for Quasimodo." *British Medical Journal*, 291 (December 21-28, 1985), 1801-03.

The author suggests that Victor Hugo's description of Quasimodo in *Notre-Dame de Paris*—multiple soft-tissue tumors, skeletal abnormalities, and bilateral deafness—is consistent with the symptoms of a patient suffering from von Recklinghausen's neurofibromatosis.

RADETZKY, JOSEPH

Belloni, L. "Il 'tumore' endorbitario del Feldmaresciallo Radetsky guarito della terapía omeopatica." *Gesnerus*, 42 (1985), 35-46.

Field Marshall Joseph Radetsky (1766-1858) spent his career as an Austrian soldier. He fought against Napoleon, served as chief-of-staff for Prince Schwarzenberg, and in 1856 was promoted to the rank of Field Marshall. After the war against the Sardinians, Radetsky was governor-general of Lombardy-Venetia between 1850 and 1857. He suffered from what he called a brain cancer which he claimed to have successfully treated through homeopathic medical techniques. Most likely the lesion was a benign cyst or hemangioma, which would explain the cure he achieved.

REMBRANDT

Braithwaite, Peter Allen and Dace Shugg. "Rembrandt's Bathsheba: The Dark Shadow of the Left Breast." *Annals of the Royal Academy of Surgeons of England*, 65 (1983), 337-38.

(See Chapter 11: Braithwaite and Shugg).

Dymarskii, L. Iu. "Taina 'virsavii', kartiny Rembrandta." *Voprosy Onkologii*, 30 (1984), 90-101.

(See Chapter 11: Braithwaite and Shugg).

Pytel, Ia. "Rak molochnoi zhelezy v kartine Rembrandta (K 370-letiiu so dnia rozhdeniia Rembrandta)," *Khirurgiia*, 1 (January 1976), 144-45.

(See Chapter 11: Braithwaite and Shugg).

ROOSEVELT, FRANKLIN DELANO

Goldsmith, Harry S. "Unanswered Mysteries in the Death of Franklin D. Roosevelt." *Surgery, Gynecology & Obstetrics*, 149 (December 1979), 899-908.

Most historians have concluded that President Franklin D. Roosevelt died on April 12, 1945, after suffering from a massive cerebral hemorrhage, brought on by severe hypertension and arteriosclerosis. During the last year of his life he had been treated with digitalis in an attempt to reduce his blood pressure, but he also suffered from a severe weight loss. The author, by examining photographs of Roosevelt between 1932 and 1945, makes note of the appearance of a dark lesion over his left eye, and its disappearance in 1944. He argues that Roosevelt's constant pain, weight loss, and death could have been caused by metastatic melanoma lesions. No autopsy was performed on the president and his medical records cannot be located.

SCHWEITZER, ALBERT

Denues, A. R., W. Munz, and V. Denues. "Le cancer a l'hopital du Docteur Albert Schweitzer de Lambarene (Afrique Equatoriale Occidentale) de 1929 a 1966." *Journal de medecine mondiale*, 16 (1969), 18-21.

From the medical records kept by Albert Schweitzer and his staff at the hospital in French Equatorial Africa, it is clear that most of the diseases they treated were infectious and parasitical in origin, although they occasionally had patients suffering from bone, breast, and gastrointestinal neoplasms. They also encountered a disease today known as Burkitt's lymphoma, although they had not idea of its etiology or nature.

TOLSTOY, LEO

Pytel' Ala. "O rakovoi bolezni, opisannoi v povesti L. N. Tolstogo 'Smert' Ivana Il'icha' (K 150-letiiu so dnia rozhdeniia L. N. Tolstogo)." *Urologii Nefrologii*, 4 (July-August 1978), 68-70.

The article, celebrating the 150th anniversary of the birth of Leo Tolstoy, speculates on the illness of Ivana Ilicha in the short story of the same name, suggesting that death was caused by a metastatic tumor of some kind, although the type of lesion cannot be identified.

TUTANKHAMUN

Weller, Malcolm. "Tutankhamun: An Adrenal Tumour?" *Lancet*, 2 (16 December 1972), 1312.

There is obvious breast development in the wooden and gilded statuettes of King Tutankhamun. He died suddenly between the ages of 18 and 20, probably of a hormone-producing tumor—perhaps an adrenal tumor—which would explain the breast enlargements.

WASHINGTON, GEORGE

(See Chapter 2: RUSH, BENJAMIN: Shimkin).

II THE ETIOLOGY OF CANCER

4 Carcinogenesis

Baltzer, Fritz. "Theodor Boveri. Leben und Werk eines Grossen Biologen." In *Grosse Naturforscher*. 1962.

(See Chapter 4: Grouchy).

Barclay, William R. "Asbestos: An Industrial Asset With a Health Cost." *Journal of the American Medical Association*, 252 (July 6, 1984), 96.

Between 1906 and 1928 medical journals sporadically reported pulmonary fibrosis, or asbestosis, in asbestos workers. By 1937 both United States and British public health officials saw a connection between asbestos exposure and pulmonary fibrosis and pleural plaques. By the 1940s the connection with lung cancer was noticed. Finally, in a 1964 article by Irving Selikoff, Jacob Churg, and E. Cuyler Hammond, the strong correlation was made between mesothelioma, lung cancer, and digestive cancers.

Behounek, F. "History of the Exposure of Miners to Radon." *Health Physics*, 19 (July 1970), 56-57.

In 1879 two German physicians, G. H. Härting and W. Hesse, noted that more than 75 percent of all miners working in the Black Forest mines died of lung neoplasms, now described by pathologists as bronchogenic carcinoma. Subsequent studies have also implicated uranium, radon, iron ore, chromates, and asbestos in the etiology of lung cancer among miners, and cancer control efforts now focus on protecting workers from unnecessarily high levels of exposure.

Bishop, Carole, and M. D. Kipling. "Dr. J. Ayrton Paris and Cancer of the Scrotum: 'Honor the Physician with the Honour Due Unto Him'." *Journal of the Society of Occupational Medicine*, 28 (January 1978), 3-5.

In his 1822 book *Pharmacologia*, John Ayrton Paris, an English physician, noted a connection between malignant cancer of the scrotum and work in the smelters of Cornwall and Wales. Paris also recognized the association Percivall Pott had made between soot and scrotal carcinoma among chimney sweeps, noting that the same etiological factors were probably at work. His work led to a new emphasis on hygiene among European workers exposed to soot, which greatly reduced the incidence of scrotal cancer in the nineteenth century.

Blanc, M., and P. Goldberg. "Cancer des voies respiratoires et travail dans l'extraction et le raffinage du nickel en Nouvelle-Caledonie." *Population*, 40 (January-March 1985), 166-74.

In recent years French epidemiologists have discovered statistically high rates of bronchial carcinomas and mesotheliomas among nickel miners in the Pacific colony of New Caledonia.

Blum, Harold F. "General History and Outline of the Concept." *National Cancer Institute Monographs*, 50 (December 1978), 211-12.

Although the earliest association of skin cancer with sunlight is commonly credited to P. G. Unna in the eighteenth century, the first major attempt at an epidemiological study was made by William Dubreuilh around 1900. He reported that the incidence of skin cancer was lower among urban dwellers in Bordeaux than among farmers in the rural countryside, and that skin lesions appeared on skin areas most exposed to the sun. It was not until 1928 that G. M. Findlay showed that mercury arc radiation induced skin cancer in mice, and in 1936 Funding showed that ultraviolet wave lengths shorter than 320 nm were carcinogenic in mice. Their discoveries led to new cancer control efforts at educating people into limiting their exposure to ultraviolet light.

Bogovski, P. "Historical Perspectives of Occupational Cancer." *Journal of Toxicology and Environmental Health*, 6 (November 1980), 921-39.

(See Chapter 4: Doll).

Borch-Johnsen, K. "Byliv og lungecancer. En kvantitativ og kvalitativ vurdering af den urbane faktor." *Ugeskrift for Laeger*, 144 (June 7, 1982), 1713-18.

Epidemiologists ever since the 1950s have speculated on the etiology of lung cancer, and by the mid-1970s it had become clear from studies all over the world that in addition to smoking, lung cancer was caused by the urban environment, particularly where automobile exhaust emissions, as well as industrial smoke, were extensive.

Borrel, A. "Defense et illustration du vitalisme montpellierain: La notion d⸲ reseau trophomelanique et la theorie vitale du cancer." *Monspeliensis Hippocrates*, 24 (1964), 25-28.

(See Chapter 4: Le Guyon and Chapter 4: Gurchot).

Boylan, E. "The History and Future of Chemical Carcinogenesis." *British Medical Bulletin*, 36 (January 1980), 5-10.

Ramazzini (1700) first noticed that breast tumors were more common in nuns than in the general female population. Breast carcinoma was the first cancer to be associated with a lifestyle. Hill (1761) observed the frequent occurrence of cancer of the nasal passages in men who used tobacco snuff. Rehn (1895) published evidence suggesting that exposure to aromatic amines caused bladder cancer. Today most epidemiologists believe that up to 80 percent of all cancers are environmentally induced.

Burdette, Walter J. "The Significance of Mutation in Relation to the Origin of Tumors: A Review." *Cancer Research*, 15 (May 1955), 201-26.

Oncologists have always sought a common explanation for the origins of cancer, despite the multitudinous ways in which malignancy manifests itself. The somatic mutation hypothesis has been accepted by many investigators. It simply argues that the initiating event in the appearance of any cancer is a mutation within a somatic cell. There are two principal difficulties with the hypothesis. First, critical laboratory data are difficult to obtain. Second, researchers have been unable to agree on an operative definition of mutation. The current state of the hypothesis makes the following arguments:

1. Chromogene mutation, position effect, and changes in cytoplasmic particles should be carefully distinguished in any discussion of mutation, and the biological connotation of the terminology preserved.

2. Evidence for the existence of genes for cancer susceptibility, which undoubtedly arose as mutants in germ cells, is extensive and convincing. Recombination of these genes without additional germinal mutation may alter susceptibility to tumors.

3. There is at present evidence neither for the existence of plasmagenes in mammalian cells nor for the origin of such material from antecedent genic substance.

4. A general correlation between mutagenicity and carcinogenicity cannot be proposed from present evidence.

5. Somatic chromogene mutation has not been excluded as a mode of origin of cancer, but the possibility that this is more than an unusual occurrence or that it adequately explains more than specific cases of carcinogenesis remains in doubt.

"Contribution to the Work of the Atomic Bomb Casualty
BCC)." *Archives of Environmental Health*, 21 (1970), 263-

, Jablon).

ieman, B. I. and S. L. Berger. *Asbestos: Medical and Legal Aspects.* New
York: 1984.

(See Chapter 4: Garfinkel).

"Chemical Carcinogenesis." *Cancer Bulletin*, 11 (January-February 1959), 15-17.

The first observation of chemical carcinogenesis was Percivall Pott's 1775 observation of scrotal cancer in chimney sweeps, which he attributed to their exposure to soot. In 1915 Yamagiwa and Ichikawa induced skin cancer in rabbits
by repeatedly applying coal tar to them, and in 1922 Passey used soot to induce
cancer in white mice. In the 1930s Japanese researchers induced liver tumors
by feeding animals orthoaminoazotoluene and dimethylaminoasobenzene. Ernest
Kennaway isolated the carcinogenic hydrocarbon component of coal tar in 1930.

Clemmesen, John. "Johannes Fibiger. Gongylonemia and Vitamin A in Carcinogenesis." *Acta Pathologica Microbiologica Scandinavia*, 270 (1978), 1-13.

(See Chapter 4: Clemmesen).

Clemmesen, John. *Johannes Fibiger.* 1978.

Johannes Andreas Grib Fibiger was born in Denmark in 1867. Fibiger specialized in the study of stomach carcinomas in rats, and eventually he claimed
that the lesions were caused by cockroaches. Fibiger's work was widely respected,
and in 1926 he received the Nobel Prize. Subsequent researchers, however, were
unable to duplicate his work. For a time they explained the hyperplastic reactions Fibiger observed to a vitamin A deficiency and "chronic irritation." Today
Fibiger is remembered for the most famous "false-first" in cancer research. Johannes Fibiger died in 1928.

Dodd, Charles. "Michael Williams's Contribution to Industrial Hygiene with
Reference to Cancer." *Proceedings of the Royal Society of Medicine*, 57
(1964), 1165-69.

(See Chapter 4: Doll).

Doll, Richard]. "Pot and the Prospects for Prevention." *British Journal of Cancer*, 32 (August 1975), 263-75.

Since Percivall Pott's landmark article in 1775, oncologists have identified a
variety of chemical carcinogens. They are as follows:

1. Squamous cell carcinoma of the scrotum among chimney sweeps exposed to coal dust.

2. Basal cell and squamous cell carcinomas among distillers of brown coal exposed to the polycyclic hydrocarbons in shale oil.

3. Basal and squamous cell carcinomas among workers exposed to coal gas, tar, and pitch.

4. Basal and squamous cell carcinomas in cotton mule spinners.

5. Bronchial carcinomas among miners exposed to radon.

6. Basal cell and squamous cell carcinomas among radiologists and radiographers exposed to x-rays.

7. Basal cell and squamous cell carcinomas, and melanomas, among sailors, farmers, and construction workers exposed to ultraviolet light.

8. Squamous cell carcinoma of the scrotum among arsenic smelter workers exposed to arsenic.

9. Bladder carcinomas among dye manufacturers exposed to 2-naphthylamine and 1-naphthylamine benzidine.

10. Bronchial, larynx, and naso-sinus carcinomas among mustard gas workers exposed to mustard gas.

11. Bladder carcinomas among chemical workers exposed to 4-amino-diphenyl.

12. Angiosarcomas of the liver among PVC workers exposed to vinyl chloride.

13. Bronchial carcinomas among sheep dip workers exposed to arsenic.

14. Mesothelioma among asbestos workers exposed to asbestos.

15. Bronchial carcinomas among chromate workers exposed to chromium.

16. Bronchial carcinomas among ion-exchange resin workers exposed to bis(chloromethyl) ether.

17. Bronchial and naso-sinus carcinomas among nickel workers exposed to nickel ore.

18. Naso-sinus carcinomas among furniture workers exposed to hard wood dust.

19. Myeloid and erythroleukemia among glue workers exposed to benzene.

20. Naso-sinus carcinomas among isopropanol workers exposed to isopropyl oil.

21. Bladder carcinomas among rubber workers exposed to 2- and 1-naphthylamine.

Enterline, P. E. "Asbestos and Cancer: The International Lag." *American Review of Respiratory Diseases*, 118 (December 1978), 975-78.

Since the major publication in 1964 by Selikoff, Churg, and Hammond, oncologists and epidemiologists have known of the conclusive link between exposure to asbestos and the subsequent development of mesothelioma. Legislation and federal court decisions in the United States have required protective clothing for all asbestos workers and removal of asbestos insulation from buildings. But except for the United States and several other developed countries, there has been little public health action in other areas to protect workers and the public from asbestos exposure, primarily because such protective steps appear to be initially too expensive.

Epstein, M. A. "Historical Background: Burkitt's Lymphoma and Epstein-Barr Virus." *IARC Scientific Publications*, No. 60, 17-27.

(See Chapter 17: Epstein).

Friedman, Leo. "Drugs, Food Additives, and Pesticides in Relation to Human Cancer. Historical Perspectives." *Oncology: Proceedings of the Tenth International Cancer Congress*, V (1970), 225-30.

Ever since Percivall Pott's discovery of the relationship between exposure to chimney soot and scrotal cancer, investigators have looked closely at the possible chemical etiologies of human cancer. Today it is known that cancer is caused by physical, chemical, and biological agents, but it is assumed that only 5 percent of human malignancies are caused by viruses, 5 percent by radiation, and 90 percent by chemicals in drugs, food additives, pollution, and pesticides. Since 1950 there has been an ever-growing concern with the introduction of new chemicals into the environment, and that fear has led to a series of amendments to the Food and Drug Law: the pesticide amendment of 1954, the food additives amendment of 1958, the color additives amendment of 1962, and a continuous series of scientific reviews at the federal level.

Fry, R. J. Michael. "Ionizing Radiation and Cancer. Historical Perspective." In Vincent T. DeVita, Jr., Samuel Hellman, and Steven Rosenberg. *Cancer. Principles & Practice of Oncology*. 1985. Pp. 102-06.

A. Frieban in 1902 first noticed a casual relation between exposure to radiation and cancer when he observed skin tumors in radiation workers. An association between radiation and leukemia was noticed first in 1911, and today the information about radiation-induced leukemogenesis is extensive. The high incidence of cancer in radium dial painters was first suspected by Martland in 1931. Osteosarcomas were identified first and then mastoid and nasal sinus carcinomas. The identification of ultraviolet light in the etiology of basal cell and squamous cell carcinomas and melanomas were first described by G. M. Findlay in 1928.

Gallo, Robert C., and Flossie Wong-Stall. "Current Thoughts on the Viral Etiology of Certain Human Cancers: The Richard and Hinda Rosenthal Foundation Award Lecture." *Cancer Research*, 44 (July 1984), 2743-49.

Since the first report in 1908 implicating a virus in the etiology of chicken leukosis, oncologists and virologists have speculated on the possible viral etiology of human cancers. Viral agents today have been identified as risk factors in Burkitt's lymphoma and nasopharyngeal carcinoma (Epstein-Barr virus), hepatoma (hepatitis B virus), and cervical cancers (papilloma viruses and herpes viruses). Still, proof of the existence of a human RNA tumor virus has not materialized, even though retroviruses have been linked conclusively to a number of animal leukemias and lymphomas.

Garfinkel, Lawrence. "Asbestos: Historical Perspective." *CA-A Cancer Journal for Clinicians*, 34 (January-February 1984), 44-47.

Asbestos is known as a carcinogenic agent in the rise of mesothelioma. It has been widely used since ancient times in the manufacture of paper and clothing. In 110 A.D. Pliny the Younger commented on the sickness of slaves who worked with asbestos. In 1906 English physicians described pulmonary fibrosis in asbestos workers. Reports of high rates of lung cancer in asbestos workers appeared in 1935, 1947, 1949, and 1951. The leading figure was Dr. Irving Selikoff of Paterson, New Jersey, who worked with two locals of the asbestos insulator workers union. Along with Drs. E. C. Hammond and Jacob Churg, Selikoff produced the 1964 article showing 255 deaths of 632 asbestos workers with 20 or more years working in the industry.

Gross, Ludwig. *Oncogenic Viruses.* New York: 1971.

(See Chapter 4: Rauscher and O'Connor).

Grouchy, Jean de. "Theodor Boveri et la theorie chromosomique de la cancerogenese." *Nouvelle revue: French Hematology and Blood Cells*, 18 (1977), 1-4.

Theodor Boveri (1862-1915) was a professor of zoology at the University of Wurzberg in Germany. Boveri studied mitosis in sea urchins, and in 1902 he reported that cancer was due to abnormal chromosomes. Boveri's theory at the time competed with the infectious disease theory, but subsequent research has shown that Boveri's theories were closer to reality than the infectious approach.

Gurchot, Charles. "The Trophoblast Theory of Cancer (John Beard, 1857-1924) Revisited." *Oncology*, 31 (1975), 310-33.

John Beard was a zoologist and embryologist at the University of Edinburgh who claimed that the etiology of cancer could be found in aberrant germ cells and trophoblasts. For Beard cancer was primarily trophoblastic tissue emerging either from an aberrant germ cell or from a somatic cell whose normally repressed "asexual generation" genes are abnormally reactivated. Beard called this "derepression." Except for teratomas, the variety of different types of tumor is because of a parallel chance of derepression of some genes of somatic characters. This represented a defensive reaction against intramural parasitization by trophoblasts and would result in the differentiation and hyperplasia of normally present more primitive somatic cells. Beard felt his theory was a variation of Julius Cohnheim's "embryonic-rest" theory. Although Beard's theory did not gain much of a following during his lifetime, more recent oncologists have been intrigued with the idea of derepression, since modern ongene theory holds to a somewhat similar point of view about the transformation of normal cells into malignant structures.

Havender, William R. "The Science and Politics of Cyclamates." *Public Interest*, 71 (Spring 1983), 17-32.

Cyclamate was discovered in 1937 and introduced as a sweetener in diet foods in 1953. Late in the 1960s Abbott Laboratories, a cyclamate manufacturer, reported a high incidence of bladder tumors in rats exposed to large doses of cyclamates. In 1969 the FDA banned its use. In 1980, even though subsequent, replicated studies showed no bladder cancer incidence in rats, the FDA refused to reapprove use of cyclamates.

Haynes, Harley A., Kevin W. Mead, and Robert M. Goldwyn. "Historical Background of Skin Cancer." In Vincent P. DeVita, Jr., Samuel Hellman, and Steven A. Rosenberg. *Cancer. Principles & Practice of Oncology*. 1985. Pp. 1343-44.

There are three primary, known causes of basal and squamous cell carcinomas of the skin: chemicals, ultraviolet light, and ionizing radiation. The knowledge of chemical carcinogenesis began with Percivall Pott's association of scrotum cancer in chimney sweeps in 1775. A century later researchers linked skin cancers to exposure to parrafin, pitch, and coal tar. In 1915 Yamagiwa and Ichikawa produced skin cancer experimentally in rabbits by exposing them to coal tar. In 1941 Peyton Rous suggested that skin cancer appeared in two stages after longtime exposure to a carcinogenic agent: from a benign papilloma to a malignant tumor. In the 1890s the association of skin cancer and ultraviolet light first began to be understood. J. N. Hyde published a landmark article entitled "On the Influence of Light in the Production of Cancers of the Skin" in 1906. In 1928 Findlay produced skin cancer experimentally by exposing mice to ulraviolet light in a mercury vapor lamp. These experiments were repeated conclusively again and again in the 1930s, 1940s, and 1950s. That man could affect the stratospheric ozone which filters out much of the carcinogenic wavelengths of ultraviolet light was first presented by McDonald in 1971 in relation to emissions from high-flying planes. Subsequent research has also implicated chlorofluoromethanes and nitrogen fertilizers. As for ionizing radiation, roentgen radiation-induced squamous cell carcinomas of the skin were first reported by Frieben in 1902, soon after the discovery of x-rays. Before the development of modern dosimetry, radiation therapy of the lymph nodes and underlying tissues resulted in heavy skin doses and subsequent carcinomas. Modern radiotherapy has significantly reduced skin doses and, consequently, radiation-induced carcinomas.

Henschen, F. "Yamagiwa's Tar Cancer and Its Historical Significance." *Gann*, 59 (December 1968), 447-51.

Katsusaburo Yamagiwa was a medical professor at the Tokyo Imperial University who had studied pathology under Rudolf Virchow. In 1914-1915 Yamagiwa painted a coal tar-benzene solution on the ears of experimental rabbits and observed the formation of "folliculoepitheliomas." It was the first clearly proven case of a chemically-induced cancer. The first clinical description of an occupationally-induced disease was Percivall Pott's 1775 account of scrotal cancer in chimney sweeps.

Herbst, Arthur L., Howard Ulfelder, and David C. Poskanzer. "Adenocarcinoma of the Vagina: Association of Maternal Stilbesterol Therapy with Tumor Appearance in Young Women." *New England Journal of Medicine*, 284 (1971), 878-81.

(See Chapter 13: Herbst, Ulfelder, and Poskanzer).

Homburger, F. "Carcinogenesis Bioassay in Historical Perspective." *Progress in Experimental Tumor Research*, 26 (1983), 182-6.

(See Chapter 4: Shimkin and Triolo).

Honti, J., and K. Lapis. "Marek-Betegseg; Marek József Dr. A kisérletes onkológia nemzetközileg ismert úttöröje." *Orvosi Hetilap*, 118 (11 September 1977), 2223-25.

Lymphoproliferative disease of chickens has the eponym "Marek's Disease" because Josef Marek, a Hungarian scientist, first described it in 1907. Subsequent research completed in 1967 demonstrated that the disease is infectious and is associated with the herpes virus.

Hueper, W. C. "Some Comments on the History and Experimental Explorations of Metal Carcinogens and Cancer." *Journal of the National Cancer Institute*, 62 (April 1979), 723-25.

(See Chapter 4: Doll).

Hutt, M. S. R. "Historical Introduction, Burkitt's Lymphoma, Nasopharyngeal Carcinoma, and Kaposi's Sarcoma." *Transactions of the Royal Society of Tropical Medicine and Hygiene*, 75 (No. 6), 761-65.

(See Chapter 17: Hutt).

Jablon, Seymour, and Joseph L. Belsky. "Radiation Induced Cancer in Atomic Bomb Survivors." *Oncology: Proceedings of the Tenth International Cancer Congress*, V (1970), 107-21.

At the request of President Harry Truman in 1948, the National Academy of Sciences established the Atomic Bomb Casualty Commission to study the long-term effects of radiation exposure. The Commission found that the leukemia rate is extremely high in atomic bomb survivors who received large doses of radiation. Thyroid, lung, and breast carcinomas were also high. Among those survivors who were less than ten years old in 1945, after a latent period of twenty years, there is now developing much higher rates of cancer in general.

Johnston, Frank R. "Hippocrates Never Heard of It. The Anatomy of a Modern Epidemic." *The American Surgeon*, 51 (January 1985), 1-7.

In 1984 one million people died of a disease which was almost unheard of five hundred years ago—cancer. As early as 1500 some people began observing high death rates from respiratory illnesses among miners in Bohemia and Saxony. But not until 350 years later did any real understanding of the nature of their illness emerge. In 1879 Härting and Hesse speculated that they were dying of bronchial malignancies. In 1913 Arnstein-Wien classified their tumors as oat cell carcinoma. Not until the 1940s did physicians understand that the disease was caused by radiation.

Kenez, J. "A kisérletes rakkutatas es Johannes Fibiger." *Orvosi Hetilap*, 108 (12 August 1967), 1567-70.

(See Chapter 4: Clemmesen).

King, D. Friday and Debra Eisenberg. "Russell's Fuchsine Body. 'The Characteristic Organism of Cancer'." *The American Journal of Dermatopathology*, 3 (Spring 1981), 55-58.

(See Chapter 2: RUSSELL, WILLIAM: King and Eisenberg).

Kipling, M. D., and H. A. Waldron. "Percivall Pott and Cancer Scroti." *British Journal of Indian Medicine*, 32 (August 1975), 244-50.

(See Chapter 4: Potter).

Kipling, M. D., R. Usherwood, and R. Varley. "A Monstrous Growth: An Historical Note on Carcinoma of Scrotum." *British Journal of Indian Medicine*, 27 (October 1970), 382-84.

(See Chapter 2: Potter).

Koprowski, Hilary. "Cell-Virus Interaction: Biological Aspects. Historical Review and Perspectives." *Oncology: Proceedings of the Tenth International Cancer Congress*, I (1970), 110-18.

For more than two decades the term "vertical transmission" was used to represent the concept of hereditary transmission of oncogenicity engendered by tumor viruses. Except for the fact that milk of certain strains of mice was shown to contain mammary tumor virus, the actual mechanisms of vertical transmission remained obscure. In 1969 Roger Weil suggested researchers focus on the early events following adsorption and penetration of the virus. The eternal unanswered question is why cells infected with oncogenic virus become cancer cells. Using SV40 and permissive AGMK cells, Hummeler, Sokol, Barbanti-Brodano, and Swetly (1971) performed morphologic studies on the initiation of the infectious process, and they showed that following viral penetration by monopinocytosis and acquisition by the virus of an extra membrane, the virus then proceeded, possibly within ten minutes after infection, to the nucleus, reaching maximum concentration at two hours after infection. During penetration of the nucleus, the newly acquired envelope is shed, and viral uncoating takes place in the nucleus.

Korbler, Johannes. "Der Tabak in der Krebslehre zu Anfang des 19. Jahrhunderts." *Proceedings of the Twenty-First International Congress of the History of Medicine*, 2 (1969), 1179-83.

John Hill, a surgeon in London, published the first report of an association between tobacco use and cancer in a 1761 study of nasal carcinomas in snuff users. In 1795 the Polish physician Samuel Thomas von Soemmering noticed an association between lip carcinomas and pipe smokers. Throughout the nineteenth century a host of physicians confirmed the connections between tobacco use and some types of cancer.

Larsen, David L. and James E. Bennett. "Chimney Sweeper's Disease Revisited:
     First Case Reported in a Black." *Plastic and Reconstructive Surgery*, 61
     (February 1978), 281-83.

Percivall Pott first reported scrotum carcinoma in 1775 in chimney sweeps.
The first reported case in a black was in 1977 at the Veterans' Hospital in In-
dianapolis. He was a 62 year old furnace cleaner who died six weeks later of
metastatic squamous cell carcinoma. Occupationally-induced squamous cell carcinomas of the scrotum have also been identified in paraffin workers (1871 by
Ogston), tar workers (1910 by Green), and mulespinners (1928 by Hoffman).

Le Guyon, Rene. "Borrell et la theorie virusale des cancers." *Bulletin de le
     Academie National de Medecine*, 151 (21 November 1967), 585-93.

Amédee Borrel was born in France in 1867 and spent his professional career as
a professor of bacteriology, hygiene, and public health at the University of Strasbourg. Although experiments on the transmission of neoplasms through cell-free
filtrates had not been formulated yet, Borrel postulated in 1907 that cancer resulted from viral invasions of normal cells. He strongly, and incorrectly, disagreed
with prevailing German views that cancer came from internal cellular changes.

Logan, W. P. "Cancer Mortality by Occupation and Social Class 1851-1971."
     IARC Science Publications, 36 (1982), 1-253.

In the nineteenth and twentieth centuries researchers have learned a great deal
about occupations, social class, and cancer. They have learned that lower class
women, particularly those with early coitus and multiple sexual partners, have
higher rates of cervical cancer. On the other hand, women who do not have children have higher rates of breast cancer. In terms of occupations, scientists have
associated high exposure to sunlight as a cause of skin cancer, aniline dyes as a
cause of bladder cancer, asbestos exposure as a cause of mesothelioma, radiation
exposure as a cause of lung cancer, and exposure to coal tar and various hydrocarbons as causes of squamous cell carcinomas.

McKusick, V. A. "Marcella O'Grady Boveri (1865-1950) and the Chromosome
     Theory of Cancer." *Journal of Medical Genetics*, 22 (December 1985), 431-
     40.

(See Chapter 1: Gallucci).

Melicow, M. M. "Percivall Pott (1713-1788): 200th Anniversary of the First
     Report of Occupation-Induced Cancer of the Scrotum in Chimney Sweepers
     (1775)." *Urology*, 6 (December 1975), 745-49.

(See Chapter 4: Potter).

Melnick, Joseph L. "Viruses and Human Cancer: Modern Historical Perspectives." *Oncology: Proceedings of the Tenth International Cancer Congress,* V (1970), 129-34.

Avian and urine leukemias induced by RNA viruses have served as a model for the study of leukemia in man. The infectous virus can readily be identified *in vivo* throughout the life span of the diseased animal, either circulating in the blood or in the malignant cells themselves. Also, the malignant cells can be propagated *in vitro*, and the resulting cultures continue to produce infectious virus. And the virus can be detected directly or by its ability to interfere with the multiplication of related viruses in susceptible cells. Electron microscopic examinations reveal particles resembling the avian and murine leukemia RNA viruses in the cells or plasma of leukemia patients. Still, actual isolation of an active biologic agent etiologically related to human leukemia has not yet been found. Recent electron microscopy has also revealed particles resembling papovaviruses in patients suffering from progressive multifocal leukoencephalopathy. The Epstein-Barr virus is now expected in patients with Burkitt's lymphoma and nasopharyngeal carcinoma. The vast majority of human solid tumors appear free of infectious virus or infectious nucleic acid. Finally, recent research indicates a connection between the herpes virus and malignancies in lower animals: neurolymphoma of chickens, adenocarcinoma of the frog kidney, rabbit lymphoma, and monkey and marmoset lymphomas.

Mesle, France. "Cancer et alimentation: Le cas des cancers de l'intestin et du rectum." *Population*, 38 (Juillet-Octobre 1983), 733-62.

Between 1950 and 1978 the incidence of colorectal cancer more than doubled in France, primarily because of increased consumption of pork and beef, as well as processed sugar and flour, and reductions in the consumption of bulk foods: vegetables and grains. Epidemiological research in the various regions of France confirms this hypothesis.

Miller, Elizabeth C. "Reactive Forms of Chemical Carcinogens: Interactions with Tissue Components. Historical Review and Perspectives." *Oncology 1970: Proceedings of the Tenth International Cancer Congress,* I (1970), 23-38.

It has been forty years since Kennaway and Hieger demonstrated the induction of skin tumors in mice upon application of 1,2,5,6-dibenzanthracene. Three years later Yoshida demonstrated the carcinogenic power of o-aminoazotoluene for the livers of rats. Soon after Hueper demonstrated that 2-naphthylamine was carcinogenic for the urinary bladders of dogs. In recent years it has become increasingly clear that many chemical carcinogens are not active as such, but require conversion *in vivo* to metabolites which are the ultimate carcinogenic forms. Regardless of the structure of the compound administered, all or nearly all chemical carcinogens yield electrophilic reactants *in vivo*, and these ultimate carcinogens induce cancer through interaction with one or more cellular constituents, particularly DNA, specific RNAs, specific proteins, or combinations thereof.

Miller, Elizabeth C., and James A. Miller. "Milestones in Chemical Carcinogenesis." *Seminars in Oncology*, 6 (December 1979), 445-56.

Three eighteenth century observations launched the field of chemical carcinogenesis: John Hill's 1761 argument that there was a connection between snuff use and nasal carcinoma; Percivall Pott's 1775 claim of a relationship between exposure to soot and the incidence of scrotal cancer in chimney sweeps; and Samuel von Soemmering's report in 1794 of a relationship between lip carcinoma and clay-pipe smoking. During the nineteenth century subsequent research by other physicians confirmed their suspicions. In 1895 Rehn pointed out the high incidence of bladder cancer among aromatic amine workers. The first metal carcinogen was identified in 1932 as nickel, which caused nasal carcinomas in nickel refinery workers. In 1915 Yamagiwa and Ichikawa demonstrated the carcinogeneity of coal tar when applied to rabbit ears, and Kennaway later identified hydrocarbons as the active agent. Lacassagne induced mammary carcinoma in mice treated with estrone in 1932.

Research after World War II implicated a wide variety of chemicals as cancer-causing agents. They are: 1) 2-Naphthylamine in urinary bladder cancer; 2) Benzidine in urinary bladder cancer; 3) 4-Aminobiphenyl and 4-nitrobiphenyl in urinary bladder cancer; 4) Bis(chloromethyl) ether in lung cancer; 5) Bis(2-chloroethyl) sulfide in respiratory tract carcinomas; 6) Vinyl chloride in liver carcinoma; 7) Hydrocarbons (tars, soots, oils) in squamous cell and lung carcinoma; 8) Chromium compounds in lung cancer; 9) Nickel compounds in lung, nasal, and sinus carcinomas; 10) Asbestos in mesotheliomas; 11) Chlornapthazine in urinary bladder cancer; 12) Diethylstilbestrol in vaginal carcinoma; 13) Inorganic arsenic compounds in skin cancer; 14) Cigarette smoking in lung, urinary tract, and pancreatic carcinoma; and 15) Betel nut and tobacco quids in buccal mucosa carcinoma.

Molieri, I. J., and O. Donato, and H. I. Scherwkopf de Gulbins. "Comentarios a la tésis doctoral de Angel H. Roffo: 'El Cancer: Contribución a su estudio', Buenos Aires, 1909." *Seminario en Medicina*, (1973), 227-31.

Angel H. Roffo, a graduate student in biology at the University of Buenos Aires in 1909, presented a Ph.D. thesis in which he evaluated the major existing theories on the etiology of cancer: the environmental irritation theory popularized by Percivall Pott, the chromosomal theory of Theodor Boveri, and the viral theory of Amédee Borrel. Roffo also speculated on the possible bacteriological origins of the disease and called for more extensive research into the nature of cancer.

Oiso, Toshio. "Incidence of Stomach Cancer and Its Relation to Dietary Habits and Nutrition in Japan between 1900 and 1975." *Cancer Research*, 35 (November 1975), 3254-58.

The Japanese have high rates of stomach cancer, probably due to a diet heavy in rice consumption, such highly salted foods as seaweed, shellfish, and soybean sauce, and the practice of burning fish when cooking. In recent years, as dietary habits change with the introduction of more western foods, stomach cancers seem to be starting to decline in incidence, while colorectal cancers are on the rise.

Onuigbo, Wilson I. B. "The Paget Cell: Mistaken for a Parasite in the 19th Century." *The American Journal of Dermatopathology*, 8 (December 1986), 520-21.

In 1874 James Paget described the carcinoma of the mammary areolae which now bears his name, but he did not understand the histology of the disease. Because the Paget cell was large and ovoid, with an opaque cytoplasm, most researchers thought it had a parasitic etiology. But by 1900 most pathologists had abandoned that theory in favor of a more nebulous, but inherently more accurate, assumption that the disease was caused by internal cellular changes. That point of view proved to be scientifically correct.

Pantoja, Enrique, and I. Rodríguez-Ibañez. "Sacrococcygeal Dermoids and Teratomas." *The American Journal of Surgery*, 132 (September 1976), 377-82.

Teratomas are among the oldest known tumors, the earliest reference being a Babylonian document from Chaldea four thousand years ago describing the tumor in an infant. The first unquestionable report of a teratoma came from a seventeenth century French obstetrician. In 1863 Rudolf Virchow introduced the term teratoma to describe the tumor. In 1841 Stanley described in detail a typical sacrococcygeal teratoma. That same year a German surgeon, W. Blizard, reported the first successful surgical removal of such a tumor when he operated on a 2 year old girl. Virchow referred to the external sacrococcygeal growths as "soft tails" in 1884, and in 1885 Middledorpf published his classic report of an intestine containing a teratoma. Theories as to the etiology of such tumors have varied greatly. In the 1920s M. A. Perlstein, E. R. Le Count, and J. Bland-Sutton argued that teratomas were actually suppressed twins or parasitic fetuses because teratomas occasionally have well-developed anatomical features, such as fingers and toes. In the 1950s and 1960s people like R. E. Gross, H. W. Clatworthy, I. A. Meeker, and G. V. Brindley claimed that teratomas originated from totipotential cells of Henson's node. A third common theory about the etiology of teratomas has existed in one form or another for more than a century, and it proposed a germ cell theory—the tumor comes from haploid germ cells through a process of autofertilization. In 1922 A. A. Law warned of the frequent malignant degeneration of sacrococcygeal teratomas and called for their surgical removal. Paul Kraske perfected the surgical technique for removing the tumors in the 1920s.

Pariza, Michael W., and Roswell K. Boutwell. "Historical Perspective: Calories and Energy Expenditure in Carcinogenesis." *American Journal of Clinical Nutrition*, 45 (1987), 151-56.

In the 1940s researchers first began to address the relationship between caloric intake, dietary fat level, and cancer incidence. In 1914 Peyton Rous showed that underfeeding slowed the growth of transplanted tumors in rats, as did excess exercise on transplanted fibrosarcomas. Caloric restriction also reduced the onset of spontaneous tumors in rats. In 1940 Albert Tannebaum showed that caloric restriction greatly reduced the incidence of spontaneous mammary tumors and primary lung adenomas in mice, as well as chemically-induced skin tumors. Subsequent research by investigators at the National Cancer Institute in the 1940s confirmed Tannebaum's results. Researchers like M. G. Mulinos and R. K. Boutwell believed that overfed laboratory animals produce excess hormones, which might lead to higher rates of cancer.

Pascarella, F. "L'Evoluzione della teoria traumatica nella genesi dei tumori." *Medicina nei Secoli*, 4 (January-March 1967), 3-9.

(See Chapter 1: Schulze).

Petrakis, Nicholas L. "Historic Milestones in Cancer Epidemiology." *Seminars in Oncology*, 6 (December 1979), 433-44.

(See Chapter 5: Petrakis).

Pitot, Henry C. "Principles of Cancer Biology: Chemical Carcinogenesis." In Vincent T. DeVita, Jr., Samuel Hellman, and Steven A. Rosenberg. *Cancer. Principles & Practice of Oncology*. 1985. Pp. 79-82.

A carcinogen is an agent whose administration to previously untreated animal tissue leads to a statistically significantly increased incidence of neoplasms of one or more histogenetic types as compared with the incidences in appropriate untreated animals. In 1775 Percivall Pott, the English physician, observed the occurrence of scrotum cancer in chimney sweeps. Pott claimed that the large amount of soot they were exposed to led to the tumors. His discovery inspired the Danish Chimney Sweeps Association in 1778 to recommend daily bathing to all of its members. In 1892 H. T. Butlin then explained that European chimney sweeps had much lower rates of scrotal cancer, compared to their English counterparts, because of daily bathing. In 1915 the Japanese pathologists Yamagiwa and Ichikawa reported the first production of skin cancer in animals treated with coal tar applications. Sir Ernest Kennaway in 1932 isolated out hydrocarbons as the carcinogenic agents in the coal tar. In 1935 Sasaki and Yoshida demonstrated that the feeding of the azo dye, o-aminoazotoluene, to rats resulted in the development of liver tumors.

Potter, Michael. "Percivall Pott's Contribution to Cancer Research." *National Cancer Institute Monograph No. 10*, (1963), 1-13.

In 1775 Percivall Pott, a surgeon at St. Bartholomew's Hospital in London, described cancer of the scrotum in chimney sweeps and recognized it as an occupational neoplasm. His work was the beginning of the theory of chemical carcinogenesis and the supposition that neoplasms are environmentally-produced in most cases.

Powell, Peter C. "Cytogenetics and Cell Hybridization. Historical Perspectives in Cytogenetics and Cell Hybridization as Applied to Neoplasia." *Oncology: The Proceedings of the Tenth International Cancer Congress*, I (1970), 358-363.

Mammalian cytogenetics and mammalian cell hybridization are relatively new fields. From Von Hansemann in 1890 and Boveri in 1914 came suggestions that abnormalities of the mitotic apparatus and of chromosome constitution might play an essential role in the neoplastic process. But not until the 1950s, when modern cytogenetic techniques developed, were detailed studies possible. Mammalian somatic cell hybridization is an even newer field, dating back only to the studies of Barski in 1960. The research today has reached three general conclusions: 1) neoplastic cells of most, but not all, mammalian tumors contain demonstrable chromosome change; 2) those chromosomal changes are frequently clonal in nature; and 3) although cytogenetic abnormalities in mammalian neoplasms are clonal in nature, they generally differ from case to case.

Rauscher, Frank J., and Timothy E. O'Connor. "Virology." In J. F. Holland and E. Frei, III. Eds. *Cancer Medicine*. Philadelphia: 1973. Pp. 15-44.

During the twentieth century researchers have identified twenty viruses which induce neoplasms in animals. They are: Ellerman and Bang's identification of the chicken leukemia virus in 1908; Rous's identification of the chicken sarcoma virus in 1911; Shope's identification of virally-induced rabbit skin carcinomas in 1933; Lucke's isolation of the frog kidney carcinoma virus in 1934; Bittner's identification of the mouse breast carcinoma virus in 1936; Gross's identification of the mouse leukemia virus in 1951; Stewart's identification of a multiple carcinoma-inducing virus in mice, rats, and rabbits in 1957; Eddy's isolation of a monkey-to-hamsters sarcoma virus in 1961; Trentin's identification of a man-to-hamster sarcoma virus in 1962; Harvey's isolation of a mouse sarcoma virus in 1964; Jarrett's identification of the cat leukemia virus in 1964; Hull's isolation of a monkey-to-hamster sarcoma-lymphoma virus in 1965; Sarma's isolation of a chicken-to-hamster fibrosarcoma virus in 1965; Darbyshire's bovine-to-hamster sarcoma virus in 1966; Opler's guinea pig leukemia virus in 1967; Sarma's dog-to-hamster fibrosarcoma virus in 1967; Melendez's monkey lymphoma virus in 1968; Graffi's hamster lymphoma virus in 1968; Snyder and Theilen's cat fibrosarcoma virus in 1969; and Wolfe's monkey fibrosarcoma virus in 1970.

Redmond, D. E. "Tobacco and Cancer: The First Clinical Report, 1761." *New England Journal of Medicine*, 282 (1970), 18-23.

The first report on the relationship between tobacco use and carcinoma came from the English physician John Hill in 1761, when he noted high rates of oral and nasal cancer among snuff users. Hill advised moderation in the use of snuff as a means of preventing such cancers.

"The Rubber Industry." *IARC Monographs*, 28 (April 1982), 31-46.

Rubber was used anciently but the commercial rubber industry did not appear in Europe until the eighteenth century. In 1844 Charles Goodyear vulcanized rubber by mixing it with sulphur and heating it. The birth of the automobile industry dramatically increased the size of the rubber industry. In 1954 R. A. M. Case and M. E. Hosker noted an unusually high rate of bladder cancer among rubber workers.

Rubin, Henry. "Historical Perspectives: Avian Tumor Viruses." *Oncology 1970: The Proceedings of the Tenth International Cancer Congress*, I (1970), 763-68.

Just before the turn of the century, when viruses were first being discovered, Sanarelli found that a tumor of rabbits called myxoma was caused by an agent which Moses proved in 1911 to be a virus. Then, in 1908, Ellermann and Bang reported that a virus was responsible for fowl leukemia. Rous discovered the chicken sarcoma virus in 1911. In 1914 Fujinami and Inamoto proved that chicken myxosarcoma was caused by a virus.

Saffiotti, Umberto. "Carcinogenesis, 1957-1977: Notes for a Historical Review." *Journal of the National Cancer Institute*, 59 (August 1977), 617-22.

Before the 1950s, polycyclic aromatic hydrocarbons, azo dyes, aromatic amines, carbamates, some alkylating agents, some metals, and some hormones were the main known classes of carcinogens. Since then, carcinogenic activity has been well documented in nitrosomines and nitrosamides, substituted hydrazines, chlorinated and other halogenated hydrocarbons, chlorinated pesticides, halo ethers, epoxides, mycotoxins, and tobacco smoke.

Salsburg, David and Andrew Heath. "When Science Progresses and Bureaucracies Lag—The Case of Cancer Research." *Public Interest*, No. 65 (1981), 30-39.

(See Chapter 7: Salsburg and Heath).

Schottenfield, D., and J. F. Haas. "The Workplace as a Cause of Cancer." *Clinical Bulletin*, 8 (1978), 54-60.

(See Chapter 4: Doll).

Schulze, H. E. "Zur Geschichte der Traumatischen Tetraplegie." *Beitrage zur Neurochirurgie*, 15 (1968), 293-96.

Another prominent theory concerning the etiology of cancer was the trauma idea of Hugo Ribbert, a German physician, in the early twentieth century. He argued that cancer cells have no unusual powers of proliferation; they have merely been freed from the restraints of "tissue tension" by mechanical isolation. Trauma exposes and then isolates predisposed epithelial cells by newly formed connective tissue. The isolated cells have altered growth tendencies that have been increased by irritation. Although subsequent research generally repudiated the trauma theory, it still survived as an explanation for cancer among lay practitioners, and some oncologists in the 1970s and 1980s still felt there might be a trauma connection in the etiology of some soft-tissue sarcomas.

Shabad, L. M. "Evoliutsiia poniatiia o khimicheskikh kantserogenakh." *Voprosy Onkologii*, 22 (1976), 15-22.

The article discusses the evolution of the scientific notion of chemical carcinogenesis, beginning with the early twentieth century Japanese research on coal tar and cancer and continuing through research on the carcinogenic nature of the hydrocarbons and other chemical compounds.

Sharpe, William D. "The New Jersey Radium Dial Painters: A Classic in Occupational Carcinogenesis." *Bulletin of the History of Medicine*, 52 (Winter 1979), 560-70.

In 1910 a radium-activated luminous paint was used on some of the more expensive Swiss and German watches, and in 1913 a cheaper version was developed in the United States. The water-based paint contained radium-226 and radium-228 placed in a zinc phosphor with trace metals added to provide color. The zinc sulfide decomposed because of alpha bombardment and the radium-228 served as a luminizer. The use of radioluminous paint was a fad that was largely over with by 1926, but at its peak between 1917 and 1924, more than a thousand people worked at radium extraction and dial painting in Orange, New Jersey. In 1931 Harrison S. Martland, the Essex County Medical Examiner, began to report unusually high rates of aplastic anemia and osteogenic sarcoma among former radium workers. Area dentists also reported unusually high rates of refractory mandibular and maxillary osteomyelitis, as well as oral cavity lesions. Martland defined radium intoxication as a new occupational disease—aplastic anemia, osteonecrosis, and osteogenic sarcoma.

Shear, M. J. "Yamagiwa's Tar Cancer and Its Historical Significance—From
   Yamagiwa to Kennaway." *Gann*, 60 (April 1969), 121-27.

In 1915 Katsusaburo Yamagiwa first described the process of chemically inducing a malignant lesion by applying coal tar solutions to the ears of experimental
rabbits. Other researchers gradually built upon Yamagiwa's work until 1955 when
Ernest Kennaway of the Royal Cancer Hospital in England actually isolated the
five-ring hydrocarbon responsible for inducing the squamous cell carcinomas.

Shevlyaghin, V. Y. "The Scientific Heritage of Professor Zilber and His Contribution to Virus-Genetic Theory of Malignant Tumours." *Neoplasma*, 26
   (1979), 113-23.

Lev Alexandrovich Zilber was born in 1894 and graduated from the University
of Moscow in 1919. He was a professor of immunology and virology at the Gema-
leya Institute of Epidemiology and Microbiology in Moscow and the founder of the
Soviet school of viral oncology. He was a brilliant researcher who described the viral antigens of a number of specific tumors. Lev Alexandrovich Zilber died in 1964.

Shimkin, Michael B., and Victor A. Triolo. "History of Chemical Carcinogenesis:
   Some Prospective Remarks." *Progress in Experimental Tumor Research*, 11
   (1969), 1-20.

There are a variety of historical landmarks in chemical carcinogenesis, and
they include: 1) Percivall Pott's 1775 identification of the connection between
chimney sweeps and the "soot wart," a squamous cell carcinoma of the scrotum;
2) Clunet's successful 1908 stimulation of sarcomas in rats exposed to x-rays; 3)
Yamagiwa and Ichikawa's 1915 report on the successful induction of skin tumors
on the ears of rabbits receiving repeated coal tar applications and lymph node
metastases in several of the animals; 4) Ernest Kennaway's isolation of polycyclic
hydrocarbons from coal tar and their implication as the causative agent in chemical carcinogenesis; 5) Wynder's role in the 1940s and 1950s in identifying tobacco
smoking as a major culprit in the development of lung, oral cavity, laryngeal,
esophageal, and perhaps bladder carcinomas; 6) Ludwig Rehn's 1895 description
of bladder cancer among aniline dye workers and Hueper's 1938 discovery that
2-naphthylamine was the chemical culprit; 7) Fischer's 1906 report that aminoazo
dyes were carcinogenic when injected into rabbit ears and Yoshida's identification of o-aminoazotoluene as the carcinogenic agent; 8) E. K. Weisberger and
J. K. Weisberger's identification of N-2-fluorenylacetamide as a carcinogenic compound in many insecticides; 9) the 1943 discovery by Henshaw and Nettleship that
urethane (ethyl carbamate) was carcinogenic in producing pulmonary tumors in
experimental animals; 10) the 1961 identification of the aflatoxins in causing liver
tumors in animals; and 11) the role of cycasin in causing liver and kidney tumors
in mice.

Shope, Richard E. "Evolutionary Episodes in the Concept of Viral Oncogenesis." *Perspectives in Biology and Medicine*, 9 (Winter 1966), 258-74.

Within the last twenty years oncologists have become especially excited about the possibility that filterable viruses may be of basic etiological importance in explaining the causes of cancer. Research into animal tumors has revealed much about the viral origins of cancer. In 1896 G. Sanarelli of Uruguay proved that infectious myxomatosis in rabbits was caused by a filterable virus. Danish researchers V. Ellerman and O. Bang demonstrated in 1908 that chicken leukemia was caused by a virus, and Peyton Rous, an American researcher, reported in 1911 that chicken sarcoma had viral origins. Since then scientists have developed six models explaining how animal tumor viruses function to cause neoplasia. 1) There are those that are directly infective for the hosts in which they naturally occur—the Rous sarcoma virus of chickens and the papilloma virus of cottontail rabbits. 2) Some viruses native to one host are oncogenic in a foreign host, such as the polyoma of mice, the papilloma of cottontail rabbits, the adenovirus of man, and the simian virus 40 of monkeys. 3) There is one virus, which causes the Bittner mouse mammary cancer, that is transmitted through the milk and infects soon after birth, although the tumors do not appear until middle age. 4) The Gross virus causing mouse lymphatic leukemia is transmitted naturally by way of the ovum and can be passed experimentally by injecting mice within a few hours of birth. Like the Bittner mouse mammary cancer, however, the tumors do not appear until middle age. 5) The polyoma virus in its natural host, the mouse, has important epidemiological considerations for the possible viral etiology of human cancers. The virus is a widespread infectious agent in mouse stocks but only rarely manifests itself as a parotid tumor. If a similar condition prevailed for human beings, one could expect certain human tumors to be caused, under certain conditions, by a virus which is widespread and usually harmless in the human population. 6) In the rabbit fibroma and papilloma, viral agents often act in concert with chemical carcinogens to cause tumors.

Simopoulos, Artemis P. "Obesity and Carcinogenesis: Historical Perspective." *American Journal of Clinical Nutrition*, 45 (1987), 271-76.

Hippocrates first made the connection between obesity and reduced lifespans, and after World War II a variety of life insurance companies and academic researchers came to similar conclusions, primarily because of the relationship between obesity and cardiovascular disease. In 1930 F. L. Hoffman first made a connection between obesity and cancer incidence, as did A. Tannebaum in 1940. Their work, however, was primarily epidemiological, not experimental. Between 1959 and 1972 the American Cancer Society conducted a study on obesity and cancer and found that individuals more than 40 percent overweight had increased cancer risks: colon and rectal cancer for men and gallbladder, breast, cervical, endometrial, ovarian, and uterine cancer in women. Subsequent research has confirmed those conclusions. The etiology of the disease is not clear, although obese individuals have elevated levels of prolactin, androgens, estrogens, and cortisol in their systems, which may play a role in triggering cancer of the reproductive system in women.

Steinfeld, Jesse L. "Smoking and Lung Cancer. A Milestone in Awareness." *Journal of the American Medical Association*, 253 (May 24-31, 1985), 2995-97.

The article provides a retrospective look at the landmark article in the 1950 *Journal of the American Medical Association* by Evarts Graham and Ernest Wynder. Entitled "Tobacco Smoking as a Possible Etiologic Factor in Bronchiogenic Carcinoma," the article led to the Surgeon General's 1964 report on the dangers of tobacco smoking and all subsequent legislation concerning smoking and health.

Stockwell, Richard M. "Irradiation Related Thyroid Cancer. History and Current Recommendations." *Connecticut Medicine*, 43 (February 1979), 63-67.

(See Chapter 14: Stockwell).

Stockwell, Serena. "Isaac Berenblum, M.D." *CA-A Cancer Journal for Clinicians*, 31 (July/August 1981), 239-40.

(See Chapter 2: BERENBLUM, ISAAC: Stockwell).

Strong, Leonell C. "Genetic Concept for the Origin of Cancer: Historical Review." *Annals of the New York Academy of Sciences*, 71 (1958), 810-38.

The genetic concept of the origin of cancer was first formulated in 1926 when it was discovered that alterations in the transplantability characteristics of cancerous tissue underwent sudden and unpredictable periodic changes that were relatively permanent from the point of origin. Leading investigators were Leonell C. Strong in the United States, who was working with mice, and K. H. Bauer in Germany, who studied human material. The change they postulated applied to any formed constituent of the cell, either nuclear or cytoplasmic, that could duplicate itself, affect the physiology of the cell specifically, and be transmitted by cell division. Subsequent research has revealed the potential of chemical, radiation, or environmentally-induced mutations as a source of carcinogenesis. Future research will focus on cytoplasmic inheritance and mutations, particularly in microbiology, the bacteriophage, bacteria, and viruses.

Strong, Leonell C. "Mother's Milk and the Offspring." *Journal of the History of Medicine*, 8 (April 1953), 210-14.

In 1936 J. J. Bittner discovered the milk agent in the etiology of adenocarcinoma of the mammary gland in mice, opening up the proposition that viruses, antibodies, bacteria, and hormones—and carcinogens—can be passed from mother to her offspring through nursing.

Supady, J. "Doświadczalne badania lekarzy polskich nad rakotwórczym działłaniem smoły pogazowej i jej pochondnych (do 1939 r.)." *Polski Tygodnik Lekarski*, 36 (March 2, 1981), 357-59.

During the 1920s and 1930s a number of Polish researchers and physicians followed up on the work of Japanese researcher Katsusaburo Yamagiwa in producing cancer in animals, especially rabbits, by regular applications of coal tar to the skin. The experiments demonstrated carcinogenesis through exposure to a pollutant.

Supady, J. "Poglady na temat patofenezy i etologii nowotworów w medycynie europejeskiej na prezelomie XIX i XX wieku." *Polski Tygodnik Lekarski*, 34 (18 June 1979), 1009-11.

At the turn of the nineteenth and twentieth centuries oncology was emerging as a medical discipline. Its experimental basis had been established by the transplantation studies launched by M. A. Novinsky; the principles of cellular pathology had been established by Rudolf Virchow; Wilhelm Roentgen had discovered the x-ray and treatment of tumors had already begun on an experimental basis; and surgeons like Theodor Billroth had performed complicated abdominal surgeries with reduced mortality rates, while other surgeons like William Halsted had promoted the notion of *en bloc* resection of tumors to prevent local recurrences. An extraordinary but naive sense of hope pervaded the scientific community in 1900 about the possibility of conquering cancer. The disease would prove to far more tenacious than they imagined.

Takahashi, T. "Historical Review of Cancer Research in Japan. Chemical Carcinogenesis and Biochemistry." *Protein Nucleic Acid Enzyme*, 15 (January 1974), 1-4.

(See Chapter 4: Shear and Chapter 4: Doll).

Thouez, J. P., and D. Godon. "La géographie du travail et la sante: Le cas de la mortalité par cancers selon les secteurs d'activite et les bassins d'emplois au Québec." *Espace, Population et Societie*, 3 (1984), 47-58.

(See Chapter 4: Thouez and Godon).

Trentin, John J., Yoshiro Yabe, and Grant Taylor. "The Quest for Human Cancer Viruses." *Science*, 137 (14 September 1962), 835-41.

(See Chapter 4: Shope).

Triolo, Victor A., and B. Giovanella. "Francesco Durante and the Cohnheim Theory of Oncogenesis." *Physis*, 8 (1966), 199-219.

(See Chapter 1: Rather).

Weisburger, Elizabeth K. "History of the Bioassay Program of the National Cancer Institute." *Progress in Experimental Tumor Research*, 26 (1983), 187-201.

(See Chapter 7: Weisburger).

Westcott, W. B. "Pioneers in the Study of Carcinogenesis." *Bulletin of the History of Dentistry*, 19 (December 1971), 1-11.

(See Chapter 5: Shimkin).

Wilde, J. "Historische Aspekte zum Schneeberger Lungenkrebs." *Zentralblatt arztl Fortbild*, 76 (February 1982), 118-20.

(See Chapter 4: Behounek).

Wold, William S. M., and Maurice Green. "Historic Milestones in Cancer Virology." *Seminars in Oncology*, 6 (December 1979), 461-78.

(See Chapter 4: Rauscher and O'Conner and Chapter 4: Shope).

Wynder, Ernst L. "A Corner of History. Microepidemiology (Evarts A. Graham and David Karnofsky)." *Preventive Medicine*, 2 (November 1973), 465-71.

(See Chapter 4: Wynder).

Wynder, Ernst L. "Some Reflections on Smoking and Lung Cancer." *Journal of Thoracic and Cardiovascular Surgery*, 88 (November 1984), Suppl., 854-57.

Wynder reviews his work at Washington University with Evarts Graham in the late 1940s and their landmark article in the 1950 issue of the *Journal of the American Medical Association* proposing tobacco smoking in the etiology of lung carcinoma. In 1953 they showed that tobacco smoke condensate was carcinogenic to mouse skin. Their work led to the famous 1964 Surgeon General's Report and legislation forcing warning signs on all cigarette packages, as well as subsequent legislation banning cigarette advertising on television.

Zimmerman, Michael R. "An Experimental Study of Mummification Pertinent to the Antiquity of Cancer." *Cancer*, 40 (September 1977), 1358-62.

There are few references in the literature to the antiquity of cancer. It must have been a rare disease, and this is confirmed by experiments on mummified tissue, which yield only rare evidence of carcinoma and sarcoma. The ability to identify soft-tissue tumors in mummified tissue has been achieved by contemporary researchers through the mummification of soft-tissue tumors and the subsequent examination of them pathologically. When those examination techniques are applied to ancient mummies, soft-tissue tumors are still extremely rare, although some have been identified. The natural conclusion is that cancer is a disease of modern, industrial society, with most tumors either environmentally-induced or the by-product of aging and longer lifespans.

5 Epidemiology

Blanc, M., and P. Goldberg. "Cancer des voies respiratoires et travail dans l'extraction et le raffinage du nickel en Nouvelle-Caledonie." *Population*, 40 (January-March 1985), 166-74.

(See Chapter 4: Blanc and Goldberg).

Bock, G. B. "Un contributo alla ricerca epidemiologica sui tumori: Domenico Rigoni-Stern (1810-1855)." *Acta Médica Historica Patav*, 20 (1973-74), 35-55.

(See Chapter 5: Scotto and Bailar).

Boice, John D., Jr., et al. "Multiple Primary Cancers in Connecticut, 1935-1982." *The Yale Journal of Biology and Medicine*, 59 (1986), 533-545.

The National Cancer Institute recently completed a study of multiple primary cancers among the Connecticut population. When compared with the general Connecticut population, cancer patients had a 31 percent increased risk of developing a second cancer and a 23 percent elevated risk of a second cancer at a different site from the first. Common environmental exposures seem responsible for the excess occurrence of many second cancers, especially those related to cigarette smoking, alcohol consumption, or both. Persons with epithelial cancers of the lung, larynx, esophagus, buccal cavity, and pharynx were particularly prone to develop new cancers in those contiguous areas. Cancers of the colon, uterine corpus, breast, and ovary frequently occurred together, suggesting underlying hormonal or dietary influences. Radiotherapy may have caused rectal cancer among patients with gynecological cancers, and chemotherapy with alkylating agents contributed to acute non-lymphocytic leukemia following multiple myeloma or cancers of the breast or ovary. Finally, genetic factors may be present, since victims of retinoblastoma often fall victim to bone cancers.

Borch-Johnsen, K. "Byliv og lungecancer. En kvantitativ og kvalitativ vurdering af den urbane faktor." *Ugeskrift for Laeger*, 144 (June 7, 1982), 1713-18.

(See Chapter 4: Borch-Johnson).

Breckinridge, C. J. "A Statistical Study of Sarcoma Complicating Paget's Disease of Bone in Three Countries." *British Journal of Cancer*, 49 (August 1979), 194-200.

(See Chapter 9: Breckinridge).

Celestino, D., and L. Curi. "Rilievi statistici sulla mortalita per cancro laringeo in Italia dal 1881 al 1962." *Clinica Oto-Rino-Laringoiatrica*, 17 (1965), 329-41.

Between 1881 and 1962 the incidence of laryngeal carcinoma has risen dramatically in Italy, probably because of increased rates of smoking as well as more effective reporting of the disease by Italian cancer registries. At the same time, survival rates have also increased, primarily because of earlier diagnosis, improved surgical techniques, and the use of radiotherapy to destroy occult disease.

Clemmesen, Johannes. "Role of Registries in Cancer Control." *Oncology: Proceedings of the Tenth International Cancer Congress*, V (1970), 335-39.

The first attempt to develop a cancer registry came in London in 1927 when city medical officials attempted a cancer census. The first successful registration of cancer cases was published by Antonio Rigoni-Stern in 1844; he reported on cancer deaths in Verona between 1760 and 1839. The modern era of cancer registration began in Hamburg, Germany, in 1927, Massachusetts and Connecticut in 1927 and 1935 respectively, and New York in 1940. Today twenty-four countries have well-organized, functioning cancer registries and cooperative programs to share the information.

Cutler, S. J., and S. S. Devesa. "Trends in Cancer Incidence and Mortality in the U.S.A." In R. Doll, J. Vudopija, and W. Davis, eds. *Host Environmental Interaction in the Etiology of Cancer in Man.* Lyon, France: 1973. Pp. 15-34.

(See Chapter 5: Greenberg).

Davies, J. N. P. "Cancer Demography. Historical Considerations." *Oncology: Proceedings of the Tenth International Cancer Congress*, V (1970), 275-79.

By 1870 cancer investigators were aware of the following epidemiological data: 1) soot causes squamous cell carcinomas in the scrotum, fingers, and other parts of the body; 2) high rates of abdominal and thigh skin cancers in Kashmir, India, are due to the Kangri pots; 3) high rates of oral cancer occur in India because of betel nut chewing; 4) high rates of penile cancer occur in India, and those rates can be reduced through the protective influence of circumcision; and 5) a high frequency of leg cancers develop in India because of tropical ulcerization of the skin.

Duchene, J., and M. Van Houte-Minet. "Le cancer en Europe." *Espace, population et societie*, 3 (1984), 59-85.

The incidence of cancer is rising in Europe, in accordance with epidemiological patterns worldwide. Lung cancer rates are increasing, especially in women, because of continuing use of tobacco, as well as because of environmental pollution. Oral cancers as well as cancers of the larynx are on the rise because of tobacco use. Cancers of the colon and rectum are also on the rise, particularly in urban areas, perhaps because of increased consumption of red meat, fats, and processed foods, and decreased consumption of grains. The incidence of uterine and cervical cancer is increasing, probably because of early detection through use of the Pap smear. Skin cancers, including melanoma, are also increasing, primarily because of increased exposure to ultraviolet sunlight.

Frigerio, N. A., and J. R. Wutzke. "Malignant Mortality in North and South Dakota, 1950-1967." *South Dakota Journal of Medicine*, 26 (November 1979), 33-37.

Mortality rates for cancer in North Dakota and South Dakota are among the lowest in the United States, except for cancer of the stomach in males and females and cancer of the kidney in females, which are slightly higher than the national average.

Greenberg, E. Robert, Theodore Colton, and Curtis Bayne. "Measurement of Cancer Incidence in the United States: Sources and Uses of Data." *Journal of the National Cancer Institute*, 68 (May 1982), 743-50.

The first large-scale surveys of cancer incidence in the United States began with the establishment of the National Cancer Institute in 1937. The second national survey took place in 1947-1948 and the third in 1969-1971. At the same time, local population-based tumor registries increased dramatically. In 1973 the National Cancer Institute established the SEER program of nine regional tumor registries. Each registry determined the incidence of cancer and the survival rates of cancer patients within its geographical boundaries. The available data is useful to physicians in advising patients about cancer risk, prevention, and public health planning.

Greenberg, Michael R. "A Note on the Changing Geography of Cancer Mortality Within Metropolitan Regions of the United States." *Demography*, 18 (August 1981), 411-20.

In the early 1950s central city counties had substantially higher cancer mortality rates, especially for respiratory and digestive neoplasms, than did suburbs. By early in the 1970s differences between central cities and suburbs had narrowed and sometimes disappeared. Possible explanations for the change are rural underreporting of disease in the 1950s and 1960s; migration of urban inhabitants to the suburbs; and the spread of industrialization and urbanization to the suburbs.

Greenberg, Michael R. "Changing Cancer Mortality Patterns in the Rural United States." *Rural Sociology*, 49 (Spring 1984), 143-53.

Because of urban pollution, improved disease reporting, smoking, alcohol consumption, nutrition similarities, and population migration, there has been a strong trend toward convergence of cancer mortality rates between urban and rural areas from 1950 to 1975.

Greenberg, Michael R. *Urbanization and Cancer Mortality. The United States Experience, 1950-1975.* New York: 1983.

(See Chapter 5: Greenberg).

Haenszel, William, and Mary G. McCrea Curnen. "The First Fifty Years of the Connecticut Tumor Registry: Reminiscences and Prospects." *The Yale Journal of Biology and Medicine*, 59 (1986), 475-84.

In the early 1930s a group of concerned physicians, health professionals, and laymen in New Haven, Connecticut, observed an alarming increase in the incidence of cancer in their city and low survival rates for victims of the disease. Between 1900 and 1934 the cancer mortality in New Haven had jumped from 66 to 180 per 100,000 people, and the average five-year survival rate for cancer patients was only 20 percent. They formed the Cancer Committee of New Haven, lobbied in the state legislature, and succeeded in establishing in 1935 the Connecticut Tumor Registry, which for the past half-century has collected cancer data from around the state.

Harrington, J. S., and N. D. McGlashan. "Migrant Workers and Cancer Patterns in South Africa." *Journal of South African Studies*, 3 (1976), 92-101.

For nearly a century black workers have migrated from rural areas in South Africa to work at the diamond and gold mines, and the records of their medical history provide an excellent data base for epidemiological studies. In the early 1930s Charles Berman first tapped that data base in studying malignant disease patterns in the mine workers. George Oettle followed up Berman's work with studies of his own in the 1950s. During these years, among South African white men, lung cancer accounted for 20 percent of all malignancies, with stomach cancer at 13.5 percent, prostatic cancer at 9 percent, and colon cancer at 5 percent. Among the miners, however, 52.8 percent of malignancies were liver cancers, 12.1 percent were esophageal cancer, 5.4 percent were lung and bronchial cancer, and 4.8 percent were bladder cancer. But liver cancer predominates in Mozambique miners and cancer of the esophagus for miners from the Xhosa homelands, the Transkei, and Ciskei. Mozambique has the highest rate of bladder cancer but lower rates of esophageal and bronchial carcinomas. The Xhosa territories have lower rates of liver and esophageal carcinoma. It appears that each locally recruited group retains a liability to the cancer most common in that group's territory of origin.

Higginson, John. "Cancer Incidence and Migrant Studies. Historical Perspective." *Oncology: Proceedings of the Tenth International Cancer Congress*, V (1970), 300-09.

Migrant studies have been very useful in confirming the role of hereditary and environmental factors in cancer etiology. The first real migrant studies on cancer were done at the Tan Tock Seng Hospital in Singapore between 1907 and 1912, where investigators concentrated on the incidence of nasopharyngeal cancer. In 1944 Ernest Kennaway proved that African liver cancer was not caused genetically when his studies of blacks in the United States indicated a low incidence. Migrant studies have confirmed that most cancers are not hereditary in origin but are environmental and therefore theoretically preventable. They have also shown that the cancerous process may be initiated early in life. Finally, migrant studies have demonstrated the importance of nonviral exogenous agents as predominant causative factors for most human cancers. If vertically transmitted viruses are important, they clearly require a second factor for activation.

Hill, Gerry B. "Counting Cancers." *Canadian Medical Association Journal*, 129 (December 15, 1983), 1262-63.

Statistical summaries of cancer incidence had tentative beginnings in England in the early eighteenth century, but it was not until the mid-twentieth century that systematic attempts were being made in Canada. Hill argues, however, that there is still a need for a complete, unduplicated count for every new case of cancer in Canada. Uniformity is also important so that distinctions can be made between malignant and benign disease, especially for disease of the breast, prostate, and thyroid. He suggests the need for legislation requiring such reporting.

Kaplan, H. S., and P. J. Tsuchitani. *Cancer in China.* New York: 1978.

(See Chapter 5: Shanmugaratnam and Chapter 5: Yeh).

Kasperski, A. "Występowanie raka krtani u chorych na obszarze byłego województwa bydgoskiego w latach 1955-1975 z uwzględnieniem niektórych
czynników epidemiologizcnych." *Otolaryngologia Polska*, 34 (1980), 125-26.

The article provides a statistical study of the incidence of cancer of the larynx
and its positive correlation with smoking.

Kessler, Irving I. "Cervical Cancer Epidemiology in Historical Perspective."
Journal of Reproductive Medicine, 12 (May 1974), 173-85.

Cervical cancer has been a recognized disease for 150 years. Nineteenth century clinicians recognized a number of etiological factors, including viruses, sexual
excess, syphilis, and multiparity. The infrequency of cervical cancer among Jewish
women was long believed to be attributable to their ritual sexual habits. Spouse
circumcision as a protective factor was first suggested to explain differences in disease occurrence between Moslem and Hindi women in the Fiji Islands. A clear-cut
reduction in death rates from cervical cancer has been evident since the 1950s,
with a paradoxical rise in incidence, accounted for by *in situ* cases detected from
cytologic screening. Survival rates increased with the widespread use of cervico-
vaginal smears. Today the herpes virus etiology theory is the most exciting area
of research. Cervical cancer today is viewed as a venereal disease.

Krokowski, E. "25 Jahre Stagnation der Kurativen Krepstherapie—Eine Wende
in Sicht." *Chirurgie*, 50 (January 1979), 39-44.

Although chemotherapy has improved survival rates for such malignancies as
choriocarcinoma, embryonic testicular carcinoma, acute lymphocytic leukemia,
and some of the lymphomas, cure rates for the solid tumors have not improved in
the last quarter of a century. And the modest improvements in cure rates can be
attributed not so much to improved therapeutic modalities but to earlier diagnosis
because of active public health programs in the industrialized societies.

La Vecchia, Carlo, and Adriano Decarli. "Decline of Childhood Cancer Mortality
in Italy, 1955-1980." *Oncology*, 45 (March/April 1988), 93-97.

Between 1955 and 1980 childhood cancer mortality in Italy dropped substantially: 35 percent for leukemia, 90 percent for Hodgkin's disease, 30 percent for
non-Hodgkin's lymphoma, 40 percent for bone sarcomas, 30 percent for Wilms'
tumors, and 65 percent for retinoblastoma. The primary reason for the change in
survival rates is early diagnosis, new, more effective radiotherapeutic techniques,
and the development of new chemotherapeutic regimens.

Levi, Fabio, and Carlo La Vecchia. "Childhood Cancer in Switzerland: Mortality
from 1951 to 1984." *Oncology*, 45 (July/August 1988), 313-17.

Between 1951 and 1984 childhood cancer mortality in Switzerland dropped dramatically, primarily because of advances in chemotherapy and the aggressive use of megavoltage radiotherapy. Certified mortality fell 60 percent for leukemias, 21 percent for lymphomas, 66 percent for Wilms' tumors, 40 percent for bone sarcomas, and 30 percent for other tumors. The overall childhood cancer mortality rate declined by 45 percent.

Lips, C. J. M., et al. "Central Registration of Multiple Endocrine Neoplasia Type 2 Families in The Netherlands." *Henry Ford Hospital Medical Journal,* 32 (1984), 236-37.

Since 1981 the Dutch have been conducting, through the Danish Tumor Registry, a long-range study on inherited tendencies to develop Multiple Endocrine Neoplasias of the Type 2 variety. They predict that eventually they will identify 500 to 700 high-risk individuals and offer those people cyclical diagnostic examinations to catch the disease at an early stage.

Madai, L. "Le premier enregistrement statistique des malades cancereux dan l'anee 1904, en Hongrie." *Genus,* 37 (1981), 227-40.

The article describes the beginning of systematic collection and creation of a cancer data base in Hungary in 1904 and the realization that although mortality rates from infectious diseases were declining, both the incidence and the death rates for cancer were increasing.

Mason, T. J. Ed. *Atlas of Cancer Mortality for U. S. Counties: 1950-1969.* Bethesda, Maryland: 1975.

The author has provided maps and tables for each county in the United States, demonstrating changes in cancer mortality between 1950 and 1969. (See Chapter 5: Greenberg).

Merabishvili, V. M. "Statistika zlokachestvennykh novoobrazovanii i organizatsiia protivorakovoi bor'by v SSSR v pervye desiatiletiia sovetskoi vlasti." *Voprosy Onkologii,* 32 (1986), 89-94.

The development of a sophisticated and complete cancer registry throughout the Soviet Union had to wait until after World War II. Until then the disruptions of World War I, the Bolshevik Revolution and civil war, and World War II prevented the systematic collection of cancer data. Since World War II it has become clear that epidemiological studies indicate that the incidence of cancer is increasing in the Soviet Union in similar patterns to other areas in the industrialized world.

Mercer, Alexander. "Risk of Dying from Tuberculosis or Cancer: Further Aspects of a Possible Association." *International Journal of Epidemiology*, 10 (December 1981), 377-80.

Early in the 1900s scientists began to notice that the decrease in the death rate from tuberculosis appeared to be offset by an equivalent increase in the death rate from cancer. At first some people suggested a direct causal link between tubercle bacillus and the development of cancer, but later a general hypothesis emerged arguing that improved natural immunity and resistance to tuberculosis has been a precondition for the increase in age specific death rates from cancer, so that this only occurs after death rates from tuberculosis have started to decline. C. B. Goodhart in 1959 speculated that there might be a genetic predisposition, such that as people became increasingly able to survive contact with the tuberculosis, a common genetic proneness to cancer and tuberculosis would mean that they became susceptible to cancer later in life.

Mesle, France. "Cancer et alimentation: Le cas des cancers de l'intestin et du rectum." *Population*, 38 (Juillet-Octobre 1983), 733-62.

(See Chapter 4: Mesle).

Miller, Robert W. "Cancer Epidemics in the People's Republic of China." *Journal of the National Cancer Institute*, 60 (1978), 1195-98.

(See Chapter 5: Shanmugaratnam and Chapter 5: Yeh).

Miller, Robert W. and Frank W. McKay. "Decline in US Childhood Cancer Mortality, 1950 to 1980." *Journal of the American Medical Association*, 251 (March 23, 1984), 1567-70.

There have been dramatic changes in cancer mortality among children since 1950, especially between 1965 and 1979. The number of deaths of persons under fifteen, as compared with the number expected at 1950 rates, fell 50 percent for leukemia, 32 percent for non-Hodgkin's lymphoma, 80 percent for Hodgkin's disease, 50 percent for bone sarcoma, 68 percent for kidney cancer, and 31 percent for all other cancers. There were 15,411 fewer deaths from childhood cancer from 1965 through 1979 than expected at 1950 rates. The major reason for the decline is improved therapies.

Moertel, C. G. "Multiple Primary Malignant Neoplasms: Historical Perspectives." *Cancer*, 40 (October 1977), 1786-92.

(See Chapter 5: Schoenberg).

Mustacchi, P. "Ramazzini and Rigoni-Stern on Parity and Breast Cancer." *Archives of Internal Medicine*, 108 (1961), 639-42.

(See Chapter 5: Scotto and Bailar).

Newitt, Guy R. "Epidemiology of Cancer. Historical Highlights." In Vincent T. DeVita, Jr., Samuel Hellman, and Steven A. Rosenberg. *Cancer. Principles & Practice of Oncology.* 1985. Pp. 152-53.

Hippocrates (460-370 B.C.) first described cancer by the terms "carcinos" and "carcinoma." Hippocrates and later Galen both agreed that cancer was caused by an excess of "black bile" and should be left untreated. In England local governments began recording vital statistics consistently in the sixteenth century, but they were not used statistically until 1772, with John Graunt's study. Graunt found a higher rate of male than female births, a high rate of infant and child mortality, and a higher rate of urban over rural deaths. In the nineteenth century Fanchou collected cancer statistics for Paris between 1830 and 1840, and Rigoni-Stern did the same for Verona, Italy, for the years between 1760 and 1839. In 1915 the Prudential Life Insurance Company published a monumental study of world cancer statistics. Michael Greenwood, a British epidemiologist, in 1926 analyzed the data from untreated cancer patients and developed the concept of the five-year survival rate.

Olakowski, T., H. Rudzinska, and H. Gadomska. "Epidemiologia raka płuca w Polsce do roku 1977." *Pneumonologia Polska*, 47 (August-September 1979), 553-64.

The article discusses the epidemiology of lung cancer in Poland up to 1977 and correlates its occurrence with smoking.

Oiso, Toshio. "Incidence of Stomach Cancer and Its Relation to Dietary Habits and Nutrition in Japan between 1900 and 1975." *Cancer Research*, 35 (November 1975), 3254-58.

(See Chapter 4: Oiso).

Panzer, D., and G. P. Wildner. "Zur Geschichte der Krebsstatistik in Deutschland bis 1949." *Zeitschrift fur Arztliche Fortbildung*, 79 (1985), 41-44.

In 1949 East Germany established a nationwide cancer registry to collect enough data to determine morbidity and mortality statistics for the entire country. Since 1949 the system has gradually become more complete and more sophisticated, indicating that at least some of the increased incidence of cancer is due to more accurate reporting of disease.

Pejovic, M. H., and M. Thuaire. "Etiologie des cancers du col de l'uterus. Le point sur 150 ans de recherche." *Journal de gynecologie, obstetrice, biologie, et reproduction*, 15 (1986), 37-43.

In the nineteenth and early twentieth centuries physicians frequently connected cervical cancer with sexual habits, since nuns and Jewish women had such low rates, and they also attributed the disease to multiparity and the trauma of childbirth to the uterus and cervix. But in 1931 Smith noted a higher incidence of cervical cancer in poor women. Late in the 1940s epidemiological research demonstrated that socioeconomic status was relevant and that single women had lower rates of the disease than married and widowed women. In 1962 Rotkin showed that low socioeconomic status and early first coitus were closely connected to cervical cancer. Contemporary data clearly implicates a sexual factor in the etiology of cervical carcinoma.

Peron, Y. "La mortalité adulte par cancer in Amerique du Nord." *Espace, population et societie*, 3 (1984), 33-45.

(See Chapter 5: Greenberg).

Petrakis, Nicholas L. "Historic Milestones in Cancer Epidemiology." *Seminars in Oncology*, 6 (December 1979), 433-44.

Epidemiological research rests on the assumption that cancer is not randomly distributed in the human population and seeks to determine the agent, host, and environmental factors explaining that distribution. Although an epidemiological approach has been employed for centuries, it did not become important for cancer research until the early 1900s when mortality rates for infectious diseases declined and those for cancer increased. The early knowledge of human carcinogens came from clinical observations of workers exposed to occupational substances associated with unusually high rates of cancer. In 1775 Percivall Pott noted the connection between chimney soot and scrotal cancer in chimney sweeps. Volkman reported several cases of scrotal cancer in 1894 among paraffin and tar workers. These malignancies were squamous cell carcinomas.

Although the modern period of epidemiological study of lung cancer is commonly considered to begin in the 1950s, there were many earlier reports. In 1937 Roffo claimed a connection between smoking and lung cancer, and Müller confirmed that notion with his own study in 1939. The classic epidemiology study was that of Wynder and Graham in the 1950s which positively correlated smoking in hundreds of individuals with lung cancer. In 1965 Selikoff reported high rates of mesothelioma in asbestos workers. That tumor almost never occurs in the general population.

In 1713 Ramazzini noticed that nuns had unusually high rates of breast cancer. Stevenson observed in 1913 that breast cancer rates were markedly higher after the age of 45 in single women than among married women. Lane-Claypon's important study in 1926 demonstrated a positive correlation of breast cancer among women who had never had children or who had borne their first child at a later age.

As for cervical cancer, researchers over the years noted a higher incidence of the disease among women with multiple sexual partners and among women who had experienced intercourse at an early age. Single women have much lower rates of cervical cancer than married women, and cervical cancer is an almost unknown disease among nuns. Epidemiological studies have clearly shown a sexual etiology for the disease.

Schmautz, R., and M. Holm-Hadulla. "Cancer Mortality in Württemberg, 1910 and 1970." *Zentralblatt fur Krebsforschung*, 87 (24 September 1976), 101-13.

During the twentieth century the cancer mortality rate has increased dramatically, consistent with similar declines in mortality rates from infectious diseases. Environmental pollution, consumption of chemicals, longer lifespans, and much improved reporting systems account for the increase in the cancer mortality during the sixty years between 1910 and 1970.

Schoenberg, Bruce S. "Multiple Malignant Primary Neoplasms." *Recent Results in Cancer Research*, 58 (1977), 1-173.

Epidemiologists today know that individuals suffering from cancer have approximately a 30 percent higher chance of acquiring a second primary neoplasm than the population at large has of falling victim to a first primary malignancy. Although there is evidence of a genetic predisposition to some tumors, the vast majority of the subsequent neoplasms are environmental in their origins, usually traceable to the same carcinogen as the first tumor. Heavy smokers with oral cavity cancer, for example, are still vulnerable to lung cancer. Individuals with a history of basal cell carcinoma from excess exposure to ultraviolet light are more vulnerable than the general population to melanomas.

Schoenberg, Bruce S. "Multiple Primary Malignant Neoplasms: The Connecticut Experience, 1935-1964." *Recent Results in Cancer Research*, 58 (1977), 1-23.

(See Chapter 5: Boice).

Scotto, Joseph and John C. Bailar. "Rigoni-Stern and Medical Statistics. A Nineteenth Century Approach to Cancer Research." *Journal of the History of Medicine and Allied Sciences*, 24 (January 1969), 65-75.

Domenico Antonio Rigoni-Stern (b. 1810) was a professor of clinical medicine at the University of Padua. He collected medical statistics about cancer and in 1842 reached several important conclusions about cancer: cancer incidence increases with age, especially for uterine cancer; the frequency of breast cancer is inversely related to the incidence of uterine cancer for different age groups; the incidence of breast cancer increases with age, especially ten to fifteen years after the usual time of menopause; unmarried women have higher rates of breast cancer; married women get more uterine cancer; cancer incidence is higher in the cities than in rural areas; hardship and anxiety increase the incidence of breast and stomach cancer; and skin cancer occurs at the same rates for men and women. Most of his findings still hold true today.

Seeger, P. G. *Krebs—Problem Ohne Ausweg? Tribut an die Zivilisation?* Heidelberg: 1974.

Cancer mortality rates continue to climb in modern societies for a variety of reasons, all of which indicate the characteristics of what contemporary historians call civilization. First, lifespans in industrial societies have improved dramatically in the twentieth century, primarily because of successful elimination of high death rates from infectious diseases, leaving increased death rates from chronic illnesses. The longer people live, the more likely they are of contracting cancer. Second, industrial pollution in urban areas has greatly increased cancer rates. Finally, dietary changes—increased consumption of animal fats and reduction in the intake of vegetables and bulk grains—have increased gastrointestinal cancer rates.

Shanmugaratnam, K. "Patterns of Cancer Occurrence in the Far East." *Oncology: Proceedings of the Tenth International Cancer Congress,* V (1970), 282-91.

The incidence and mortality rates of cancer are far lower in the Far East than in the United States, but the differences are probably due to underreporting. Still, there are distinctive differences in cancer occurrence between the two regions. The differences are as follows:

1. Cancer of the oral cavity is high among Indians and Thais, probably because of chewing betel-quid containing tobacco and other additives.

2. Nasopharyngeal carcinoma, a rare cancer in most of the world, has a very high incidence in Southern China and Southeast Asia, probably because of some environmental factor or biological entity.

3. Cancer of the esophagus occurs at very high rates in most countries of the Far East, as does cancer of the stomach in Japan.

4. Liver cancer occurs at very high rates in Southeast Asia, Southern China, and Japan. Most of the liver neoplasms are hepatocellular carcinomas caused by liver fluke infestation.

5. Lung cancer rates are lower in the Far East than in the United States and Europe.

6. Cervical cancer is by far the most common neoplasm in females throughout the Far East, and malignant trophoblastic disease is more common there than in Europe and the United States.

7. Tumors of the colon, rectum, breast, prostate and skin occur less frequently in the Far East than in the West.

Shimkin, Michael B. "Some Historical Landmarks in Cancer Epidemiology." In David Schottenfeld. *Cancer Epidemiology and Prevention.* 1975. Pp. 60-75.

In 1713 Bernardino Ramazzini of Padua, Italy, launched the era of epidemiology when he noted that breast cancer occurred more frequently among Roman Catholic nuns than in the female population at large. Domenico Rigoni-Stern confirmed those observations in 1844. In 1775 Percivall Pott observed high rates of cancer of the scrotum in chimney sweeps; Pott knew that coal soot was the carcinogenic agent. Yamagiwa and Ichikawa in 1915 reported the carcinogenic nature of coal tar on rabbit skin, and in 1930 Kennaway isolated benzpyrene as a carcinogenic polycyclic hydrocarbon. In 1879 F. H. Härting reported high rates of bronchogenic carcinoma among miners in the Black Forest of Germany. Ludwig Rehn, a German physician, reported in 1895 the occurrence of bladder cancer among workers in the aniline dye industry. The first socioeconomic study on the etiology of cancer came in 1912 when Wilhelm Weinberg of Stuttgart reported higher rates of uterine cancer among poor women. Cancer of the nose in snuff users was reported by John Hill in 1761, and the association of lung cancer and cigarette smoking was suspected clinically by 1940 but not demonstrated in controlled studies until 1950. By 1964 the evidence for carcinogenic association had become overwhelming. In the 1940s researchers established higher rates of uterine cancer among women with lower economic status, early first coitus, and multiple sex partners. In 1865 Charles Thiersch established the connection between skin carcinomas and exposure to sunlight.

Steinfeld, Jesse L. "Smoking and Lung Cancer. A Milestone in Awareness." *Journal of the American Medical Association*, 253 (May 24-31, 1985), 2995-97.

(See Chapter 4: Steinfeld).

Supady, J. "Ankieta statystyczna z 1931 r. na temat występowania nowotworów
złośliwych w populacji II rzeczpospolitej." *Wiadomosci Lekarskie*, 34 (February 15, 1981), 351-55.

The article provides a statistical survey of the incidence of malignant tumors
in Poland since 1931, focusing on the general increase in tumors of the breast,
lung, colon, and rectum.

Supady, J. "Pierwsze Polskie statystyki sekcyjne na temat występowania nowotworów." *Wiadomosci Lekarskie*, 32 (September 1, 1979), 1263-67.

Late in the nineteenth century the Polish government and Polish medical societies began attempting the systematic collection of statistical data on the appearance of malignant neoplasms.

Thouez, J. P., and D. Godon. "La géographie du travail et la sante: Le cas de
la mortalité par cancers selon les secteurs d'activite et les bassins d'emplois
au Québec." *Espace, Population et Societie*, 3 (1984), 47-58.

During the twentieth century industrial development in the province of Québec
had led to cancer mortality rates similar to those in other industrial areas of the
world, with pronounced rates of mesothelioma among asbestos workers, bronchial
and lung cancers among miners and metal workers, and bladder cancers among
dye workers.

Wagner, G. "Cancer Registration: Historical Aspects." *IARC Science Publications*, (1986), 3-12.

(See Chapter 5: Clemmesen).

Walsh, Brendan M. "Health Education and the Demand for Tobacco in Ireland,
1953-1976: A Note." *Economic and Social Review*, 11 (January 1980), 147-51.

In 1962 the Royal College of Physicians published its report linking tobacco
smoking with lung cancer. In Ireland the cancer scare received widespread press
coverage. Television advertising of cigarettes was phased out by 1971, a warning
was placed on all cigarette packages, and several publicly financed antismoking
campaigns were launched. In the last twenty-three years there has been a modest
decline in tobacco smoking, but it is due more to rising tobacco prices than the
antismoking campaigns.

Wynder, Ernst L. "Some Reflections on Smoking and Lung Cancer." *Journal of
Thoracic and Cardiovascular Surgery*, 88 (November 1984), Suppl., 854-57.

(See Chapter 4: Wynder).

Yeh, Samuel D. J. "Experimental and Clinical Oncology in the People's Republic of China." *American Journal of Chinese Medicine*, 1 (1973), 193-94.

(See Chapter 5: Yeh).

Yeh, Samuel D. J. "Nuclear Medicine and Cancer Research in the People's Republic of China." *American Journal of Chinese Medicine*, 7 (1979), 149-55.

Most imaging equipment and radionuclides are made in China and a number of excellent textbooks on nuclear medicine and radiotherapy are available in Chinese. Precautions on radiation safety are heavily stressed. Chinese medicinal plants are always added in order to improve the therapeutic effects of classical chemotherapeutic agents or to lessen their side effects. High rates of nasopharyngeal cancer are probably caused by the Epstein-Barr virus; high rates of lung cancer by cigarette smoking and atmospheric pollution; high rates of liver hepatomas because of exposure to aflatoxins; and high rates of esophageal carcinoma because of low intakes of vitamins A and C as well as high levels of nitrates and nitrosomines in preserved food.

6 Pathology

Ackerman, Lauren V. "Tumor Pathologists I Have Known." *American Journal of Clinical Pathology*, 77 (April 1982), 385-90.

In this H. P. Smith Award Lecture, the author reviews his personal association with Charles Oberling (the pioneer in electronmicroscopy and in the ultrastructure of tumor cells and tumor viruses); Rupert Willis (human and animal tumor pathologist), and Cuthbert Dukes (pioneer in the pathology of intestinal tumors).

Agamova, K. A. "Razvitie tsitologicheskoi diagnostiki opukholi cheloveka." *Sovetskoi Medicine*, 6 (1982), 65-69.

The article reviews the early history of pathology, particularly the pioneering work of Rudolf Virchow and the birth of cellular pathology, as well as a review of the post-World War II rise of exfoliative cytology.

Anderson, C. Th. "Robert Remak and the Multinucleated Cell: Eliminating a Barrier to the Acceptance of Cell Division." *The Bulletin of the History of Medicine*, 60 (1986), 523-43.

(See Chapter 22: Aterman).

Aterman, Kurt, Wolfgang Remmele, and Muriel Smith. "Karl Touton and His 'Xanthelasmatic Giant Cell'," *The American Journal of Dermatopathology*, 10 (Summer 1988), 257-69.

In 1838 Johannes Müller offered the first description of multinucleated giant cells. Five years later Jules Vogel noticed similar cells in a fungating tumor of the uterus. In the 1850s Robert Remak and Rudolf Virchow began theorizing on cell division and Virchow offered his theory that all cells came from other cells. In

1868 Langhans described the presence of multinucleated giant cells in tubercular lesions and the tendency of the nuclei to be located on the periphery of the cell. In 1885 Karl Touton, a German physician, first described the "xanthelasmatic giant cell" that now bears his name. Touton noted that the cells were characterized by a sharply defined membrane, a finely granular or threadlike content, a large, rounded or oval nucleus, and dense arrangements of lipid drops. Today we suspect that Touton cells develop when the stimulus to cell fusion is accompanied also by a factor stimulating lipid uptake.

Bode, U. K. *Fruhe Histologische Krebsforschung in Deutschland, Frankreich und Oesterreich.* Köln: 1979.

(See Chapter 6: Fisher and Hermann).

Bracegirdle, Brian. "J. J. Lister and the Establishment of Histology." *Medical History,* 21 (1977), 187-91.

There were three main problems with the late eighteenth and early nineteenth century microscopes: chromatic and spherical aberrations, and coma. Joseph Jackson Lister, a wine merchant in England, solved the problem of the spherical aberrations. A lens brings axial rays to a different focus from marginal ones and causes poor image quality especially when it is associated with coma, where what should be a small circle in the image occurs as a smear of light resembling a comet. Lister was intrigued with microscopes and discovered that an achromatic lens has two aplanatic foci. If a second lens is arranged at the aplanatic focus of the first, higher magnifications are obtained without chromatic or spherical defects, and with the coma eliminated. A rigid stand was necessary to minimize vibrations and lens displacement. In 1826 Lister had such a microscope designed. Widespread manufacture of his microscope was underway by the 1840s, and German pathologists used it to study normal and pathological tissues. J. J. Lister's microscope was the technological breakthrough which paved the way for the development of histology.

Carmichael, Erskine. "Dr. Papanicolau and the Pap Smear." *The Alabama Journal of Medical Science,* 21 (January 1984), 101-04.

(See Chapter 2: PAPANICOLAU, GEORGES: Carmichael).

Candiani, G. B. "The Classification of Endometriosis: Historical Review and Present Status of the Art." *Acta European Fertility,* 17 (March-April 1986), 85-92.

The type of hyperplastic change in the endometrium, today called adenomatous hyperplasia, was first described by Thomas S. Cullen, a physician at Johns Hopkins University Medical School, in 1900. Ten years later I. C. Rubin of New York provided an excellent description of the cellular changes in the endometrium which lead to uterine cancer. By the 1930s and 1940s the work of people like S. R. Gusberg, A. T. Hertig, and S. C. Sommers had all confirmed the premalignant stage of endometrial carcinoma and the use of hysterectomy as a treatment to prevent development of the disease.

Identification of carcinoma *in situ* of the cervix also came from I. C. Rubin, even though a number of his contemporaries in Europe denied the possibility of identifying the beginning stages of cervical carcinoma. Working in Vienna early in the 1900s, Rubin established *in situ* carcinoma as a distinct pathological entity. In the 1920s Georges Papanicolaou and Aurel Babes independently developed early diagnosis of cervical carcinoma through cytological examination of vaginal smears.

Churchill, Frederick B. "Rudolf Virchow and the Pathologist's Criteria for the Inheritance of Acquired Characteristics." *The Journal of the History of Medicine and Allied Sciences*, 31 (April 1976), 117-48.

(See Chapter 6: Fisher and Hermann and Chapter 6: Krumblaar).

"Cuthbert Esquire Dukes (1890-1977)." *European Journal of Surgical Oncology*, 13 (February 1987), 77.

Cuthbert Dukes, the prominent British pathologist, pioneered the modern staging of rectal carcinomas. In 1930 Dukes divided the lesions into Stage A where the growth is confined to the rectal wall; Stage B where the growth has spread by direct continuity to the extra-rectal tissues; and Stage C, where there are lymph node metastases. In 1935 Dukes revised the system by dividing Stage C into Stage C1, where the involved nodes are confined to the near proximity of the tumor, and Stage C2, where there is a continuous chain of nodes containing tumor deposits up to the main ligature on the superior hemorrhoidal or inferior mesenteric vessels.

Dehner, Louis P. "Classic Neuroblastoma: Histopathologic Grading as a Prognostic Indicator. The Shimada System and Its Progenitors." *The American Journal of Pediatric Hematology/Oncology*, 10 (1988), 143-54.

(See Chapter 10: Dehner).

Douglass, L. E. "A Further Comment on the Contributions of Aurel Babes to Cytology and Pathology." *Acta Cytologica*, 11 (1967), 217-24.

(See Chapter 13: Douglass).

Fels, E. "Remarks on a Commentary on the Discovery of the Histogenesis of the Chorionepithelioma." *American Journal of Obstetrics and Gynecology*, 131 (July 15, 1978), 704-05.

(See Chapter 13: Ober and Fess).

Fisher, Edwin R., and Cecelia M. Hermann. "Historic Milestones in Cancer Pathology." *Seminars in Oncology*, 6 (1979), 428-32.

The Greek physician Hippocrates first identified a series of disorders characterized by noninflammatory, hard swellings and ulcers with a tendency to become generalized and fatal, and called it "karkinos," or cancer in Latin. The Roman physician Galen believed cancer was one of the four basic humors, or fluids, of the body, and that view prevailed for almost two millenia. Despite the development of the microscope beginning in the late sixteenth century, there was little progress in a conceptual understanding of cancer until the end of the eighteenth century. Real understanding of the cellular nature of cancer did not come until the nineteenth century improvements in the optical microscope. In 1825 Raspail first developed the technique of frozen sections for slide analysis of malignant tissue, and in 1871 Rutherford gave birth to the field of surgical pathology by developing the quick diagnosis of frozen sections. Cytologic techniques for cancer diagnosis were first suggested by Walshe in 1844, but it was not until the work of Georges Papanicolaou in the 1920s and 1930s that the field of exfoliative cytology greatly improved cancer diagnosis. Johannes Müller and his student Rudolf Virchow provided the first confirmed research on the cellular nature of malignant tissue in the 1830s. Thiersch and Waldeyer later demonstrated the epithelial nature of carcinomas and the embolic nature of metastases. In 1897 Hansemann proposed that the clinical behavior of neoplasms might be related to their degree of differentiation. In 1920 Broder published an article on the histologic grading of squamous cell carcinoma and its prognostic implications. Dukes provided a similar process for rectal carcinomas in 1932.

Gold, Michael. *A Conspiracy of Cells: One Woman's Immortal Legacy and the Medical Scandal It Caused*. Albany: 1986.

In 1950 researchers at Johns Hopkins University took cervical cells from Henrietta Lacks, who died of cervical carcinoma a year later. The scientists succeeded in getting her cancer cells to grow successfully *in vitro*. Scientists around the world requested samples of the cells, which were then widely distributed for research. Almost immediately, the "HeLa" cell cultures contaminated other tissue cultures. In 1968 researchers determined that twenty-four of the thirty-four cell lines at the American Type Culture Collection were contaminated by HeLa cells. Walter Nelson-Rees, head of the Cell Culture Laboratory at the University of California at Berkeley, discovered in 1973 that some Russian tissue cultures were also contaminated, and he spent the next eight years working to discover other contaminated cell cultures and the impact of the contamination on research results.

Hertig, Arthur T. "Early Concepts of Dysplasia and Carcinoma *In Situ* (A Backward Glance at a Forward Process)." *Obstetrical and Gynecological Survey*, 34 (November 1979), 795-803.

The relationship between carcinoma *in situ* of the cervix and a full-blown invasive carcinoma was first hinted at in 1886 by Williams in England, and other pathologists like Cullen (1900), Rubin (1910), and Novak (1929) were aware of the disturbing changes which could occur in the cellular structure of the cervix. Still, pathologists did not recognize the preinvasive stages of cervical cancer as a biologic entity until the 1930s. In 1933 Schiller introduced the iodine test for non-glycogenated squamous epithelium. During the 1930s at the Free Hospital for Women in Boston, Frank A. Pemberton, George V. Smith, and Paul A. Younge clarified the relationship between carcinoma *in situ* and invasive carcinoma. Younge coined the term "carcinoma *in situ*."

Hunter, John A. A. and Karl Holubar, eds. "In Praise of Alexander Breslow." *American Journal of Dermatopathology*, 6 (Summer 1984), Suppl. 1, 151-57.

(See Chapter 18: Hunter and Holubar).

Hutter, Robert V. P. "Lobular Carcinoma *in Situ*." *CA-A Cancer Journal for Clinicians* , 32 (July-August 1982), 232-33.

(See Chapter 11: Hutter).

Jewett, Hugh J. "Historical Development of the Staging of Bladder Tumors: Personal Reminiscences." *Urological Survey*, 27 (April 1977), 37-40.

(See Chapter 20: Jewett).

Koprowska, I. "Concurrent Discoveries of the Value of Vaginal Smears for Diagnosis of Uterine Cancer." *Diagnostic Cytopathololgy*, 1 (July-September 1985), 245-48.

In 1928 Aurel A. Babes of the University of Bucharest in Romania and Georges Papanicolaou of the Cornell Medical College in the United States simultaneously announced the relationship between cytological abnormalities in vaginal smears and the likelihood of cervical and uterine carcinoma. See Chapter 13: Douglass and Chapter 3: PAPANICOLAOU, GEORGES: Carmichael.

Kramer, W. "On the Classification of Tumours of the Peripheral Nervous System." *Psychiatria, Neurologia, Neurochirurgia*, 72 (1969), 65-75.

(See Chapter 10: Kramer).

Krumblaar, E. B. "The Centenary of the Cell Doctrine." *Annals of the History of Medicine*, 1 (1939), 427-37.

In 1839 Theodor A. Schwann, a German physiologist and student of Johannes Müller, founded modern histology when he wrote "Mikroskopische Untersuchungen." The year before, Matthias J. Schleiden, the German botanist, had proposed the cellular theory for all plant tissues, and Schwann then argued that all animal tissues, including embyros, were also composed of cells. In 1840 Müller then applied that understanding to cancer in his book *On the Nature and Structural Characteristics of Cancer.*

Maulitz, Russell C. "Schwann's Way: Cells and Crystals." *Journal of the History of Medicine and Allied Sciences*, 26 (October 1971), 422-37.

(See Chapter 22: Krumblaar).

Melicow, M. M. "Carcinoma *in Situ*: An Historical Perspective." *Urology Clinic of North America*, 3 (February 1976), 5-11.

(See Chapter 13: Douglass).

Mildner, T. "Versuche zur Krebs-Diagnostik und Therapie vor 200 Jahren." *Deutsch Medizinische Journal*, 17 (5 March 1966), 141-44.

(See Chapter 6: Fisher and Hermann).

Naylor, B. "The History of Exfoliate Cancer Cytology." *Medical Bulletin*, 26 (1960), 289-96.

(See Chapter 13: Douglass and Chapter 2: PAPANICOLAOU, GEORGES: Carmichael).

Rather, L. J. "Who Discovered the Pathognomonic Giant Cell of Hodgkin's Disease?" *Bulletin of the New York Academy of Medicine*, 48 (August 1972), 943-50.

What actually happened in regard to the discovery of the pathognomonic cell of Hodgkin's disease was that many investigators, beginning in the 1860s, recognized and described one or more varieties of large cells in patients with a disease characterized especially by enlargement of the lymph nodes and spleen in the absence of a leukemic blood picture, a disease usually referred back to Hodgkin's report in 1832. Virchow in Germany and Cornil and Ranvier in France described a large cell with only a few nuclei and another, the true giant cell of Virchow, containing ten or twenty or more nuclei. In Great Britain Murchison and Tuckwell described the smaller of the two kinds of cells in 1870, and in the same year Bristowe and Pick gave an excellent description of that cell in tissues from Tuckwell's patient, calling attention to the prominent nucleoli probably for the first time. Two years later Langhans noted both kinds of cells and distinguished the larger, the so-called true giant cell, from another highly multinucleated cell seen in tubercles (now called Langhan's cell). The presence of peculiar large cells in the involved tissue was by now common knowledge.

Later in the 1870s the reports of Greenfield, Coupland, and Turner appeared. In 1892 Goldmann, using Ehrlich's staining procedures, described the nucleolar acidophilia of the smaller "giant" cells (whose presence he took for granted). Good descriptions of the smaller cell were also given by de la Hausse in 1890 and Glockner in 1895. In 1898 Sternberg, using the new staining procedures, gave his outstanding description of the cell now regarded as pathognomonic of Hodgkin's disease. In 1902 came Dorothy Reed's equally good description and superior illustrations of that cell. The elevation of the Sternberg-Reed cell to its present status of *sina qua non* took place only a few decades ago.

Russell, K. "Tissue Culture—A Brief Historical Review." *Clio Medica*, 4 (1969), 109-19.

The art of growing tissue *in vitro* has been practiced for many years but perfected only recently. Ross Granville Harrison (1870-1959) of Yale University in 1907 succeeded in growing tadpole nerve cells on a microscope slide. It was the beginning of tissue culture research. The development of antibiotics in the late 1930s and 1940s greatly reduced the problem of contaminated tissue cultures, and the use of new culture media composed of proteins, salts, vitamins, and hormones also advanced the work. The impact of tissue cultures on cancer research was enormous. In 1930 Fischer was the first to obtain cell lines of malignant cells: the Rous chicken sarcoma and the Ehrlich carcinoma which he kept for 12 years. In 1954 Leighton showed that if sarcoma or carcinoma cells are grown in close association with normal fibroblasts, the tumor cells invade and destroy the normal cells. In the 1950s Woods and Eagle demonstrated the different metabolic levels between normal and malignant cells. The tissue culture has also been used to evaluate selective chemotherapeutic drugs.

Rywlin, Arkadi M. "Non-Hodgkin's Malignant Lymphomas. Brief Historical Review and Simple Unifying Classification." *The American Journal of Dermatopathology*, 2 (Spring 1980), 17-24.

(See Chapter 17: Rywlin).

Schlumberger, Hans G. "Origins of the Cell Concept in Pathology." *Archives of Pathology*, 37 (1944), 396-407.

The origins of the cell concept in pathology go back to the development of the first reliable microscopes in the late eighteenth and early nineteenth centuries. In 1838 Matthias Schleiden, a German botanist, first published his studies on the cellular composition of plant tissue. That same year Johannes Müller of the University of Berlin noted the dramatic differences between the cellular structures of normal and malignant tissues. A year later Theodor Schwann, a student of Müller, proposed the theory that all living tissue was composed of cells which divide and replace themselves.

Stetson, Chandler A. "Pathology." In John Z. Bowers and Elizabeth F. Purcell, eds. *Advances in American Medicine: Essays at the Bicentennial.* New York: 1976. Volume 2. Pp. 536-51.

Pathology began as a discipline when Giovanni Morgagni in 1761 argued that manifestations of disease can frequently be explained in terms of pathological changes in organs or tissues. With the advent of the microscope in the 1830s, people like G.S. Schleiden, F. T. Schwann, and Johannes Müller explained the cellular composition of plant and animal tissue. In 1858 Rudolf Virchow published his *Cellularpathologie* and took pathology well beyond morbid anatomy to its modern existence as a discipline of cellular structures. By the end of the nineteenth century Robert Koch had published his influential paper on anthrax; Louis Pasteur was explaining the significance of his studies on beer and micro-organisms; Joseph Lister was perfecting his notions on antisepsis; and Julius Cohnheim had performed his studies on the pathophysiology of inflammation. In oncology the leading pathologists in the early twentieth century were Peyton Rous, James Ewing, and Aldred Warthin. In the 1920s and 1930s, Aurel Babes in Romania and Georges Papanicolaou in the United States developed the vaginal cytology techniques for early diagnosis of carcinoma *in situ.* The revolution in experimental biology and the birth of molecular biology came after World War II when people like Oswald T. Avery at the Rockefeller Institute, Albert Claude at the Jules Bordet Institute, and James Watson and F. H. Crick at Cambridge unraveled human genes and the DNA molecule. All these trends had a dramatic effect on oncology, leading to a new research focus. Around the world researchers by the 1960s and 1970s became convinced that the riddle of cancer would be solved only when the riddles of molecular biology at the cell level were solved.

von Haam, Emmerich. "The Historical Background of Oral Cytology." *Acta Cytologica*, 9 (1965), 270-72.

The first attempt at the cytologic diagnosis of pharyngeal cancer by oral smears was made in 1860 by L. S. Beale. In 1949 L. F. Morrison made the first modern application of oral cytology to diagnose nasopharyngeal lesions. During the late 1950s and 1960s researchers like R. A. Cawson, E. S. Hopp, S. Silverman, and W. O. Umiker developed the criteria for determining malignancy from oral smears: 1) large nucleus with an increased nuclear/cytoplasmic ratio; 2) hyperchromatic nucleus; 3) irregular size and shape of nucleus; 4) increase in the amount of coarsely granular cytoplasm; 5) dense and prominent nuclear membrane; 6) multinucleation; 7) multiple and/or large nucleoli; 8) cytoplasmic vacuoles; 9) phagocytic activity; 10) altered staining quality of the cytoplasm; and 11) cytoplasmic inclusions.

Witkowski, Jan A. "Experimental Pathology and the Origins of Tissue Culture: Leo Loeb's Contribution." *Medical History*, 27 (July 1983), 269-88.

(See Chapter 7: Witkowski).

Wood, David A. "Clinical Classification of Cancer. Purposes and Methods: Historical Perspective." *Oncology: Proceedings of the Tenth International Cancer Congress*, IV (1970), 128-33.

Clinical staging systems are reliable only if certain basic rules are observed. First, the clinical classification for a given cancer location must be applicable to all cases, regardless of the treatment used. Second, all classifications must be based on clinical examination of the patient before treatment; otherwise there can be no comparison of the results of treatment. Third, a classification cannot be changed once it is made. Finally, clinical staging cannot be merged or combined with other sorts of staging, or the integrity of the clinical staging is violated.

During the twentieth century oncologists from around the world have worked to develop an international system of clinical classification. A number of organizations and congresses were involved, including the Cancer Commission of the Health Organization of the League of Nations in the 1920s; the International Committee for Stage-Grouping in Cancer and for Presentation of the Results of Treatment of Cancer (ICPR), which began meeting in London in 1950; and the International Union Against Cancer in the late 1950s. What emerged was the "TNM System," in which "T" represented the degree of local extension of the tumor, "N" the condition of the regional lymph nodes, and "M" the presence or absence of distant metastases.

Wright, James R., Jr. "The Development of the Frozen Section Technique, the Evolution of the Surgical Biopsy, and the Origins of Surgical Pathology." *Bulletin of the History of Medicine*, 59 (Fall 1985), 295-326.

In the nineteenth and early twentieth centuries surgeons often had to decide about lesions simply from their gross appearance. Surgeons had to proceed knowing that the wrong diagnosis on the malignancy of a tumor could result either in unnecessary disfigurement or the death of the patient. Today a biopsy with a rapid frozen section diagnosis is a standard diagnostic tool for a surgeon who has exposed a tumor. The invention of the frozen section technique greatly increased the number of surgical biopsies being performed, and at the same time gave rise to the field of surgical pathology as a subspecialty. Three developments in the nineteenth century made all this possible. First, the rise of anesthesia and aseptic technique allowed surgeons to perform longer and more extensive procedures requiring improved diagnostic skills. Second, the resolution and magnification capabilities of new microscopes improved analysis of cellular morphology. And third, preparation techniques of tissue specimens for microscopic analysis improved greatly.

The key to histologic success is the preparation of thin and uniform tissue sections which can then be stained to show nuclear and cytoplasmic detail. For surgical pathology the need was for immediate production of tissue slides so surgeons could know how to proceed during an operation on a tumor. Thomas Cullen at Johns Hopkins University, Henrique Plenge of Heidelberg, Ludwig Pick of Berlin, Alfredo Kanthack at Cambridge, Ernest H. Shaw of London, and Louis B. Wilson at the Mayo Clinic all developed techniques in the late 1890s and early 1900s for immediately freezing soft tissues, slicing them, staining them, and analyzing them while surgery was actually proceeding.

Although the technique of frozen sections appeared in the early 1900s, it took a full generation before most pathologists would accept it. Conservatives simply doubted the efficacy of the technique. Nevertheless, by the 1920s it was becoming increasingly used and some pathologists were beginning to describe themselves as "clinical pathologists," meaning that they specialized in the new technique and considered themselves part of the surgical team. In 1922 the American Society of Clinical Pathologists was formed and by the end of the decade the technique of the frozen section was well accepted.

Late in the 1920s the field of "surgical pathology" then emerged from clinical pathology, primarily because in 1926 the American College of Surgeons began requiring that all accredited hospitals guarantee that each surgical specimen be examined by a pathologist and that a report be made on each specimen. The standard led to the creation of a surgical pathology laboratory in every hospital seeking accreditation.

Zulch, K. J. "Historical Development of the Classification of Brain Tumours and the New Proposal of the World Health Organization (WHO)." *Neurosurgical Review*, 4 (1981), 123-27.

In 1911 Bielschowsky first devised a classification system for tumors of the neuronal cells, and in 1918 Ribbert first described the different stages of maturation of the gliomas: spongioneuroblastoma to spongioblastoma to glioblastoma to neuroblastoma. In the 1920s Bailey began describing the cell types present in brain tumors.

7 Research and Control

Beliaev, I. I. "M. A. Novinskii i problema profilakiti raka (k 100-letiiu eksperi-mental'noi onkologii." *Gigiena i Sanitaria*, 6 (June 1977), 47-48.

(See Chapter 7: Shabad).

Breslow, Lester. "From Cancer Research to Cancer Control." *Progress in Clinical and Biological Research*, 120 (1983), 1-19.

When Congress established the National Cancer Institute in 1937, it gave the new agency a triple charge to implement intramural research, extramural research, and cancer control measures. Although the first two objectives have been achieved, the goal of establishing effective cancer control programs has lagged badly. There are three apparent reasons for the inability of the United States to sustain an effective, long-term program of cancer control. Only dramatic political action can overcome these problems.

1. Physicians generally did not historically view cancer as requiring any as-sumption of public responsibility. Organized medicine opposed the 1937 anti-cancer legislation, warning "that the danger of putting the government in a dominant position in relation to medical research is apparent," and gen-erally resisted governmental action for cancer control as an encroachment on the domain of private practice.

2. The long latent period in cancer development made it difficult to identify etiologic factors, permitting the development of economic resistance to con-trol measures. Even after cigarettes were found to be responsible for most lung and oral cancers, as well as cardiovascular diseases, powerful corpo-rate forces strongly opposed action to control the disease agent, as did their political representatives in Congress. The complex way which occupational factors influence cancer occurrence has obscured any obvious links and al-lowed industry to resist control.

3. The large public investment in biomedical research and training created another potent force—at the corporate, academic, and political levels—with special interests and substantial influence. That force early began to resist public expenditures for cancer control as a threat to its own sustenance and profit levels.

Although many of these attitudes have changed in recent years, especially the negative attitude toward federal government grants, the early resistance prevented significant improvements in cancer control programs until the 1970s.

Bud, R. F. "Strategy in American Cancer Research After World War II." *The Social Study of Science*, 8 (November 1978), 425-29.

Since World War II oncology research in the United States has focused on the level of molecular biology, particularly the nature of oncogenesis, the viral etiology of tumors, and the genetic component of neoplastic disease. On the clinical level, research into chemotherapy was at its peak in the 1950s, 1960s, and 1970s. In the 1980s a new interest has been shown in immunotherapy. At the institutional level, cancer funding has been dramatically augmented by the National Cancer Act of 1971 and the enhanced research budget of the National Cancer Institute.

Clarkson, B. D. "The Elusive Goal." *Cancer Research*, 41 (December 1981), 4865-84.

In the last half century physicians and researchers have made dramatic strides in treating cancer. In surgery, the most important development in the twentieth century has been the notion of *en bloc* resection, which has reduced local recurrences of disease. The rise of radiotherapy, especially the megavoltage technologies, has assisted surgeons by providing post-operative therapy to destroy occult malignancies and pre-operative therapy to reduce large tumors and make them resectable. In the field of chemotherapy, the development of the nitrogen mustards, the antifolic acid treatments, and the antibiotic therapies have brought on marked improvements in survival rates for patients with choriocarcinomas, testicular cancers, Wilms' tumors, leukemias, and lymphomas. Nevertheless, progress against adult solid tumors has been slow in recent years, and the most promising therapies in the future will involve new technologies in immunology, genetic engineering, and basic biological research at the molecular level.

Clowes, G. H. A. "Cancer Research Fifty Years Ago and Now." *Cancer Research*, 16 (1956), 2-4.

It was not until 1903 when Gaylord brought the Jensen mouse carcinoma to the United States that experimental material became available and stimulated a boom in research. In 1904 investigators discovered that mice which had recovered spontaneously from tumor transplants were immune to subsequent transplants. This led to sophisticated attempts to determine the nature of the immune mechanism involved and the biochemical nature of tumors. Their work led to the founding of the American Association for Cancer Research. In the past fifty years cancer research has evolved from a scientific stepchild to the major area of biomedical research in the world.

Endicott, Kenneth M. "Trends in the Support of Cancer Research in the United States." *Canadian Cancer Conference*, 8 (1969), 1-8.

Early in the 1900s the American Medical Association and the American Gynecological Society appointed committees to study the rising cancer mortality rate in the United States. The first formal organization to fight cancer was formed in 1913—the American Society for the Control of Cancer. Congress created the National Cancer Institute in 1937 to promote basic research, inform the public about the danger of cancer and the importance of early diagnosis, and procure a reliable radium source for cancer treatment. After World War II the American Society for the Control of Cancer became the American Cancer Society. By 1950 the combined research grants of the American Cancer Society and the National Cancer Institute totaled approximately $35 million annually. As public concern over cancer grew in the 1950s and 1960s, the volume of research money available increased commensurately. By 1968 the American Cancer Society was providing $45 million for research and the National Cancer Institute $185 million. What oncologists must guard against, however, is growing public frustration with the pace of success in cancer therapy. The disease is extraordinarily complex and tenacious, and oncologists must educate the public and legislators about the importance of basic research and a long-term commitment to the struggle against the disease.

Furth, Jacob. "An Historical Sketch of Experimental Leukemia." In Marvin A. Rich. *Experimental Leukemia.* New York: 1968. Pp. 1-11.

Extensive research on viral leukemia began with V. Ellerman's 1908 discovery of a filterable agent in chickens capable of producing "systemic" leukemia as well as solid tumors of lymphoid cells. In 1911 Peyton Rous isolated the chicken sarcoma virus. In 1926 and 1927 E. P. Snidjers and Tio T. Gie transplanted malignant lymphomas through fifty-eight passages of guinea pigs. In 1930 C. H. Krebs demonstrated that radiation exposure led to a higher incidence of leukemia. The chemical carcinogenesis of leukemia was shown with benzol (Lignac, 1932), trypan blue (Gillman, 1949), and polycyclic aromatic hydrocarbons (Shay, 1956).

Heller, John R. "The Impact of Research Upon Clinical Cancer." *Progress in Clinical Cancer*, 1 (1965), 15-25.

Over the centuries a number of scientists have contributed to major advances in the understanding of cancer. The first observation in epidemiology was made by

Ambroise Paré in the sixteenth century when he concluded that cancer was more common in women than in men. In 1775 Percivall Pott made his historic contribution to carcinogenesis when he described squamous cell carcinoma in chimney sweeps. Biopsy of cancer began to be accepted at the turn of the twentieth century. In 1895 Cullin described the frozen section technique, but not until the 1940s have pathological studies been accepted as the only reliable way of diagnosing malignancy. Exfoliative cytology began in 1837 with Dunne's microscopic studies of body fluids, and in 1847 Pouchet published the first study of the exfoliative cytology of the female genital tract. The first report of the usefulness of the smear technique as a diagnostic aid in cancer of the cervix came with the work of Georges Papanicolaou in 1928. Cytological diagnoses for cancer of the stomach and respiratory tract were developed late in the 1950s and early in the 1960s.

"History of Experimental Oncology (On the Centenary of Publication of the Article by M. A. Novinsky.)" *Arkhiv Patologii*, 38 (1976), 104-07.

(See Chapter 7: Shabad).

Kalberer, J. T., and G. R. Newell. "Funding Impact of the National Cancer Act and Beyond." *Cancer Research*, 39 (October 1979), 4274-84.

The National Cancer Act of 1971 had a dramatic impact on funding for cancer research in the United States. President Richard M. Nixon assumed personal responsibility for achieving "the conquest of cancer," and with his support, as well as a growing public concern about cancer mortality rates, the National Cancer Institute received a real legislative boost in 1971 from Congress. The National Cancer Act of 1971 gave the National Cancer Institute the power to submit its annual proposed budget directly to the president for approval, independently of the budget of the Department of Health, Education, and Welfare in general and the National Institutes of Health in particular. With that bureaucratic independence, the National Cancer Institute experienced rapid increases in funding. In 1971 its annual budget stood at $230 million, but that figure increased to $937 million in 1979 and promised to increase even more in the future.

Meyer, P. A. "The Last Per Se: The Delaney Cancer Clause in United States Food Regulation." Ph.D. Dissertation. University of Wisconsin. 1983.

(See Chapter 7: Salsburg and Heath).

Mike, Valerie. "Clinical Studies in Cancer: A Historical Perspective." In Valerie Mike and Kenneth E. Stanley. *Statistics in Medical Research. Methods and Issues, with Applications in Cancer Research*. New York: 1982. Pp. 111-55.

In the twentieth century the major developments in effective cancer therapy programs have been: 1) the development of *en bloc* resection in surgery, first systematized by William Stewart Halsted late in the nineteenth century; 2) the discovery of X-rays by Wilhelm Roentgen in the 1890s and the subsequent development of radiotherapy; 3) the development of inbred systems of experimental animals, the transplantation of tumors into these animals, and the testing of systematic modes of therapies on them; 4) the development of randomized clinical trials in the late 1950s; 5) the demonstration that the fractional-kill hypothesis is applicable to cancer, as it is to the action of antiseptics on bacteria; and 6) the birth of modern chemotherapy and its antitumor capabilities.

Morris, Harold F., and Lynnard J. Slaughter. "Historical Development of Transplantable Hepatomas." *Advances in Experimental Medicine and Biology,* 92 (1977), 1-19.

One of the most important considerations in the test of malignancy among tissues produced by experimental carcinogenesis is the transplantability of the lesion. A stock of inbred rats was acquired by the National Institutes of Health in 1940, and after several more years of inbreeding, transplantation experiments were launched. By the early 1950s researchers achieved successful transplantation of induced tumors. N-2-fluorenyldiacetamide was found to induce liver tumors in the rats, especially adenocarcinomas and cholangiocarcinomas. Liver tumors developed rapidly in normal male rats but the chemical's carcinogenic activity was almost completely inhibited in the female rat and in the castrated male rate receiving diethylstilbestrol in addition to the carcinogen.

Neiman, I. M. "K stoletiiu eksperimental'noi onkologii." *Patologii Fiziologii Eksperimental,* 6 (November-December 1976), 3-5.

(See Chapter 7: Shabad).

Pasqualini, C. D. "Veinte años de leucemia experimental en Argentina." *Sangre,* 23 (1978), 69-71.

(See Chapter 7: Furth).

Pitot, Henry C. "The Rous Sarcoma Virus." *Journal of the American Medical Association,* 250 (September 16, 1983), 1447-48.

In 1911 the pathologist Peyton Rous first reported the transmission of a solid tumor by a cell-free filtrate. At the time most researchers believed there was an infectious process at work. Not until 1951 and the discovery by L. Gross that leukemia could be transmitted in mice by inoculation of newborn animals with cell-free extracts of the neoplasm from mice did medical scientists begin to consider the possibility that viruses could be a cause of cancer. Since then the question of viral etiology, especially in the 1960s and 1970s, has become one of the most exciting research areas in oncology.

Rosen, George. "Nicholas Senn's Experimental Work on Cancer Transmissibility." *The American Journal of Surgical Pathology*, 1 (March 1977), 85-87.

Nicholas Senn was born in Switzerland in 1844 and immigrated to Wisconsin in 1852. He received a medical degree from the Chicago Medical College in 1868, studied subsequently at the University of Munich, and then spent his career as a surgeon at the Rush Medical College in Chicago and at the University of Chicago. Late in the nineteenth century, scientists were preoccupied with the transmissibility of cancer, suspecting that the disease had a microbial origin. Experimental research focused on inoculating human cancers in laboratory animals. But in 1901 Senn inoculated himself with a piece of tissue from a human lip carcinoma. The small tumor was placed in his arm, and it disappeared in about four weeks. Senn concluded that the etiology of cancer was not microbial. Nicholas Senn died in 1908.

Salsburg, David and Andrew Heath. "When Science Progresses and Bureaucracies Lag—The Case of Cancer Research." *Public Interest*, No. 65 (1981), 30-39.

The hunt for chemical carcinogens began in earnest in the 1950s with formation of the International Union Against Cancer. At the same time Berenblum and Schubik developed the cancer "initiator/promoter" concept, and in 1958 the Delaney clause amended the Food, Drug, and Cosmetic Act, which prohibited use of any additives shown to cause cancer in laboratory animals. The National Cancer Institute and FDA then developed four operative assumptions in testing chemicals suspected of being carcinogenic.

1. Only a few chemical compounds cause cancer.

2. Because of the long latency for human cancers, it is necessary to follow treated animals for their entire lifetimes. That naturally confines research to short-lived mice and rats, whose tumors may or may not be analagous to human lesions.

3. In order to catch "weak" carcinogens, it is necessary to treat animals with huge doses.

4. Every known human carcinogen causes cancer in animals. Recent research, however, has shown that 184 chemical compounds cause cancer in laboratory animals and many others actually reduce the incidence of certain types of cancer. Yet, the FDA is unable to respond to this new knowledge with innovative public policies.

Sorkin, IuE. "'Bolenz' N. A. Nekrasova i khirurg E. I. Bogdanovskii." *Vestnik Khirurgiia*, 111 (July 1973), 135-38.

The article explains the work of scientist N. A. Nekrasova and surgeon E. I. Bogdanovskii in the transplantation of skin tumors as part of their research in experimental oncology.

Shabad, L. M. "Centennial of Experimental Cancer Research (M. A. Novinsky). *International Journal of Cancer*, 18 (15 July 1976), 130-31.

In 1875 and 1876, Mistislav Novinsky, a graduate student at the Medical-Surgery Academy of St. Petersburg, Russia, successfully transplanted a nasal carcinoma from a dog to another dog, proving that tumors could be transplanted in animals of the same species.

Shabad, L. M. "On the History of Experimental Oncology." *Neoplasma*, 23 (1976), 569-75.

The history of experimental oncology began in 1876 with M. A. Novinsky's successful transplantation of a nasal carcinoma from one dog to another. As early as 1777 James Nooth, an English surgeon, had inoculated himself with some tumor from a patient and observed several days of immunological reaction in his arm. In 1808 a French surgeon, Jean Louis Alibert, injected himself with some tissue from a breast carcinoma. He developed an inflammatory reaction which he observed for several days. Unsuccessful attempts to transplant tumors from one species to another were made by Guillaume Dupuytren in 1807 and Bernard Langenback in 1840. In the 1880s Arthur Hanau of Zürich successfully transplanted rats with an epidermoid carcinoma. Henry Morau of Paris successfully transplanted mammary tumors in mice.

Shabad, L. M. "O nekotorykh putiakh razvitiia sovetskoi eksperimental'noi onkologii." *Eksperimental'Naia Khirurgiia i Anestezioilogia*, 12 (July-August 1967), 3-6.

(See Chapter 7: Shabad, "On the History of Experimental Oncology").

Shabad, L. M. "Sto let eksperimentl'noi onkologii." *Voprosy Onkologii*, 23 (1976), 15-26.

(See Chapter 7: Shabad: "On the History of Experimental Oncology").

Shabad, L. M. "Znachenie issledovanii N. N. Petrova v razvitii eksperimental'noi onkologii." *Voprosy Onkologii*, 18 (1972), 104-11.

(See Chapter 7: Shabad).

Shabad, L. M. "Zum Hundertjahrigen Jubilaum der Experimentellen Onkologie." *Archiv Geschwulstforsch,* 47 (1977), 1-6.

(See Chapter 7: Shabad).

Shabad, L. M. and L. Graciute. "Le centenaire de la première transplantation de tumeur." *Bulletin cancer,* 63 (July-September 1976), 305-08.

(See Chapter 7: Shabad).

Shimkin, Michael B. "A. E. C. Lathrop: Mouse Woman of Granby." *Cancer Research,* 35 (1975), 1597-98.

Abbie E. C. Lathrop owned a commercial mice colony in Granby, Massachusetts, in the late 1800s and early 1900s, to supply scientists with research animals. Along with famed pathologist Leo Loeb, Lathrop demonstrated that mammary carcinomas in mice usually occurred in family lines and were hormone-dependent. Reductions in tumor size were achieved by ovariectomies in the diseased mice.

Shimkin, Michael B. "An Historical Note on Tumor Transplantation in Man." *Cancer,* 35 (1975), 540-41.

The first recorded attempt to transfer cancer from one person to another in order to measure the transmittability of the disease is attributed to Jean Louis Alibert (1768-1837), a French dermatologist who served as physician to Louis XVIII. In 1808 Alibert allowed himself to be injected with tumor tissue from a breast cancer patient. Several medical students underwent the same experiment at the same time. After an initial inflammatory reaction at the site of the injection, there were no long-term consequences of the experiment, allowing Alibert to conclude that cancer was not contagious.

Shimkin, Michael B. "Arthur Nathan Hanau: A Further Note on the History of Transplantation of Tumors." *Cancer,* 13 (1960), 211.

In the 1880s Arthur Hanau of Zürich successfully transplanted epidermoid carcinomas in rats.

Shimkin, Michael B. "Committee on Growth, 1945-1956: Another Noble Experiment." *Cancer Research,* 39 (January 1979), 262-68.

(See Chapter 30: Shimkin).

Shimkin, Michael B. "M. A. Novinsky: A Note on the History of Transplantation of Tumors." *Cancer,* 8 (1955), 653-55.

Although Arthur Hanau has been generally credited with the first success in transplanting tumors from one animal to another of the same species with his work on rats, M. A. Novinsky actually was the first to do so when he transplanted nasal carcinomas from one dog to another in 1875-1876.

Shishkov, V. P. "M. A. Novinskii (K 100-letiiu eksperimental'noi onkoligii." *Veterinariia*, 6 (June 1976), 100.

(See Chapter 7: Shabad).

Stewart, Harold L. "Perspectives in Comparative Oncology." *National Cancer Institute Monograph No. 32: Hematopoietic Neoplasms*, August 1969, 1-5.

Although some concern was expressed early in the nineteenth century about cancer in animals, it was not until 1858 that the French physician Leblanc reported a variety of animal tumors, recognizing that cancers do occur in animals. Not until 1900, in Germany and England, did systematic research in animal neoplasms begin. Transplantation from one rodent to another began in 1876. In 1908 came the discovery of the viral transmission of chicken leukemia and chicken sarcoma in 1911. In the 1920s and 1930s there was widespread research into the nature of animal virology and cancer. Contemporary questions to be answered include why cancer is so much more frequent in the mammary glands of mice than in women and practically unknown in the utters of cows; why does mammary cancer in women metastasize so early to the regional lymph nodes when it will not spread there at all in mice. Does a species exist whose mammary cancers resemble histologically human cancer and can serve as a model?

Supady, J. "Doświadczaine transplantacje nowotworów w pracach lekarzy Polskich na przełomie XIX i XX wieku." *Wiadomosci Lekarskie*, 32 (June 15, 1979), 887-90.

Along with people like Arthur Hanau in Zürich and Mistislav Novinsky in St. Petersburg, Polish researchers worked on the problem of transplanting tumors from animal to animal and animal to man. During much of the nineteenth century they believed they were transplanting a tumor-producing agent of some kind rather than tumor cells themselves. It was not until the twentieth century and the rise of cellular pathology that they began to understand the real nature of the disease.

Supady, J. "Serologia nowotworów w badaniach Ludwika Hirszfelda i jego współpracownikow w okresie II rzeczypospolitej." *Wiadomosci Lekarskie*, 34 (February 1, 1981), 257-62.

The article recounts the contributions of Polish scientist Ludwika Hirszfelda to the study of tumor serology.

Triolo, Victor A. "Nineteenth Century Foundations of Cancer Research. Origins of Experimental Research." *Cancer Research*, 24 (January 1964), 4-27.

The first experimental system to achieve organized status, because of its foundation in classical microbiology, was founded upon the concept of cancer as an infectious disease. After 1900 this "parasitic theory" rested on the concept of viral origins. The theory of biological irritation received its foundation in the discovery of the environmental influence of tar and certain dyes as carcinogenic agents in the late nineteenth and early twentieth centuries. In the early 1900s, the idea of cancer as a product of cellular pathology gained currency. The theory of cell autonomy advanced the concept that the neoplastic process fell into the category of abnormal physiology.

Weisburger, Elizabeth K. "History of the Bioassay Program of the National Cancer Institute." *Progress in Experimental Tumor Research*, 26 (1983), 187-201.

In 1961, at the urging of Michael Shimkin, director of biometry, diagnostic research, epidemiology, and carcinogenesis for the National Cancer Institute, the NCI established a Carcinogenesis Studies Branch to analyze the carcinogenic affects of various chemicals on experimental animals. In 1962 the Carcinogenesis Studies Branch began issuing research contracts to business and academic researchers. Paul Kotin headed the branch beginning late in 1962. Its funding remained limited until 1971, when passage of the National Cancer Act greatly expanded research appropriations. By 1972 more than 400 compounds were being tested on 100,000 animals in the system. In the mid-1970s it became known as the Carcinogenesis Testing Program of the National Cancer Institute.

Wienhouse, Sidney. "Prometheus and Pandora—Cancer Research on Our Diamond Anniversary: Presidential Address." *Cancer Research*, 42 (September 1982), 3471-74.

Sidney Weinhouse offers his presidential address to the American Association for Cancer Research. Cancer researchers today are caught in a firestorm, especially in their animal studies of environmental carcinogens. If a substance is carcinogenic to animals, it is a potential carcinogenic hazard to some people, even if vested interests ridicule the methodology and the results. Clinical oncologists are also caught on the horns of a dilemma—although major strides have been made in fighting cancer, such common neoplasms as those of the colon, lung, breast, and prostate still elude control, giving ammunition to quacks and pseudoscientists promoting alternative therapies. Finally, there is considerable belief in the public sphere that science is "out of control," and oncologists must confront that public fear and skepticism.

Witkowski, Jan A. "Experimental Pathology and the Origins of Tissue Culture: Leo Loeb's Contribution." *Medical History*, 27 (July 1983), 269-88.

Born in Germany in 1869, Leo Loeb immigrated to the United States in 1897, where he taught pathology at the medical schools of the Johns Hopkins University, McGill University, the University of Pennsylvania, and Washington University. Loeb is best remembered for his work on the transplantation of tumors in rats. Through dozens of generations of rats, Loeb transplanted spindle-cell sarcomas and malignant thyroid lesions and demonstrated that new tumors arose from the peripheral cells of the transplants and not from cellular fluids. Along with Abbie E. C. Lathrop, Loeb also demonstrated that mammary carcinomas in mice were more disposed to occur in family lines and were hormone-dependent.

Yeh, Samuel D. J. "Nuclear Medicine and Cancer Research in the People's Republic of China." *American Journal of Chinese Medicine*, 7 (1979), 149-55.

(See Chapter 5: Yeh).

8   Tumor Metastasis

Braverman, Irwin M. "Commentary: Migratory Necrolytic Erythema." *Archives of Dermatology*, 118 (October 1982), 796-98.

Today migratory necrolytic erythema is associated with metastatic pancreatic carcinoma. S. Rothman first wrote about cutaneous eruptions and internal cancer in 1925. The skin lesions were characterized by flaccid vesicles and bullae on the surface of the skin. They broke quickly, leaving behind denudation and crusts. The individual lesions run their course in seven to fourteen days, and lesions are found in all stages of development. In 1966 McGavran described a woman with a bullous and eczematous eruption of the extremities. She was also suffering from a pancreatic glucagonoma. In 1971 Wilkinson bestowed on the disease the name "necrolytic migratory erythema."

Grundmann,   E.   "Die   Vorstellungen   von   Julius   Cohnheim   zur Geschwülstentstehung und Metastasierung im Blickwinkel Neuer Forschungsergebnisse." *Zentralblatt für Allgemeine Pathologie und Pathologische Anatomie*, 130 (1985), 323-31.

Julius Cohnheim was born in Pomerania in 1839. He studied medicine at the University of Berlin and worked with the famed pathologist Rudolf Virchow. Before his death in 1884, Cohnheim was a professor of pathology at universities in Kiel, Breslau, and Leipzig. Cohnheim's major contribution to oncology was his belief that malignant tumors developed from immature embryonic cells left in tissues. Cohnheim was also among the earliest pathologists to postulate that metastatic tumors were extensions of the original localized tumor.

Haneveld, G. T. "Compression as a Treatment of Cancer: A Historical Survey." *Archivum Chirurgicum Neerlandicum*, 3 (1979), 1-8.

(See Chapter 28: Haneveld).

Onuigbo, Wilson I. B. "A History of Hematogenous Metastasis." *Cancer Research*, 30 (December 1970), 2821-26.

The metastatic process involves five steps: liberation of cells from the primary tumor; transportation of the liberated material; deposition of the transported tumor tissue; establishment of the deposits in their new surroundings; and growth of the established deposits. Liberation is assisted by the poor cohesive state of cancer cells. In 1856 S. Van Der Kolk noted that the vein wall may be penetrated but the artery is rarely attacked. J. D. Bryant in 1888 observed that ulceration or penetration of the blood vessels probably opened a passage for malignant cells into the bloodstream. Much earlier, W. H. Walshe had claimed that each cancer cell set free is potentially a new tumor in embryo.

By the second half of the nineteenth century, the use of the bloodstream to transport malignant cells was clear to many observers. James Paget, Theodor Billroth, William Jenner, and Bernard Langenback all observed cancerous thrombi in the veins and pulmonary arteries on autopsy. Joseph Coats was convinced that metastasis was primarily a lymphatic process, with the lymphatic system transporting cancer cells by way of the large lymphatic collecting trunks into the bloodstream. In 1900 A. Monti also observed malignant cells in the process of mitosis while moving through the bloodstream. An irony of Rudolf Virchow's life is that he did not understand the nature of cellular metastasis because of the possibility of transpulmonary passage. He was committed to the idea of metastasis not through cellular transportation but to the transfer of what he called "morbid juices" from the tumor into the bloodstream. New tumor deposits then evolved from those morbid fluids.

In the 1840s J. Bell and W. Budd argued that the malignant cells are ultimately deposited in the capillaries because they are too large to traverse these vessels freely. Thomas Hodgkin, Theodor Billroth, and Nicholas Senn all agreed with that conclusion.

In 1878 Joseph Coats argued that the malignant cells are active when passing through the bloodstream or lymphatic system, and as soon as they are deposited a microscopic tumor begins because the process of accelerated mitosis continues. Colomatti in 1877 described the process of liberation, transportation, deposition, establishment, and new growth as the stages of metastasis. In the 1880s James Paget then described the process of tertiary metastasis from secondary, metastatic tumors.

Onuigbo, Wilson I. B. "An Historical Criticism of Tumor Metastasis." *Journal of the History of Medicine and Allied Sciences*, 13 (October 1958), 529-31.

The mechanism of metastasis was not understood before the nineteenth century. Later pathologists believed that local and lymph node metastases were lymph-borne. They did not believe that distant metastases were lymphogenous. Instead, they indicted the bloodstream. The dominant view of the nineteenth and early twentieth centuries was that local spread of carcinoma was predominantly by lymphatic routes, but that distant metastases denoted embolic spread by the bloodstream. Only recently have pathologists started arguing that distant lymphogenous metastases are possible.

Onuigbo, Wilson I. B. "Joseph Coats (1846-1899) of Glasgow and the Theory of Cancer Metastasis." *Scottish Medical Journal,* 15 (August 1970), 281-84.

Joseph Coats, a physician and pathologist in Glasgow, Scotland, argued that metastasis occurred through the lymphatic system and through the bloodstream. Writing in the 1870s, Coats emphasized that tumor cells can gain immediate entry into the venous radicles within the lymph nodes. As for the bloodstream, Coats observed not only embolized pulmonary vessels but also evidence of radical extension and formulation of small nodules.

Onuigbo, Wilson I. B. "The Age-Old Dictum on the Spread of Tumours." *Centaurus,* 8 (1963), 263-68.

Since the early twentieth century, the consensus about metastasis has been that carcinomas spread through the lymphatic system and sarcomas through the bloodstream. Actually, the old writings demonstrate clearly that physicians believed that carcinomatous invasion of the organs occurred after the lymph nodes had been involved, whereas sarcomatous invasion of the organs occurred in the absence of lymph node involvement. The old masters held that carcinomas usually first invade the lymph nodes before invading the organs, but that sarcomas from the first are apt to invade the organs.

Onuigbo, Wilson I. B. "A History of the Cell Theory of Cancer Metastasis." *Gesnerus,* 20 (1963), 90-95.

In the late eighteenth century, the theory of humoral metastasis reached its apogee. Physicians believed that the blood contained a "poisonous fluid" in which cancerous tissue fixed itself somewhere else in the body. By the early nineteenth century surgeons in Europe had become convinced that the cause of metastasis was the leaving behind of clinically occult malignant tissue, and that in removing a tumor surgeons should make a wide excision to make sure no cancerous tissue was left behind. Those remaining tissues would inevitably cause a recurrence of the disease. The advent of the microscope in the 1830s soon proved the minute structure of living tissues. By the last third of the nineteenth century a large number of physicians believed that each cancerous cell was actually a tumor in embryo capable of spreading and causing new tumors. In the 1880s Cohnheim speculated that secondary tumor growths came from the lymphatic and vascular spread of tumor cells. Since then the cell theory has been dominant.

Onuigbo, Wilson I. B. "Historical Data on the Dynamics of Lymphatic Metastasis." *Oncology*, 26 (1972), 505-14.

(See Chapter 8: Onuigbo, "An Historical Criticism of Tumour Metastasis").

Onuigbo, Wilson I. B. "Patterns of Metastasis in Lung Cancer: A Review." *Cancer Research*, 21 (October 1961), 1077-85.

He argues that the contemporary hematogenous theory of lung carcinoma metastasis through the bloodstream follows the tradition of nineteenth century medicine. He disagrees with that hypothesis, in favor of a lymphogenous route in metastasis, primarily since blood-rich lungs do not seem to more frequently produce distant metastases than the lymphatic route.

Onuigbo, Wilson I. B. "The Paradox of Virchow's Views on Cancer Metastasis." *Bulletin of the History of Medicine*, 36 (1962), 444-49.

Rudolf Virchow is widely considered to be the father of cellular pathology. But for most of his life, he held to a humoral theory of cancer metastasis, arguing that "morbid juices" from the primary tumor, not cells, spread through the bloodstream, infected a new site, and the infection led to a secondary tumor. What confused Virchow was that the lung did not filter out cancer cells, so he assumed it must be cancerous fluid passing through the lung capillaries. Not until late in his life did Virchow convert to the idea of cellular metastasis.

Onuigbo, Wilson I. B. "Secondary Skin Cancer in Nineteenth-Century Britain." *British Journal of Dermatology*, 94 (1976), 457-63.

As early as 1805 British physicians recognized metastatic lesions of primary tumors occurring in the skin, but they had no idea of the mechanism which brought the lesions to distant sites. Astley Cooper in the 1840s argued that secondary deposits of breast cancer must be transferred to their locations by the lymphatic system. In 1883 D. W. Finlay argued that secondary lesions of gastric carcinoma are carried to their new locations by the bloodstream. Nineteenth century surgeons realized that patient prognosis after the appearance of secondary skin lesions was quite poor, but they nevertheless recommended surgical excision of the new tumors.

Onuigbo, Wilson I. B. "Thomas Hodgkin (1798-1866) on Cancer Cell Carriage." *Medical History*, 11 (October 1967), 406-11.

On a primitive level Thomas Hodgkin understood the cellular nature of cancer carriage through clinical observations that tumors frequently spread from the original site along the path of lymphatic vessels to lymph nodes. Against the general opinion of the time, Hodgkin argued that metastatic tumors were directly connected to the original tumor. Most people were still loyal to the old humoral concept. Along with John Hunter, Hodgkin was the founder of the British school of the pathological anatomy of cancer. He also described the selectivity of metastasis—that certain tumors had a tendency to spread to certain sites, although he did not know why. While debate surrounded him about whether cancer originated in the lymphatic or blood systems, Hodgkin argued that it was not a question of origination but simply transportation by the lymphatic and blood systems. Hodgkin was also an early leader in the surgical pathology of cancer. He forcefully advocated wide excision of tumors with an appropriate margin so no residual tumor or tumor tissue was left behind.

Rather, L. J. "Langenback on the Mechanism of Tumor Metastasis." *Clio Médica*, 10 (September 1975), 213-25.

In 1840 Bernard Langenback of Goettingen proposed a new theory of cancer metastasis. At the time physicians did not know whether metastatic lesions were primary or secondary or just how the spread of the disease occurred. While performing autopsies on cancer patients, particularly women who had died of uterine carcinomas, Langenback noticed more deposits of tumor cells in the pelvic veins, the pulmonary artery, the heart, and the pulmonary arterial branches. He thought that cancer spread in one of two ways: that some primitive form of cancer "juice" in the bloodstream slowly evolved into cancer cells, making all metastases a type of primary tumor, or that cancer cells gained access to the bloodstream, deposited in small capillaries, and then proceeded to grow into new tumors. Excited by the new cellular theories of Schwann and Müller, Langenback actually leaned toward the latter theory as the best explanation of the mechanism of metastasis. History would prove his theory to be correct in its fundamental proposition.

Wilder, Robert J. "The Historical Development of the Concept of Tumor Metastasis." *Journal of the Mt. Sinai Hospital*, 23 (1956), 728-34.

(See Chapter 8: Onuigbo).

III MALIGNANT DISEASES

9 Bone

Allison, Marvin J., et al. "Metastatic Tumor of Bone in a Tiahuanaco Female."
Bulletin of the New York Academy of Medicine, 56 (July-August 1980), 581-
87.

A female mummy was excavated in 1978 near Arica, Chile. Archaeologists
estimate that she lived around the 8th century A.D. Skeletal remains indicate
that she was suffering from widespread bone metastases, probably from a breast
carcinoma.

Bergsagel, Daniel E., and Walter Rider. "Plasma Cell Neoplasms. History." In
Vincent P. DeVita, Jr., Samuel Hellman, and Steven A. Rosenberg. *Cancer.
Principles & Practice of Oncology.* 1985. Pp. 1753-54.

Although John Dalrymple, Henry Bence Jones, and William MacIntyre first
described the clinical features of the disease between 1846 and 1850, the term
"multiple myeloma" was coined in 1873 by Johann Rustizky. The elevated serum
protein and increased erythrocyte sedimentation rate in multiple myeloma patients was reported by Ellinger in 1899, and in 1900 Wright described the close
relationship between myeloma cells and plasma cells. That diagnosis, however,
was not experimentally proven until the 1930s when marrow aspiration and studies of serum proteins by ultracentrifugation and electrophoresis began. Treatment
was impossible until 1947 when researchers demonstrated that urethane had positive chemotherapeutic effects on the lesions. In 1958 the drug Sarcolysin produced
significant improvement. In the 1970s the beneficial effects of cyclophosphamide
and adrenocortical steroids have become apparent.

Brackenridge, C. J. "A Statistical Study of Sarcoma Complicating Paget's Disease of Bone in Three Countries." *British Journal of Cancer*, 40 (August 1979), 194-200.

Data concerning sex, age at presentation, and anatomical site of sarcoma complicating Paget's disease of the bone were compiled from the literature for white patients in Australia, Great Britain, and the United States between 1918 and 1977. The evidence suggested that sex and tumor-site distribution are free from bias, except for the skull. There was a male predominance for all sites except the skull, where the odds ratio of sarcoma compared with other locations is more than twice as high for females as for males. No national differences emerged in the sex ratio of patients. In Australia a latitudinal effect was detected, with sarcoma complications accompanying Paget's disease of the bone declining with an increase in latitude from Queensland to Victoria. Also, patients with bone involvement above the waist were younger than those suffering from tumors in the feet, legs, and pelvic girdle.

Brighetti, A. "Il morbo di Kahler-Bozzolo (Evoluzione delle conoscenze)." *Policlinio*, 74 (22 May 1967), 702-08.

Between 1846 and 1850 John Dalrymple, Henry Bence Jones, and William MacIntyre described the major clinical features of multiple myeloma. Their patient was a man named Thomas Alexander McBean. In 1873 Rustizky coined the term "multiple myeloma" because multiple bone tumors were common to the illness. In Europe it is still called Kahler's disease because O. Kahler, a German physician, published a detailed review of the lesion in 1889. Elevated serum protein and increased erythrocyte sedimentation were described by Ellinger in 1899. In the 1930s the disease became widely recognized as a plasma cell neoplasm.

Brooks, Sheilagh and Jerome Melbye. "Skeletal Lesions of Pre-Columbian Multiple Myeloma." *Paleopathology*, 1 (1967), 23-29.

They report a case of possible multiple myeloma in the skeletal remains of a 40 year old female near St. Louis, Missouri, who lived around 1200 A. D. She had multiple bone perforations of between 2 and 17 mm.

"Cancer Eponyms: Ewing's Sarcoma." *Cancer Bulletin*, 6 (September-October 1954), 105, 114.

In 1921 James Ewing, the renowned American pathologist, described the endothelioma, a bone sarcoma, but his work was greatly criticized by other pathologists, who believed that a tumor with such clinical and radiographic features was not really a pathological entity. Subsequent research has supported Ewing's contention, amd the metastatic potential of the tumor. Oncologists named the lesion after Ewing.

"Cancer Eponyms: Nelaton's Tumor." *Cancer Bulletin*, 12 (July-August 1960), 67-68.

In 1818 Sir Astley Cooper first described giant-cell bone tumors, but it was not until the writings of Auguste Nelaton in the 1860s that the benign but dangerous nature of the lesion began to be understood. Born in France in 1807, Nelaton was the physician to Napoleon III and a professor of surgery at the Hopital St. Louis. He was also the author of a five-volume text on surgical pathology. Nelaton died in 1873.

Cassidy, Claire. "Probable Malignancy in a Sadlermuit Eskimo Mandible." *American Journal of Physical Anthropololgy*, 46 (March 1977), 291-96.

The mandible of a 30 year old Sadlermuit Eskimo woman was discovered and analyzed by paleoanthropologists. She shows evidence of a metastatic carcinoma lesion in the mandible, although the source of the primary tumor cannot be determined.

Clamp, John R. "Some Aspects of the First Recorded Case of Multiple Myeloma." *Lancet*, No. 7530 (23 December 1967), 1354-56.

In a series of papers published between 1846 and 1850, John Dalrymple, Henry Bence Jones, and William MacIntyre described all the essential features of multiple myeloma. The patient was a man named Thomas Alexander McBean. They described the clinical aspects of the disease, the presence and properties of Bence-Jones protein in the patient's urine, and, after post-mortem examination, the tumors of the ribs, sternum, and the cervical, lumbar, and thoracic vertebrae, concluding that the disorder was a malignant disease of the bone. It was the first cancer in which a specific biochemical agent was identified—the Bence-Jones protein. Not until the 1930s did oncologists and hematologists recognize multiple myeloma as a plasma cell neoplasm.

Dastuge, J. "Tumeur maxillaire sur an crâne de moyen age." *Bulletin de l'Association Francais du Cancer*, 52 (January-March 1965), 69-72.

The article describes a bone tumor in the jaw of the skeleton of a medieval French male.

Gadomska, H. "Ocena częstosci wyst ępowania osteosarcoma na tle innych postaci nowotdworow zosliwych kości, Warszawa 1963-1974." *Nowotwory*, 1979, Suppl., 13-21.

The article is a study of the frequency of osteosarcoma and other malignant bone tumors in Warsaw between 1963 and 1974.

Garcia-Alejo, R. H. "Enfermedad osea de Paget: Comentarios a sus primeras descripciones y evolución histórica de su etiopatogenía." *Asclepio*, 34 (1982), 181-97.

(See Chapter 9: "Paget's Disease of Bone").

Gladykowka-Rzeczycka, J. "Mandibular Tumor in a Male Skeleton from a Medieval Burial Ground in Czersk." *Folia Morphologica*, 37 (1978), 191-96.

Paleoanthropologists located the skeletal remains, including the skull, of a man who died in Czersk, Poland, approximately 800 years ago. Examination of the skull indicated that the individual probably died of a malignant bone tumor of the jaw.

Gladykowka-Rzeczycka, J. and M. Urbanowicz. "Mnogie wyrśla kostne szkieletu z przedhistorycznego cmentarzyska dawnej ludności pruszcza Gdanskiego." *Folia Morphologica*, 29 (1970), 317-29.

Paleoanthropologists discovered numerous bone lesions, probably due to a case of multiple myeloma, in the skeletal remains of a medieval male living in the Gdansk area.

"History of Bone Tumors." *Cancer Bulletin*, 16 (March-April 1964), 36.

Bone tumors have been found in the skeletal remains of ancient dinosaurs as well as in pre-modern human beings. In 1845 Lebert described the histological criteria for differentiation between sarcoma and carcinoma of the bone, and in the 1850s Rudolf Virchow published widely on the morphology of bone tumors. In terms of surgical treatment, Cooper performed the first well-planned hip-joint disarticulation; Berger standardized the interscapulothoracic amputation in 1887; and Girard performed the first successful hempelvectomy in 1895. Surgical mortality rates for such extensive procedures gradually dropped in the twentieth century with the development of antibiotics and blood transfusion technologies.

Houghton, P. "Cancer and the Pre-Historic Maori." *New Zealand Medical Journal*, 80 (28 August 1974), 185-86.

Skeletal remains from Maori tribesmen indicate that even a thousand years ago people suffered from such primary bone diseases as multiple myeloma and osteosarcoma, localized nasopharyngeal carcinoma, metastatic melanoma, and probably a variety of metastatic carcinomas which had spread as secondary tumors to the bones.

Kelln, E. E., et al. "A Seventeenth Century Mandibular Tumor in a North American Indian." *Oral Surgery, Oral Medicine, Oral Pathology,* 23 (1967), 78-81.

The skeleton of a 20 year old female was found near the Kanawha River in Putnam County, West Virginia. She was probably a member of the Shawnee tribe. She had a large osseous tumor on the right mandible. Roentgenographic examination indicated it was a solid tumor. The tumor was most likely an osteogenic sarcoma.

Lagier, R., C. A. Baud, and G. Arnaud. "Lesions Characteristic of Infection or Malignant Tumor in Paleo-Eskimo Skulls. An Anatomical and Radiological Study of Two Specimens." *Virchow's Archives,* 395 (1982), 237-43.

Cancer was a disease of ancient as well as modern society. Among the skeletal remains of Alaskan Eskimos from the Paleolithic Era, paleoanthropologists have identified lesions confirming the presence of metastatic disease.

Lichenstein, L. "Progressi nella diágnosi e terapía del tumori scheletrici negli Ultimi 30 Anni." *Chirurgía degli Organi di Movimento,* 59 (1971), 313-31.

Until recently the only useful treatment against bone tumors was surgical amputation, and even then the disease had often already metastasized to other sites, particularly the lungs. In terms of diagnostic improvements, the development of CT scans, bone scintigraphy, and angiography have assisted in locating polyosotic disease, metastatic lesions, and intraosseous tumor extension. New histological grading systems have also been developed by pathologists and clinicians. As a result of these trends in diagnosis and grading, the use of limb-sparing surgical resection rather than amputation has become a possibility, especially for low-grade, intracompartmental lesions showing no evidence of metastasis.

McCarthy, E. F. "Giant-Cell Tumor of Bone: An Historical Perspective." *Clinical Orthopedics,* 153 (November-December 1980), 14-25.

Until the early twentieth century giant-cell tumors of the bone were considered dangerous, potentially metastatic sarcomas which were just as dangerous to patients as osteosarcoma, chondrosarcoma, and the soft-tissue sarcomas. The recommended treatment for "giant-cell sarcoma" was amputation whenever possible. But in 1912 Joseph C. Bloodgood of Johns Hopkins University published an influential article entitled "The Conservative Treatment of Giant-Cell Sarcoma." He advocated dropping the word sarcoma from the description of the lesion, because it only rarely metastasized, and argued that more conservative, tissue-saving surgical excision could be used without threatening the long-term survival of the patient. Since then that has been the approach, combined with megavoltage radiotherapy, for giant-cell tumors of the bone.

Morse, Dan, R. C. Dailey, and Jennings Bunn. "Prehistoric Multiple Myeloma."
   Bulletin of the New York Academy of Medicine, 50 (April 1974), 447-58.

Archaeologically, a diagnosis of multiple myeloma requires first an osteolytic
carcinomatous metastasis, as well as discreteness of individual lesions and extensive distribution. They present four cases of possible prehistoric multiple myelomas from skeletal remains of Indians in Mississippi and Florida. The tumor originates in bone marrow and histologically is a plasma cell neoplasm.

Ninomiya, S., and M. Abe. "Historical Review of Ewing's Sarcoma." *Orthopedic
   Surgery*, 20 (August 1969), 1092-96.

(See Chapter 2: EWING, JAMES: Stewart and Chapter 9: "Cancer Eponyms:
Ewing's Sarcoma").

Onuigbo, Wilson I. B. "Cancerous Pathologic Fractures. Concepts in the Nineteenth Century." *New York State Journal of Medicine*, 76 (May 1976), 771-
   72.

During the nineteenth century knowledge of cancerous bone fractures increased
dramatically. Prominent European and American physicians like John Warren,
James Paget, and Charles Bell recognized the association between malignant lesions and weakening of the bone. For a long time the relationship between the
primary tumor and the fractured bone was poorly understood. Many physicians
thought the fracture occurred first and then a tumor developed at the site of the
break. Toward the end of the nineteenth century a consensus began to emerge
among physicians that pathologic fractures could be secondary manifestations of
primary tumors.

"Paget's Disease of Bone." *Cancer Bulletin*, 14 (May-June 1962), 52.

In 1876 James Paget (1814-1899) first described osteitis deformans, a disease
causing the enlargement and deformation of large body bones. The most serious
complications of the disease are pathological fractures and a tendency to develop
osteosarcoma.

Peltier, Leonard F. "Historical Note on Bone and Soft-Tissue Sarcoma." *Journal
   of Surgical Oncology*, 30 (December 1985), 201-05.

(See Chapter 19: Peltier).

Ritchie, William and Stafford Warren. "The Occurrence of Multiple Bony Lesions Suggesting Myelomas in the Skeleton of a Pre-Columbian Indian." *American Journal of Roentgenology*, 28 (1932), 622-28.

They report a case of possible multiple myeloma from an elderly male who lived near Binghamton, New York, around 800 A.D. The skeletal bones are riddled with small and large perforations.

Schultz, M. "Ein Knochentumor an Einem Präkolumbischen Indianerschädel aus Peru. Ein Beitrag zur Differentialdiagnose Knocherner Schadeltumoren." *Virchow's Archives*, 378 (2 June 1978), 121-32.

The author reports discovery of a malignant tumor, probably an osteosarcoma, in the skeletal remains of an ancient Incan from Pre-Columbian Peru.

Sienski, W. and M. Dabska. "Mięsaki kościotworcze w materiale zakładu patologii nowotworów Instytutu Onkologii w Warszawie w latach 1948-1977." *Nowotwory*, 1979, Supp. 47-52.

The article surveys bone tumors and bone marrow tumors–multiple myeloma–in the Department of Pathology at the Institute of Oncology in Warsaw between 1948 and 1977.

Sjovold, T. "A Pregnant Woman from the Middle Ages with Exostosis Multiplex." *OSSA*, 1 (1974), 3-23.

(See Chapter 13: Sjovold).

Strouhal, Eugen. "Tumors in the Remains of Ancient Egyptians." *American Journal of Physical Anthropology*, 45 (November 1976), 613-19.

A survey of the tumors found in the remains of ancient Egyptians shows evidence of osteomas, chondromas, chondrosarcomas, osteosarcomas, multiple myelomas, and metastatic carcinoma lesions in the bone. Only rarely do soft-tissue lesions appear in the mummified remains, although the multiple myelomas can leave behind evidence of their presence in the form of bone scarring and perforations.

Tkocz, Izabella and Franz Bierring. "A Medieval Case of Metastasizing Carcinoma with Multiple Osteosclerotic Bone Lesions." *American Journal of Physical Anthropology*, 65 (December 1984), 373-80.

Anthropologists in 1977 exhumed the skeletal remains of a man who died in 1470 in Svendborg, Denmark. He was an elderly man at the time of death and suffered from a widespread series of metastatic bone lesions, probably caused by prostate cancer.

Wells, Calvin. "Ancient Egyptian Pathology." *Journal of Laryngology and Oto-laryngology*, 77 (1963), 261-65.

The article describes the paleopathologic examination of the skull of a young Egyptian man who lived around 3,000 B. C. Radiologic analysis of the skull reveals widespread destruction of the maxillary, palatal, and pterygoid parts of the skull and metastatic lesions at other sites on the skull. The only conclusion can be that the young man suffered from a destructive nasopharyngeal carcinoma.

Wells, Calvin. "Two Mediaeval Cases of Malignant Disease." *British Medical Journal*, 5398 (1964), 1611-12.

Among paleopathologists evidence of neoplastic disease in ancient skeletons is rare, although most of the lesions discovered appear to have been nasopharyngeal in origin. The article describes two cases of multiple myelomatosis in the remains of fifteenth and sixteenth century individuals from Kent and Suffolk counties in England.

Werner-Brzezinska, H. "Pierwotne mięsaki kościopochodne leczone w Instytucie Onkologii w latach 1947-1970." *Nowotwory*, 1979, Supp. 117-21.

The article surveys the use of surgery, radiotherapy, and chemotherapy in the treatment of osteosarcomas, chondrosarcomas, Ewing's sarcoma, various soft-tissue sarcomas, and multiple myeloma at the Oncological Institute in Warsaw, Poland, between 1947 and 1970.

Williams, G. D., William A. Ritchie, and P. F. Titterington. "Multiple Bony Lesions Suggesting Myeloma in a Pre-Columbian Indian Aged 10 Years." *American Journal of Roentgenology*, 46 (1941), 351-55.

They report a possible case of multiple myeloma in the skeletal remains of a 10 year old American Indian boy living near Binghamton, New York, around 1200 A. D.

Vyhnanek, L. "Osteoma Ostoideum. Eine Kasuistik aus dem Fruhmittelalter-lichen Skelettmaterial." *Zeitsschrift für Orthopaedia und ihre Grenzgebiete*, 109 (November 1971), 922-23.

German paleoanthropologists have been able to identify tumor lesions in medieval skeletal remains. Most likely the afflicted individuals suffered from osteosarcomas and multiple myelomas.

Yamada, F. "A Story Inscribed in the Mandible." *Shikai Tenbo*, 64 (September 1984), 563-65.

Cancer was a disease of the ancient Japanese people as well as in modern society. Skeletal remains from the skull of a medieval man from central Japan indicate the presence of an invasive facial carcinoma or possibly, but less likely, a metastatic lesion from a different primary neoplasm.

10 Brain and Nervous System

"An Early Account of Meningioma." *Cancer Bulletin*, 9 (July-August 1957), 65.

(See Chapter 18: Netsky and Lapresle).

Bean, William B., Benjamin Felson, and Kenneth Dolan. "A Nonletter From the Editor and a Case for all Seasons." *Seminars in Roentgenology*, XVII (July 1982), 153-62.

(See Chapter 10: "Cancer Eponyms: von Recklinghausen's Disease" and Chapter 3: MERRICK, JOSEPH: Carswell).

Borit, A. "History of Tumors of the Pineal Region." *American Journal of Surgical Pathology*, 5 (September 1981), 613-20.

(See Chapter 10: Zulch).

Bucy, Paul C. "Glioblastomas." *Surgical Neurology*, 24 (November 1985), 589-90.

In 1936 Dr. K. G. McKenzie of Toronto provided the first surgical approach to glioblastomas, previously considered inoperable, terminal lesions. McKenzie's procedure was only palliative. He recommended removal of enough of the tumor to relieve intercranial pressure and allow the brain to settle back away from the dura. This would give the patient a few extra months of comfort and life. By the 1940s the advent of megavoltage radiotherapy techniques had given surgeons another approach to the glioblastoma, both pre-operatively to reduce a tumor and post-operatively to destroy occult tumor tissue and provide the margin of healthy tissue.

"Cancer Eponyms: von Recklinghausen's Disease." *Cancer Bulletin*, 7 (May-June 1955), 49.

Friedrich Daniel von Recklinghausen was born in Gutersloh, Westphalia, in 1833. He received a medical degree at the University of Berlin in 1855 and then studied under Rudolf Virchow. He was a professor of pathology and from 1872 to 1910 taught at the University of Strasbourg. Von Recklinghausen died in 1910. In 1882 he described the neurofibromatosis that now bears his name. It is an inherited disease in which tumors grow at the end of nerves, usually in the skin, and produce isolated, non-encapsulated nodules with pigmented deposits of melanin in the overlying epidermis. Tumors can also appear in the cranial cavity, spinal cord, thorax, retroperitoneal sympathetic nervous system, intestines, and pelvis. They are not only disfiguring but potentially life threatening because of damage they can do to internal organs.

"Cushing's Syndrome." *Cancer Bulletin*, 15 (May-June 1963), 45.

Harvey Cushing, the famed Harvard neurosurgeon, first described in 1932 the disease which now bears his name—hyperadrenocorticism caused by excess secretion from the pituitary gland. It is caused by a adenoma, carcinoma, bilateral hyperplasia, or unilateral hyperplasia. The clinical symptoms of Cushing's syndrome are protein depletion, shrinking of muscle mass, osteoporosis, hypertension, and peripheral edema.

Dehner, Louis P. "Classic Neuroblastoma: Histopathologic Grading as a Prognostic Indicator. The Shimada System and Its Progenitors." *The American Journal of Pediatric Hematology/Oncology*, 10 (1988), 143-54.

Classic neuroblastoma of adrenal or extra-adrenal origin is one of the most common solid tumors among children. Although neuroblastoma was first identified in the nineteenth century, histopathologic grading was a rather recent phenomenon. Until the 1960s neuroblastoma was simply viewed as an embryonal tumor arising in the sympathetic nervous system, adrenal medulla, and sympathetic ganglia from neural crest precusors. But histopathologic grading of neuroblastomas evolved as it became apparent that neuroblasts have the capacity to differentiate into ganglion cells and Schwann cells. Because most neuroblastic tumors have variable histologic features, early grading systems were subject to sampling errors and interobserver differences. It was generally acknowledged that the ganglioneuroblastomas have a better prognosis than the undifferentiated neuroblastoma, but the number and maturity of the ganglion cells in a particular tumor needed to designate a tumor as a ganglionblastoma were problematic. In 1984, however, Shimada offered a classification system to address those problems, differentiating between ganglioneuromas, ganglioneuroblastomas, and neuroblastomas by analyzing the maturity of the ganglion cells, the presence of discrete nodules of neuroblastomas, evidence of spindle-shaped cells with a pale-staining nucleus, fibrillary processes, and cellular groupings.

Ehring, F. "Geschichte der Dermatologie. Die Krankengeschichte der Abson-
    derlichen Kasslichen Haut des Johann Gottfried Rheinhardt, eines Mannes
    von 50 Jahren. Eine Neurofibromatose aus dem Jahre 1793." *Hautarzt*, 21
    (November 1970), 513-14.

(See Chapter 10: Fulton).

Emmanuel, I. G. "Symposium on Pituitary Tumours: Historical Aspects of Ra-
    diotherapy, Present Treatment and Results." *Clinical Radiology*, 17 (1966),
    154-60.

Victor Horsley in 1889 made the first unsuccessful attempt at removal of a
pituitary tumor, but between 1904 and 1906 he performed ten more operations,
and only two of the patients died. In 1907 Schloffer made the first successful partial removal of a pituitary tumor through the transsphenoidal approach. The first
successful use of radiotherapy on pituitary tumors came in 1909 when two French
physicians, Gramegna and Beclere, used an early Crooke's tube with a voltage not
exceeding 80 KV and a long glass cylinder used intraorally. They used the beam
on a 45 year old woman, treating her for one hour, twice a week, over a four-week
period. She experienced temporary regression of her tumor. Beclere later that
year used a five-field approach which looked forward to later beam directed radiotherapy. The patient, a 16 year old girl suffering from giantism, recovered and
was still alive thirteen years later. In 1925 Dott, Bailey, and Cushing advocated
post-operative radiotherapy for all pituitary patients as a means of reducing local
recurrence. They applied a radium source to the roof of the mouth. Rawlings first
reported the use of radon seeds in 1929. Although Cushing was an outstanding
surgeon, he became a strong advocate of adjuvant radiotherapy. In 1939 Henderson, after reviewing Cushing's patient records, began to advocate radiotherapy
as a necessary post-operative treatment to reduce local recurrence. By the 1940s
the treatment of choice for chromophobe adenoma was an intracranial surgical
resection followed by radiotherapy.

During the 1940s the era of megavoltage radiotherapy began. Linear accelerators, electron beams, cyclotrons, and synchrocyclotrons all had a great impact
on treatment of pituitary adenomas. By the 1960s some cancer centers were reporting a 90 percent recurrence-free rate in chromophobe adenomas treated with
surgery and radiotherapy.

"Eponym: Rathke's Pouch Tumor." *Cancer Bulletin*, 18 (March-April 1966),
    32-33.

Martin Heinrich Rathke was born in Danzig on August 25, 1793. He received
his M. D. degree at the University of Berlin in 1818. He practiced privately before
becoming a professor at the University of Dorpat in 1828. In 1835 Rathke joined
the faculty of the University of Konigsberg. He remained there until his death
on September 3, 1860. Widely considered the father of invertebrate embryology,
Rathke was responsible in 1838 for describing the congenital tumors arising from

the craniopharyngeal ducts between the pituitary and the pharynx. Not until the 1950s, with developments in surgery and endocrinology, was wide resection of the tumor feasible. Over the years the tumor has been known as Rathke's tumor, hypophyseal duct tumors, adamantinomas, ameloblastoma, and cranio-pharyngiomas.

Fulton, John F. "Robert W. Smith's Description of Generalized Neurofibromato-sis." *New England Journal of Medicine*, 200 (1929), 1315-17.

Neurofibromatosis was first observed by Johann Gottfried Rheinhardt in 1793, but its first general description came in 1849 with Robert W. Smith's observation of two cases. Smith was a physician in Dublin, Ireland. Although he had no idea of the etiology of the disease, his description of the systemic nature of the tumors was especially accurate.

Gans, Otto. "Ein Fall von Neurofibromatosis (morbus Recklinghausen) Dargestellt von J. de Ribera (1588-1656)." *Hautarzt*, 30 (July 1969), 332-33.

The author describes a seventeenth century case of von Recklinghausen's tu-mor tumor observed by the Italian physician Ribera.

German, William J., and Stevenson Flanigan. "Pituitary Adenomas: A Follow-Up Study of the Cushing Series." *Clinical Neurosurgery*, 10 (1964), 72-81.

In 1939 W. R. Henderson published a follow-up on the brain surgeries of famed surgeon Harvey Cushing. Between 1905 and 1932 Cushing performed 338 oper-ations for pituitary tumors at the Peter Bent Brigham Hospital associated with Harvard University. The series ended in 1932 before the advent of chemotherapy or blood banks. Most of the tumors were chromophobes. The surgical mortality rate was 2.4 percent in the last ten years of the series, compared to 6.3 percent in the beginning. Intracranial tumor extensions were the most common cause of op-erative deaths. Hematoma was the greatest hazard after frontal operations, while meningitis was the culprit after the transsphenoidal approach. The death rate for patients with acromegaly was higher than for the patients with chromophobes. In 1957 there were 39 patients still alive, and most of them had received a frontal surgery rather than the transsphenoidal.

Giuffre, Renato. "Successful Radical Removal of an Intracranial Meningioma in 1835 by Professor Pecchioli of Siena." *Journal of Neurosurgery*, 60 (January 1984), 47-51.

In 1835 Zanobi Pecchioli, professor of surgery and operating medicine at the University of Siena, removed a meningioma. The lesion was a large ulcerated cranial outgrowth at the level of the right sinciput, which at the time of the operation proved to originate from the dura mater and to be eroding the bone. Surgery was radical. The patient recovered and attended for follow-up review several times in the course of thirty months, with no sign of recurrence. The procedure was later selected for the competition for the chair of surgery at the University of Paris in 1840.

Horwitz, Norman H. "Sir Geoffrey Jefferson on Invasive Pituitary Adenomas." *Journal of Neurosurgery*, 42 (February 1975), 244.

In 1940 Sir Geoffrey Jefferson made his presidential address to the Royal Society of Medicine in Great Britain, in which he spoke of his experience with invasive adenomas of the anterior pituitary. His work was important for two reasons: he described the clinical symptoms of individuals suffering from this tumor, making diagnosis easier, and he showed that the operative mortality in these patients increases tenfold when compared with patients suffering from localized pituitary tumors.

Kirkpatrick, Douglas B. "The First Primary Brain-Tumor Operation." *Journal of Neurosurgery*, 61 (November 1984), 809-13.

On November 25, 1884, Dr. Rickman J. Godlee performed the first recognized resection of a primary brain tumor. He was at the Hospital for Epilepsy and Paralysis in London. Godlee found an encapsulated glioma and removed it, although the patient died nearly a month later of meningitis and secondary complications. An autopsy revealed no remnant of the excised glioma. The operation was widely reported in the British press because such surgery was extraordinary at the time. The science of neurological function and localization was quite primitive; the principles of microbiology and antisepsis were only beginning to be understood; and there was no clinical precedent for operating on a normal-appearing skull in order to manipulate the enclosed brain, and such a bold step was guaranteed to attract medical interest as well as criticism. The surgery proved to be a pioneering step in surgery as well as in the nuerosciences.

Klawans, Harold L. "The Acromegaly of Maximinus I: The Possible Influence of a Pituitary Tumor on the Life and Death of a Roman Emperor." In F. Clifford Rose and W. F. Bynum. *Historical Aspects of the Neurosciences.* New York: 1982. Pp. 317-26.

(See Chapter 3: Maximinus I).

Kramer, W. "On the Classification of Tumours of the Peripheral Nervous System." *Psychiatria, Neurologia, Neurochirurgia*, 72 (1969), 65-75.

Rudolf Virchow in 1863 first provided a classification of nervous system tumors based on their cellular structure rather than clinical characteristics. Since then several important steps in histological studies have been taken. The first was the realization that the cells of peripheral nervous system tumors are derived from Schwann cells and not from fibrocytes of the coverings of the nerves. The second step was J. Verocay's recognition of the neuroectodermal origin of the tumors on a histological level. The third step was Verocay's realization that connective tissues are often involved in peripheral nervous system tumors. Contemporary classification systems are based on the following fundamental assumptions:

1. A regional classification in terminal and central neurinomata has little value for determining the course of the disease or the prognosis.

2. A histologic classification based on the tissues from which the tumor arises is the essential element of successful tumor classification. Currently thirteen types of tumors of the peripheral nervous system are identified: neuroma, neurinoma, neurofibroma, fibroma, melanoma, glomus tumor, leiomyoma, haemangioma, lipoma, ganglioneuroma, pheochromocytoma, paraganglioma, and glioma.

3. An etiologic classification is still not possible because of the variety of carcinogenic agents which trigger the transformation of normal tissues into neoplasms.

4. Clinical data is not really helpful in creating a useful classification system.

Ljunggren, Bengt. "The Case of George Gershwin." *Neurosurgery*, 10 (June 1982), 733-36.

(See Chapter 3: Ljunggren).

Mironovich, N. I. "Pervye operatsii meningiom golovnogo mozga v rossi." *Voprosy Nierokhirurgiia*, 30 (November-December 1966), 50-51.

The article briefly recounts the early history of neurosurgery in the Soviet Union.

Molina-Negro, Pedro. "Jules Hardy, M.D." *Surgical Neurology*, 22 (August 1984), 109-12.

(See Chapter 3: HARDY, JULES: Molina-Negro).

Netsky, Martin G. and Jean Lapresle. "The First Account of a Meningioma." *Bulletin of the History of Medicine*, 30 (1956), 465-68.

Felix Platter (1536-1614) was a professor of medicine at the University of Basel. After an autopsy on Casper Benecurtius, Platter attributed death to an encapsulated brain tumor the size of a "medium-sized apple." Physicians today would describe the tumor as a parasagittal meningioma. Platter was the first individual to describe such a tumor.

Onuigbo, Wilson I. E. "Historical Errors in Neuroblastoma Literature." *Indian Journal of the History of Medicine*, 15 (June 1970), 20-22.

Neuroblastomas usually occur in very young children and originate in the neural crest progenitors of the sympathetic nervous system and the adrenal medulla. Historically they have been very difficult to diagnose because they are characterized by a high rate of spontaneous regression in infancy. The tumor has symptoms similar to Horner's syndrome and leukemia. Histogenically the tumor is easily confused with some other small round cell childhood tumors like Ewing's sarcoma, lymphoma, soft-tissue sarcoma, and peripheral neuroepitheliomas.

Pearce, J. M. S. "The First Attempt at Removal of Brain Tumors." In F. Clifford Rose and W. F. Bynum. *Historical Aspects of the Neurosciences*. New York: 1982. Pp. 239-42.

In 1879 William Macewen, a surgeon at the Royal Infirmary in Glasgow, Scotland, removed a tumor from the left frontal lobe of 14 year old girl. She survived for eight years. In 1884 Rickman J. Godlee of the Hospital for Epilepsy and Paralysis in London, removed a tumor from the brain cortex of a 22 year old man. The patient died four weeks later of post-operative infection. Nevertheless, Rickman Godlee's operation was a landmark in the history of neurosurgery.

Satoh, O. "Transsphenoidal Surgery for Pituitary Adenomas: Historical Review and Present Trends." *No Shinkei Geka*, 12 (January 1984), 7-26.

(See Chapter 23: Satoh).

van Heerden, Jonathan A. "First Encounters With Pheochromocytoma." *American Journal of Surgery*, 144 (August 1982), 277-79.

The first successful resection of a pheochromocytoma was performed by Roux in Lausanne, Switzerland, in 1926, and the first such procedure in the United States was performed shortly thereafter by C. H. Mayo at the Mayo Clinic. The patient was Mother Joachim, a Roman Catholic nun who came to the clinic suffering from headaches, fatigue, severe hypertension, and nausea. Exploratory surgery revealed a lemon-sized tumor on the left adrenal, which Mayo felt resembled a brain tumor. He performed the resection and the tumor proved to be a malignant enlargement of the ganglion resting on a renal vessel. After the operation the patient recovered from the symptoms and survived for 18 years.

Wilkins, R. H. and I. A. Brody. "Von Recklinghausen's Neurofibromatosis." *Archives of Neurology*, 24 (April 1971), 374-77.

(See Chapter 10: "Cancer Eponyms: von Recklinghausen's Disease").

Zanca, Attilio, and Andrea Zanca. "Antique Illustrations of Neurofibromatosis." *International Journal of Dermatology*, 19 (January/February 1980), 55-58.

Friedrich Daniel von Recklinghausen gave a classic description in 1882 of neurofibromatosis, and eventually the illness became known as Recklinghausen's disease. The first description of the disease had been given by Robert William Smith in 1849, but von Recklinghausen's analysis had more scientific detail. Centuries before, however, there were descriptions of a disease which was probably neurofibromatosis. Ulisse Aldrovandi, a Bolognese physician, described a patient with the disease in 1592. Ambroise Paré, the French surgeon, wrote in 1578 about a patient with "hornlike growth and fleshy masses all over his body," which was probably a case of neurofibromatosis. Medieval literature also contains a number of descriptions of the disease. People suffering from neurofibromatosis were regularly described as "monsters."

Zulch, K. J. "Historical Development of the Classification of Brain Tumours and the New Proposal of the World Health Organization (WHO)." *Neurosurgical Review*, 4 (1981), 123-27.

In 1911 Bielschowsky first devised a classification system for tumors of the neuronal cells, and in 1918 Ribbert first described the different stages of maturation of the gliomas: spongioneuroblastoma to spongioblastoma to glioblastoma to neuroblastoma. In the 1920s Bailey began describing the cell types present in brain tumors.

Zulch, K. J. "Reflections on the Surgery of the Pineal Gland (A Glimpse Into the Past)." *Neurosurgical Review*, 4 (1981), 159-62.

The first attempt to remove a pineal gland tumor was by the English surgeon C. Brunner in 1913, who approached the tumor surgically through the corpus callosum, still the preferred technique. The first successful removal of a pineal gland tumor was also in 1913. Later studies on dogs in the 1920s improved the technique. By the 1930s the era of routine removal of pineal and quadrigeminal tumors had arrived.

11 Breast

Allison, Marvin J., et al. "Metastatic Tumor of Bone in a Tiahuanaco Female." *Bulletin of the New York Academy of Medicine*, 56 (July-August 1980), 581-87.

(See Chapter 9: Allison).

Austoker, J. L. "The 'Treatment of Choice': Breast Cancer Surgery 1860-1985." *Society for the Social History of Medicine Bulletin*, 37 (December 1985), 100-07.

(See Chapter 11: Handley).

Bloom, H. J. G., W. W. Richardson, and E. J. Harries. "Natural History of Untreated Breast Cancer (1805-1933)." *British Medical Journal*, 2 (July 28, 1962), 213-21.

The paper presents a series of 250 cases of untreated breast cancer at the Middlesex Hospital in Great Britain between 1805 and 1933; correlates the histological grade of the tumor in 86 patients for whom tissue sections survive; and compares survival rates with those of patients receiving treatment. Treatment increases the survival rate for all three stages of disease, especially in patients with high-grade malignancies.

Braithwaite, Peter Allen and Shugg, Dace. "Rembrandt's Bathsheba: The Dark Shadow of the Left Breast." *Annals of the Royal College of Surgeons of England*, 65 (1983), 337-38.

Hendrickje Stoffels, Rembrandt's mistress and model for the painting "Bathsheba at Her Toilet," may have been suffering from a breast carcinoma. The painting indicates skin discoloration, distortion of symmetry with axillary fulness, and peau d'orange. She died in 1663, nine years after the painting, perhaps of disseminated breast cancer.

Caffaratto, T. M. "Patología e clínica del carcinoma mammario." *Minerva Ginecologica*, 36 (December 1984), 891-910.

(See Chapter 11: De Moulin).

Cutter, Max. "Conservative Radical Mastectomy." *Journal of the International College of Surgeons*, 44 (December 1965), 697-701.

The modern groundwork for the radical mastectomy began in 1700 when Jean Louis Petit, first director of the French Surgical Academy, advised removal of the axilla and pectoral fascia in breast cancer cases. In 1870 Lord Lister divided the pectoralis major and minor to gain access to the axilla. At the same time the German surgeons Volkmann and Heidenhain removed both pectoral muscles. In 1894 came the Halsted mastectomy. By 1945 two opposite trends were at work. In 1947 Andreassen and Dahl-Iversen of Copenhagen and in 1949 Margottini and Bucalossi of Rome began performing superradical mastectomies by removing the parasternal lymph nodes as well. That was abandoned in 1959. The other trend was toward more conservative surgery. The author advocates the Halsted mastectomy with preservation of the pectoralis major muscle, like the conservative radical mastectomy developed by Patey. Its benefits are primarily cosmetic by eliminating the hollow deformity below the clavical. It leaves a stronger arm with less likelihood of edema, without any greater chance of local recurrence.

Dalton, Martin L. and Karl H. Grozinger. "Curt Schimmelbusch and Schimmelbusch's Disease." *Surgery*, 63 (May 1968), 859-61.

Curt Schimmelbusch was born in western Prussia in 1860. He received his medical degree from the University of Würzburg in 1882 and later specialized in bacteriology. He worked at the University of Berlin Clinic and died of tuberculosis in 1895. In 1892, Schimmelbusch created the term "cystadenoma" to describe cystic breast disease. It is characterized by multiple epithelial cysts spread over the breasts and complete mobility of the skin over the diseased breast. It can be a precancerous lesion.

d'Auteuil, Pierre and J. Lemay. "La thérapeutique endocrinienne du cancer
    du sein: Un historique." *Union médicale du Canada*, 114 (February 1985),
    139-45.

Hormonal therapy for treatment of breast cancer began in 1896 when George
Beatson of Glasgow first described the tumor regression he had achieved in women
with metastatic breast carcinoma by removing their ovaries. Beatson found the
surgery effective in premenopausal women. In 1905 H. Lett described the temporary remission of tumors in one-third of his patients suffering from inoperable
breast cancer after oophorectomy. The procedure was largely abandoned until
the 1930s, and by the 1950s it was clinically clear that endocrine therapy for
pre-menopausal breast cancer patients could be beneficial in achieving tumor regression.

De Moulin, Daniel. *A Short History of Breast Cancer*. Amsterdam: 1983.

    (See Chapter 11: De Moulin).

De Moulin, Daniel. "Historical Notes on Breast Cancer. Emphasis on The
    Netherlands. I. Pathological and Therapeutic Concepts in the Seventeenth
    Century." *The Netherlands Journal of Surgery*, 32 (1980), 129-34.

For centuries, interest in cancer in general focused primarily on breast cancer because the disease was so visible and so deadly. Not until the nineteenth
century developments in anesthesia and antisepsis, which permitted surgeons to
treat internal lesions, did concern for cancer begin to include other types of the
disease. At the beginning of the seventeenth century, the prevailing explanation
for cancer was the humoral pathology first developed by the Roman physician
Galen. He attributed cancer to an excess of "black bile." By the beginning of the
nineteenth century, belief in humoral pathology had given way to the more modern concept of cellular pathology. In the two hundred years between the belief in
humoral pathology and the belief in cellular pathology, several other theories explaining the causes of cancer competed for supremacy in the medical community.
The "iatromechanical school" argued that all physical and chemical processes in
the human body were brought on by the motion of atomic particles. Cancers
developed when blockages occurred in the motion of these particles. Friedrich
Hoffmann (1660-1742), a professor of medicine at Halle, was a leading advocate
of the iatromechanical school. The "iatrochemical school," led by Leyden professor Francois de le Boe Sylvius (1614-1672), attached great importance to the
lymphatic system, arguing that changes in the nature of lymphatic fluids toward
an acidic base caused cancer. It was called acrimony. Claude Deshais Gendron
(1663-1750), a renowned physician in Paris, argued that cancers were "nerve-
like and gland-like" parts which had turned into hard, cold masses which sent
out "roots" and grew into surrounding tissues. Gendron denied the acrimony or
lymphatic notions and argued that only removal of the mass could effect a cure.
Adrian Helvetius (1661-1741), a Dutch physician, argued that cancer was caused

by an external trauma, and he claimed that surgery was the only hope. It was widely held in the seventeenth century that cancer was contagious and the idea of metastasis was not known. As for treatment, physicians who believed in the acidic theory usually prescribed alkaline solutions topically to the tumor, especially an arsenic lotion. Those who believed in solid tumors were inclined toward mastectomies.

De Moulin, Daniel. "Historical Notes on Breast Cancer, With Emphasis on The Netherlands. II. Pathophysiological Concepts, Diagnosis and Therapy in the 18th Century." *The Netherlands Journal of Surgery*, 33 (October 1981), 206-16.

In the eighteenth century steady improvements were made in clinical diagnosis and in surgical technique, with developments in France having the greatest impact on Dutch physicians. But in terms of etiology, change was very slow. The old Galenic distinction between cancer and scirrhus still held, and most argued that cancer was caused by an external blow or humoral imbalances in the body. Boerhaave thought that a special nerve secretion mixed with mammary secretions caused breast cancer. Others attributed breast cancer to daily predisposition, childlessness, lack of exercise, and menopause. Although the concept of metastasis was not really understood, physicians were studying the relationships between primary tumors and secondary deposits. Morgagni carefully noticed the consistent axilla deposits in breast cancer victims.

Diagnosis of breast cancer was not difficult since most women with the disease went to a physician only after the tumor had ulcerated through the skin and was causing pain. Treatment involved mechanical manipulation and compression to dilute or displace the corrupting fluids, a variety of poultices and chemical applications, special diets, laxatives, and mastectomy. The leading advocate of breast surgery was L. Heister.

De Moulin, Daniel. "Historical Notes on Breast Cancer, With Emphasis on The Netherlands. III. The Growth of Scientific Surgery in the 19th Century." *The Netherlands Journal of Surgery*, 34 (December 1982), 193-200.

The introduction of anesthetics (1847) and antisepsis (1867), the use of the microscope and the rise of cellular pathology, the development of bacteriology, and a scientific attitude toward statistical data all paved the way for dramatic improvements in surgical treatment in the nineteenth century. Late in the 1830s a Leyden physician, Herman Luhrman, offered a histological description of a breast carcinoma. Johanne Schrant (1823-1864) provided a variety of descriptions of microscopic cancer tissues. Ludovicus van der Kolk in the 1850s described finding clincally occult cancer cells in healthy tissue at a distance from a primary breast tumor. He recommended that surgeons make wider excisions in removing breast tumor. After the establishment of antisepsis in the 1870s, breast cancer surgery began to increase in magnitude. In 1880 Richard Volkman recommended clearance of the whole fossa axillaris in the presence of palpable nodes, along with removal of the diseased breast. Halsted introduced his radical mastectomy in the 1890s. In The Netherlands, the most important cancer surgeon at the time was Johannes Korteweg at Leyden University. Radiotherapy of breast cancer first appeared in The Netherlands in 1903 with the work of D. H. van der Goot.

Egan, Robert L. "Evolution of the Team Approach in Breast Cancer." *Cancer; Diagnosis, Treatment, Research,* 36 (November 1975), 1815-22.

(See Chapter 22: Puretz).

Farrow, Joseph H. "Antiquity of Breast Cancer." *Cancer,* 28 (December 1971), 1369-71.

Farrow provides a brief outline history of the treatment of breast cancer, from its first discovery among the Egyptians, surgical excisions among the Greeks and Romans, the evolution of the mastectomy in the nineteenth century, and the development of the oophorectomy, radiotherapy, and hormone therapy. He praises the value of the radical mastectomy and questions current trends toward lesser procedures for which clinical evidence is incomplete.

Fiks, Arsen. "Cystosarcoma Phylloides of the Mammary Gland—Müller's Tumor." *Virchows Archives,* 392 (1981), 1-6.

In 1838 Johannes Müller provided the classical description of cystosarcoma phylloides, today classified as tumor phylloides, of the breast. The lesion has been difficult to classify, and 62 separate synonyms have been used since 1824 to describe it. Today, it is known that there are benign, premalignant, and malignant forms of the lesion. Histological evaluations must consider the degree of maturity of the mesenchymal component.

Fisher, Bernard. "The Revolution in Breast Cancer Surgery: Science or Anecdotalism." *World Journal of Surgery,* 9 (1985), 655-66.

(See Chapter 11: Fisher and Gebhardt).

Fisher, Bernard, and Mark C. Gebhardt. "The Evolution of Breast Cancer Surgery: Past, Present, and Future." *Seminars in Oncology,* 5 (December 1978), 385-94.

Although the mastectomy had been performed episodically in treating breast cancer for thousands of years, it was not until the 1890s that William Stewart Halsted of the Johns Hopkins University systematically developed the surgical procedure. He believed that metastasis in breast cancer occurred through the lymphatic system, not through the bloodstream, and that surgeons should remove the primary tumor by amputating the breast and the regional lymphatics and lymph nodes by an *en bloc* dissection. Halsted's surgery was based on two suppositions: that breast cancer was primarily a local disease until delays in treatment allowed it to metastasize, and that the lymphatic system provided an effective barrier, for a matter of time at least, to the passage of tumor cells. For the next 75 years the Halsted radical mastectomy was the "treatment of choice" for breast cancer.

But in the 1970s the zenith occurred in cancer surgery based on anatomical principles. New understanding of tumor biology and immunology have changed treatment approaches. The major new concepts are:

1. Most, if not all, patients with solid tumors have disseminated disease by the time a clinical diagnosis is established. The fact that some patients are "cured" by operation alone is no indication that the surgery eradicated every cancer cell, that the disease was completely local-regional in extent, and that dissemination had not yet taken place. The residual tumor-cell burden may have been sufficiently minimal for its eradication by host factors.

2. The lymphatic system probably does not serve as a block to the passage of tumor cells. Indeed, the lymphatic system and bloodstream are both vascular systems so intertwined that it is no longer realistic to consider them independently as routes of neoplastic dissemination.

3. Negative lymph nodes on dissection do not just mean that tumor cell dissemination had not yet occurred. It would seem that patients with negative nodes have a better prognosis than those with positive nodes because such nodal status reflects host conditions which in addition to preventing growth of tumor in nodes also prevent distant metastases.

4. Breast cancer is a heterogeneous group of cancers of the breast residing in a heterogeneous group of women. As a consequence of the multiple host-tumor permutations, consideration of the natural history of breast cancer as a single phenomenon is an anachronism.

The modern burden of surgical oncology, therefore, is to reduce the tumor burden to a number of viable cells that are entirely destroyable by host immunologic factors, chemotherapy, or a combination of both. As systemic therapy becomes more effective, it is likely that less radical surgical procedures will be employed.

Fletcher, Gilbert H. "History of Irradiation in the Primary Management of Apparently Regionally Confined Breast Cancer." *International Journal of Radiation Oncology, Biology, and Physics*, 11 (December 1985), 2133-2142.

(See Chapter 24: Fletcher).

Gilbertsen, V. A. "Beatson's Contribution to Cancer Research." *Surgo*, 32 (1964), 17-19.

(See Chapter 11: Goldenberg).

Goldenberg, Ira S. "Hormones and Breast Cancer: Historical Perspectives."
    Surgery, 53 (February 1963), 285-88.

In 1889 A. Schinzinger of Germany first noted that the prognosis was poor
in young breast cancer patients and a little better in post-menopausal women.
He advocated removal of the ovaries to "bring about breast atrophy," which he
felt would also shrink tumors. At the same time Scottish surgeon G. T. Beatson
came to the same conclusion. Soon castration was widely used for women with
inoperable lesions. In 1905 Foveau de Courmelles of France began radiation castration. After World War II Charles Huggins of Chicago used adrenalectomy and
hypophysectomy for advanced breast cancer. About 20 to 30 percent of women
with breast cancer will improve with such treatment.

Goldwyn, Robert M. "Theodore Gaillard Thomas and the Inframammary Inci-
    sion." *Plastic and Reconstructive Surgery*, 76 (September 1985), 475-77.

In 1882 Theodore Thomas wrote a landmark article first proposing use of the
inframammary incision to remove benign breast tumors because the surgery left
few visible scars or depressions and removed patient anxiety. At the time surgeons
did not perform excisions on benign tumors because of the poor cosmetic results.
Thomas argued that the new procedure would remove the lesion, relieve patient
anxiety about the presence of the tumor, and achieve acceptable cosmetic results.

Greco, T. "Rembrandt e il cancro della mammella." *Ospital Italien Chirurgia*,
    22 (February 1970), 141-44.

(See Chapter 11: Braithwaite and Shugg).

Gruber, D., R. Hofmann, and E. Ehler. "Cancer Mammarum Infructose Extir-
    patus bei C. E. Eschenbach 1755." *Zentralblatt für Chirurgie*, 96 (30 October
    1971), 1526-30.

Recognizing that the only hope for a cure of breast cancer was elimination of
the lesion, German physician, C.E. Eschenbach surgically excised a large breast
carcinoma from a young female patient in 1755. He also noticed hard masses of
tissue in the axilla, indicating lymphatic involvement.

Handley, R. S. "Gordon-Taylor, Breast Cancer and the Middlesex Hospital."
    Annals of the Royal College of Surgeons of England, 49 (September 1971),
    151-64.

Cancer research began at Middlesex Hospital in 1792 when a charity cancer
ward was opened at the suggestion of surgeon John Howard. Howard especially
wanted accurate records of each case maintained and clinical trials of new treatment methods. Breast cancer was most commonly treated. Abandoned treatments included freezing tumors, applications of condurango bark and turpentine,

and compression of the tumor. In the 1860s Dr. Charles Moore suggested that localized recurrence of breast carcinoma was the result of inadequate surgical excision, not to a general constitutional change in the patient or any special predisposition of healthy breast tissue to transform itself into tumor. He wanted wide excision of the tumor as a whole, not any cutting into the tumor, and irrigating the wound with zinc chloride. In the 1890s and early 1900s W. S. Handley argued that breast cancer spreads in a centrifugal manner by direct growth of columns of cancer cells in all directions from the primary tumor, along the lymphatics, the rear of the columns being strangled by fibrous tissue. His theory has not stood the test of time as the master process by which cancer spreads, but it is still true of the way in which carcinoma cells spread when the usual lymphatic channels have been blocked by the proliferation of cancer cells in the draining nodes. The theory led to modification of the Halsted mastectomy by suggesting that less skin and more subcutaneous tissues should be removed by fashioning skin flaps. It is still practiced today. Sir Gordon Gordon-Taylor advocated radical surgery and doubted the efficacy of radiotherapy in early stage breast carcinoma.

Helman, Paul, and M. B. Bennett. "Role Played by the Breast Clinic Groote Schuur Hospital in the Control of Breast Cancer." *South African Journal of Surgery*, 16 (June 1978), 103-09.

The article reviews the history of breast cancer treatment at the Groote Schuur Hospital in South Africa: use of the Halsted radical mastectomy, the rise of radiotherapeutic techniques, the switch to the modified radical mastectomy in the 1960s and 1970s, and the development of hormonal and chemotherapy. The hospital has also played a central role in public health education movements, encouraging breast self-examination and later mammograms for early diagnosis.

"The History of Mammography." *Cancer Bulletin*, 17 (July-August 1965), 84-85.

In 1913 Albert Salomon published his study of roentgenographic examination of 3,000 amputated breasts, hoping to identify identifiable characteristics of carcinomas. S. L. Warren published similar reports on 119 patients in 1930. In 1951 R. Leborgue of Uruguay described the multiple punctate calcifications which are almost pathognomonic of a malignant tumor. In 1960 R. L. Egan of M. D. Anderson Hospital and Tumor Institute in Houston began the modern era of mammography.

Huard, Paul. "Velpeau, cancérologue." *Congrès National des Societies Savantes.* II (1968), 159-62.

Alfred Velpeau was born in France in 1795 and eventually became one of Europe's most prominent surgeons. In 1858 Velpeau began to advocate a much wider surgical excision for breast cancer, including removal of the breast and the underlying pectoral muscle. Velpeau's assumptions and recommendations hinted at the work which American surgeon William Halsted would develop in the 1890s.

Hutter, Robert V. P. "Lobular Carcinoma *in Situ*." *CA-A Cancer Journal for Clinicians*, 32 (July-August 1982), 232-33.

In 1919 James Ewing first described premalignant changes in breast tissue, and in 1932 Broder introduced the term "carcinoma *in situ*" to describe the neoplastic transformation of epithelial cells which remain confined by a basement membrane at their site of origin. In 1941 Foote and Stewart named and described these cancerous changes of the lobules of the breast as "loublar carcinoma *in situ*" and Muir independently used the term "intra-acinar carcinoma" for them. Foote and Stewart also described the characteristic appearance of the invasive form of lobular carcinoma and nodal metastases. They also recognized the multicentricity of the lesion and said that they arose from terminal ducts. Treatment of the disease has been very controversial. Some researchers report that more than 90 percent of the cases of lobular carcinoma *in situ* are multicentric, and that more than a third are bilateral. They advocate mastectomy as the treatment of choice. Others call for less mutilating treatment, especially frequent follow-ups to make sure the lesion does not become invasive.

Jensen, Elwood V. "Hormone Dependency of Human Breast Cancers." *Cancer*, 46 (December 15, 1980), 2759-61.

Some breast cancers are hormone-dependent—growth depends on a continued supply of female sex hormones. That relationship was first suggested in 1836. In 1896 G. T. Beatson performed oophorectomies for young women with metastatic lesions and saw striking regressions in many of them. The highest incidence of breast cancer is in postmenopausal women where the ovaries no longer produce significant levels of steroid hormones. For some of them removal of the adrenal glands had similar results. In 1953 it was proven that removal of the pituitary gland was effective. Today hypophysectomy and adrenalectomy are reserved for patients with skin or lymph node metastases or long intervals between the mastectomy and the appearance of metastases. Brain and abdominal metastases do not respond. Breast cancers which show low estrogen binding or lacking cytosolic estrogen receptors rarely respond to endocrine therapy.

Kambouris, Angelos A. "The Current Controversies in Surgical Management of Early Breast Cancer." *Henry Ford Hospital Medical Journal*, 32 (1984), 39-45.

The Halsted radical mastectomy retains its primacy for 75 years, even though cure rates for breast cancer leveled out and did not improve after the early 1940s. By the 1950s debate concerning treatment of early stage breast carcinoma centered around three issues: 1) preservation of the pectoralis major and minor muscles through use of a modified radical mastectomy; 2) skepticism about the "mechanistic" theories in favor of the argument that breast cancer is essentially a systemic disease requiring systemic therapies, regardless of the surgical treatment of the primary lesion; and 3) the role of radiotherapy in association with modified mastectomies as a means of controlling local recurrences and preserving tissue. By the 1980s the following approaches were emerging: 1) modified radical mastectomy is best for Stage 1 breast cancer; 2) radiotherapy and breast-preserving procedures are equally effective in treating Stage 1 tumors, although longer follow-up periods are necessary; 3) selection of breast-preservation approaches is made for cosmetic and psychological reasons, not because of superior results; 4) patients with noninvasive, multicentric, bilateral, and familial breast cancers are not considered good candidates for breast-preserving approaches; 5) modified radical mastectomy is superior to treat Stage II breast cancers, with adjuvant chemotherapy also employed; 6) when radiotherapy is used as a primary modality for Stage II disease, local-regional failure is high, often requiring salvage mastectomies; and 7) careful patient selection is required for less radical approaches to early stage breast carcinoma.

Kleinmann, Ruth. "Facing Cancer in the Seventeenth Century: The Last Illness of Anne of Austria, 1664-1666." *Advances in Thanatology*, 4 (1978), 37-55.

(See Chapter 3: ANNE OF AUSTRIA: Kleinmann).

Lewison, Edward F. "Breast Cancer Surgery from Halsted to 1972." *Proceedings of the National Cancer Conference*, 7 (1973), 275-79.

The major developments in the history of breast cancer surgery are: 1) the appearance of the radical mastectomy by William Halsted in the 1880s; 2) the rise of the superradical mastectomy by Urban, Margottini, and Veronesi in the late 1940s and 1950s; and 3) the growing popularity of the simple mastectomy combined with radiotherapy in the 1960s and 1970s.

MacMahon, Charles E., and John L. Cahill. "The Evolution of the Concept of the Use of Surgical Castration in the Palliation of Breast Cancer in Pre-Menopausal Females." *Annals of Surgery*, 184 (December 1976), 713-16.

Astley Cooper in 1836 described the metastatic lesions of breast cancer and their likelihood of spreading to the lung, vertebra, and ovary, along with "an increase in size of the primary lesion premenstrually with some diminution in the size after cessation of the menses." A. Schinzinger of Friedborg, Germany, noted in 1889 that the survival rates for breast carcinoma were worse among younger victims, and speculated that castration might prematurely age the patient and cause a shrinkage of all breast tissue, malignant as well as normal. The birth of hormonal therapy for breast cancer, however, began with the work of George Thomas Beatson of Glasgow, Scotland. Early in his career, Beatson learned that lactating cattle, if their ovaries were removed, would continue giving milk all of their lives. He also noted histologic changes in the lactating breast after pregnancy, especially the proliferation of epithelial cells, and thought they resembled carcinoma cells. In 1895 he performed a bilateral oophorectomy on a young woman with advanced, inoperable, ulcerating breast carcinoma. She initially underwent a complete regression of the tumor, although it recurred nearly four years later and killed her. Oophorectomy became very common between 1900 and 1910, declining then when ovarian radiation became more common. Not until 1953, when Charles Huggins explained the benefits of oophorectomy and adrenalectomy, did surgical castration become common again for treatment of advanced, premenopausal breast carcinoma.

Mansfield, C. M. "Early Breast Cancer, Its History and Results of Treatment." *Experimental Biology and Medicine*, 5 (1976), 1-129.

(See Chapter 11: Kampouris).

Mendelson, B. C. "The Evolution of Breast Reconstruction." *The Medical Journal of Australia*, 9 (January 9, 1982), 7-8.

The first breast reconstruction was performed by Vincenz Czerny at the University of Heidelberg in 1895. He transplanted a lipoma from the hip. Sir Harold Gillies, the father of British plastic surgery, using the tubed abdominal flap method, began breast reconstruction in 1942, but it required six operations over the course of six months. In 1964, with the advent of the silicone gel mammary prosthesis, a one-step reconstruction was possible for simple mastectomy patients when enough skin was left. In 1973 T. D. Cronin of the United States perfected the nipple-areolar complex reconstruction using skin from a transverse thoracoepigastric flap taken from below the breast. However, there were still a series of delaying preliminary operations. By 1979 the German surgeons H. Hohler and H. Bohmert had developed a two-step procedure: transposed thoracoepigastric flap (without delay) and insertion of the mammary prosthesis as the second procedure.

Meyer, Kenneth and William C. Beck. "Mastectomy Performed by Laurence Heister in the Eighteenth Century." *Surgery, Gynecology & Obstetrics*, 159 (October 1984), 391-94.

In 1720 Laurence Heister, a Dutch physician, performed a mastectomy for removal of a large tumor. He was aware that the tumor did not adhere to other tissues and did not involve the axilla. It was probably not malignant but a cytosarcoma phylloides.

Murley, Reginald. "Breast Cancer: Keynes and Conservatism." *The British Journal of Clinical Practice*, 40 (February 1986), 49-58.

Geoffrey Keynes of the St. Bartholomew's Hospital pioneered the idea of using radiotherapy instead of or in addition to radical surgery for the treatment of breast cancer in the 1930s. One of his associates, Robert McWhirter, by the late 1930s was advocating simple mastectomy and radiotherapy instead of the Halsted radical mastectomy because he felt long-term survival rates were the same while quality of life was substantially improved. Keynes's work inspired a new approach to breast cancer treatment by the 1950s, with the radical mastectomy declining somewhat in use and simple mastectomies or local excisions combined with radiotherapy increased. The development of megavoltage external electron beam therapy in the 1950s and 1960s strengthened that approach. The routine use of oophorectomy, adrenalectomy, and hypophysectomy in pre-menopausal women also declined unless distant metastases were already clinically evident.

Murley, Reginald. "Breast Cancer: Keynes and Conservatism." *Transactions of the Medical Society*, 99-100 (1982-1984), 1-13.

(See Chapter 11: Murley).

Mustacchi, P. "Ramazzini and Rigoni-Stern on Parity and Breast Cancer." *Archives of Internal Medicine*, 108 (1961), 639-42.

(See Chapter 5: Scotto and Bailar).

Onuigbo, Wilson I. B. "Paget's 1874 Article on the Breast: Modern Misconceptions." *International Journal of Dermatology*, 24 (October 1975), 537-38.

In 1874 James Paget first described carcinoma of the nipple and areola. He believed that overt skin lesions brought about the underlying cancer, not that the cancer was the cause of the skin lesion.

Perel, Level. "Conception pathogénique et traitement du cancer du sein au 18eme siècle." In *Congrès International d'Histoire de la Medecine*. Québec: 1976. Pp. 1073-80.

(See Chapter 11: De Moulin).

Perel, Level. "Historique de la reconstruction du sein après ablation pour cancer." In *Proceedings of the XXIII International Congress of the History of Medicine*. London: 1974. Pp. 1170-71.

(See Chapter 11: Mendelson).

Popov, E. "Khronologichen analiz na terminologiiata i kliniko-morfologichnite predstavi vurkhu cystosarcoma phyllodes na mlechnata zhleza." *Khirurgiia*, 31 (1978), 210-16.

(See Chapter 11: Fiks).

Puretz, Donald H. "Mammography. History, Current Events, and Recommendations." *New York State Journal of Medicine*, 76 (November 1976), 1985-91.

Mammography has been available since 1930, but not until the work of R. L. Egan at M. D. Anderson Hospital in the 1950s did its superiority over palpation become clear in detecting early breast carcinoma. It is cost effective, widely available, and has minimal side effects. Because of its potential for giving excess radiation to patients, it should be used for high-risk women, which includes women with a family history of breast cancer, early menarche, late menopause, and a late first child, as well as women with no history of breast feeding and women over forty.

Ravitch, Mark M. "Carcinoma of the Breast. The Place of the Halsted Radical Mastectomy." *The Johns Hopkins Medical Journal*, 129 (October 1974), 202-11.

In the 1890s, through surgical experience and clinical follow-up, William Halsted of Johns Hopkins University Medical School developed the surgical procedure for breast cancer which now bears his name. By 1890 he knew that a lymph node dissection of the axilla was essential to patient survival, and by the mid-1890s he was removing the pectoralis major muscle as a means of reducing local recurrences of disease. Occasionally he also performed more radical procedures involving removal of the pectoralis minor muscle and dissection of the supraclavicular glands. In the 1940s and 1950s the radical procedure became popular for a time, with the addition of an extensive mediastinal and pleural procedure. Medical debate in the 1970s revolved around several important questions: 1) a modified radical mastectomy with excision of the breast and axillary contents but without resection of the muscles; 2) irradiation alone; 3) simple mastectomy alone; or 4) simple mastectomy combined with irradiation or just a lumpectomy. Today, nearly ninety years after Halsted began developing his procedure, medical debate still centers on his approach to breast cancer.

Robinson, James O. "Treatment of Breast Cancer Through the Ages." *The American Journal of Surgery*, 15 (March 1985), 317-33.

(See Chapter 11: De Moulin).

Rosen, Peter Paul. "Specimen Radiography and the Diagnosis of Clinically Occult Mammary Carcinoma. A Brief Historical Review." *Pathology Annual*, 15 (1980), 225-37.

(See Chapter 24: Rosen).

Ross, W. M. "Carcinoma of the Breast in the Section of Radiology." *Journal of the Royal Society of Medicine*, 73 (October 1980), 734-38.

The Section of Radiology has existed at the Newcastle General Hospital, Newcastle upon Tyne, Great Britain, for fifty years. Over the years physicians and researchers have approached breast carcinoma from the following perspectives:

1. (1930s) Concern with long term survival called for assumptions that all cases have occult or apparent metastasis and the immunological system must be boosted by injections of colloidal selenium and low X-ray doses.

2. (1940s) Radical mastectomies must be followed up by postoperative radiotherapy to prevent localized recurrences. They also began to deal with the concept that receptors in the cells of some breast carcinomas react differently to hormones, resulting in different survival rates.

3. (1950s) Concern with histologic grading of tumors to provide prognosis for individual disease and the role of metastasis, biochemical markers, axillary involvement, and steroid receptors. Also discussions began about the possibility of breast reconstruction surgery.

4. (1960s) Concern about initiating the widespread use of mammography as a means of detecting occult breast tumors.

5. (1970s) Concern about the role of cytotoxic agents in survival rates and the value of prophylactic treatment in early stage tumors. Also real doubts were expressed about chemotherapy and radiotherapy studies which claim good survival rates after only three years of clinical study, especially when survival rates for breast cancer are relevant only after 10 years.

"Sero-Cystic Disease of the Breast—Brodie's Tumor." *Cancer Bulletin*, 13 (May-June 1961), 58-59.

Benjamin Brodie (1783-1862), a physician at St. George's Hospital in London, in the 1840s delivered a series of lectures describing benign cystic lesions of the breast and the differences between them and carcinomas. The eponym "Brodie's Tumor" became the common reference to the disease.

Simmer, H. H. "Kastration Beim Mammakarzinom: Eine Retrospektive." *Muenchener Medizinische Wochenschrift*, 120 (224 November 1978), 1555.

(See Chapter 11: Simmer).

Simmer, H. H. "Oophorectomy for Breast Cancer Patients: Its Proposal, First Performance, and First Explanation as an Endocrine Ablation." *Clio Medica*, 4 (December 1969), 227-49.

In 1889 Albert S. Schinzinger of the University of Frieburg proposed a "prophylactic" bilateral oophorectomy in pre-menopausal patients with breast cancer prior to operating on the diseased breast. Schinzinger's rationale was that breasts atrophied after menopause, and that the oophorectomy, by inducing menopause, might shrink breast tumors. On June 15, 1895, George Thomas Beatson of the Glasgow Cancer Hospital performed the first bilateral oophorectomy in a premenopausal patient with inoperable recurrent breast cancer. Beatson believed, after animal observation, that removal of the ovaries prolonged lactation, which he saw as a fatty degeneration of glandular cells. He thought an oophorectomy in breast cancer patients would bring about a fatty degeneration of cancer cells. Beatson also believed the ovaries were the source of breast cancer by secreting cells or transforming breast tissue into germinal cells. In 1897 Stanley Boyd of the Charing Cross Hospital in London first explained oophorectomy as an endocrine ablation.

Stehlin, John S., Jr., et al. "Treatment of Carcinoma of the Breast." *Surgery, Gynecology & Obstetrics*, 149 (December 1979), 911-22.

William S. Halsted developed the radical mastectomy in the 1890s and until World War II it was the standard treatment for breast cancer. But in the 1940s survival rates reached a plateau and some physicians began questioning the procedure. In 1949 McWhirter, an English radiotherapist, argued that radiation therapy was as effective as mastectomy in treating patients with early stage disease. Two British surgeons also reported that a modified radical mastectomy which preserved the pectoralis major muscle achieved survival rates equal to those of the radical mastectomy. In the late 1940s and 1950s some Italian surgeons experimented with extended radical mastectomies, removing the internal mammary lymph nodes, but it was abandoned at the end of the decade because long-term survival rates were not improved. Also in the 1950s more and more advocates of minimal surgery combined with radiotherapy began to appear at oncology meetings around the world. In 1963 Auchinclos advocated preservation of both pectoralis muscles for women with fewer than four positive lymph nodes. More and more data began to accumulate that long-term survival rates for women receiving radical mastectomies and those receiving modified radical mastectomies or lumpectomies combined with external beam radiotherapy were exactly the same. By the 1970s the opposition to routine use of the Halsted mastectomy continued to increase.

Steinfeld, Alan D. "A Historical Report of a Mastectomy for Carcinoma of the Breast." *Surgery, Gynecology & Obstetrics*, 141 (October 1975), 616-17.

In 1728 Dr. Zabdiel Boylston of Boston, Massachusetts, performed what today would be called a modified radical mastectomy on Sarah Winslow, who was suffering from a carcinoma of the left breast. Ms. Winslow survived for 39 years after the surgery, which was among the first mastectomies performed in the American colonies.

Uriburu, J. V., E. T. Bernardello, and J. A. Gesualdi. "Historia de la patología y cirugía mamaria en la Argentina." *Seminario de Medicina*, (1969), 207-09.

(See Chapter 11: De Moulin).

Vaeth, Jerome M. "Historical Aspects of Tylectomy and Radiation Therapy in the Treatment of Cancer of the Breast." *Frontiers of Radiation Therapy and Oncology*, 17 (1983), 1-10.

(See Chapter 24: Vaeth).

Vasquez, Albaladejo G., and Ferrer R. Sospedra. "Evolución de las técnicas quirúrgicas en el cancer de mamá." *Revista Espania de Oncologia*, 28 (1981), 83-94.

(See Chapter 11: Lewison).

Vaubel, W. E. "Der Wandel der Operativen Behandlung des Brustdrusenkarzinoms vom Mittelalter bis zur Neuzeit." *Proceedings of the International Congress of the History of Medicine*, 2 (1968), 1728-39.

(See Chapter 11: Handley).

12 Gastrointestinal

Absolon, K. B., and M. J. Absolon, eds. "Resection of the Cancerous Pylorus Performed by Theodor Billroth (With 5 Woodcuts and 3 Lithographs)." *Review of Surgery*, 25 (November-December 1968), 381-408.

(See Chapter 23: Brunschwig and Simandi).

Absolon, K. B. "First Laryngectomy for Cancer as Performed by Theodor Billroth on December 31, 1873: A Hundredth Anniversary." *Review of Surgery*, 31 (March-April 1974), 65-70.

(See Chapter 23: Schechter and Morfit).

Bock, O. A. A. "The Relationship between Chronic Gastritis, Gastric Ulceration, and Carcinoma of the Stomach. A Historical Review." *South African Journal of Medicine*, 48 (12 October 1974), 2063-66.

Since early in the 1800s it has been known that gastric ulceration and chronic gastritis are closely connected, and by the 1920s British and American researchers had noted that carcinoma of the stomach is always associated with chronic gastritis. Usually the carcinoma originates in the area of the intestinal metaplasia.

Breen, R. E. and Garnjobst, W. "Surgical Procedures for Carcinoma of the Rectum: A Historical Review." *Diseases of the Colon and Rectum*, 26 (October 1983), 680-85.

(See Chapter 23: Polglase and Chapter 23: Hughes).

Brunschwig, Alexander and Edith Simandi. "First Successful Pylorectomy for Cancer." *Surgery, Gynecology & Obstetrics*, 92 (March 1951), 375-79.

(See Chapter 23: Brunschwig and Simandi).

Colcock, B. P. "Surgical Process in the Treatment of Rectal Cancer." *Surgery, Gynecology & Obstetrics*, 121 (1965), 997-1003.

(See Chapter 23: Polglase and Chapter 23: Hughes).

"Cuthbert Esquire Dukes (1890-1977)." *European Journal of Surgical Oncology*, 13 (February 1987), 77.

(See Chapter 22: "Cuthbert Esquire Dukes 1890-1977").

De Usobiaga, E. "Historia del cancer gastrico." *Revista Espania de Enfermidades*, 30 (15 January 1970), 226-36.

(See Chapter 23: "Evolution of Gastric Surgery").

Edelmann, G. "Le cancer de rectum par Henri Mondor il y a trois quarts de siècle." *Chirurgie*, 111 (1985), 397-400.

Early in the 1900s Henri Mondor was a French physician who specialized in diseases of the colon and rectum. Mondor was an early advocate of the extensive surgical exision of the lower colon, rectum, and adjacent lymph tissues for carcinoma of the colon and rectum, a procedure that William E. Miles perfected. Mondor also advocated studies of the lymph drainage patterns from the lower colon and rectum so that surgeons could more effectively operate to prevent local recurrences.

Ellis, H. "Eponyms in Oncology. William Ernest Miles (1869-1947)." *European Journal of Surgical Oncology*, 12 (March 1986), 85.

(See Chapter 23: Ellis).

"Eponym: Plummer-Vinson Syndrome." *Cancer Bulletin*, 16 (September-October 1964), 88-89.

In 1922 a young American physician named Vinson described the association of anemia and dysphagia in middle-aged women, and he cited the earlier work of Plummer. By the 1930s the eponym "Plummer-Vinson" was commonly used to describe the disease. It is characterized by anemia, fissures at the corner of the mouth, atrophy of the mucous membranes of the oropharynx and the tongue, glossitis, spoon-shaped nails, splenomegaly, edentia, and chronic thickening of the mucosa on either side of the cricoid. The disease often leads to carcinoma of the atrophic mucosal membrane.

"The Evolution of Gastric Surgery." *Cancer Bulletin*, 11 (January-February 1959), 2-4.

(See Chapter 23: "The Evolution of Gastric Surgery").

"Evolution of Surgical Intervention in Rectal Carcinoma." *Cancer Bulletin*, 13
    (May-June 1961), 45-48.

(See Chapter 23: "Evolution of Surgical Intervention in Rectal Carcinoma").

Fitzgerald, R. H. "What is the Dukes' System for Carcinoma of the Rectum?"
    Diseases of the Colon and Rectum, 25 (July-August 1982), 474-77.

In the 1930s C. Dukes and H. Westhues demonstrated clinically and statistically that the downward lymphatic and tissue spread of rectal carcinomas was
unusual. At the time surgical resection of rectal tumors usually required removal
of the sphincter muscle, leaving patients incontinent and necessitating colostomies.
Because of the work of Dukes and Westhues, surgical removal of the sphincter became unusual.

Gibbon, J. H., Jr. "Changing Concepts in the Therapy of Carcinoma of the
    Esophagus." *Transactions and Studies of the College of Physicians of Philadel-
    phia*, 30 (1963), 127-32.

(See Chapter 12: Watson and Goodner).

Gilbertsen, V. A. "Contributions of William Ernest Miles to Surgery of the Rec-
    tum for Cancer." *Diseases of the Colon and Rectum*, 7 (September-October
    1964), 375-80.

(See Chapter 23: Gilbertsen).

Granshaw, L. "Clinical Research: The Case of St. Mark's Hospital, London, and
    Colo-Rectal Surgery." *Society for the Social History of Medicine Bulletin*,
    37 (December 1985), 50-53.

(See Chapter 23: Polglase).

Harrison, R. Cameron and F. Miks. "Canadian Contributions Towards the Com-
    prehension of Hyperinsulinism: The First Successful Excision of an Insuli-
    noma." *The Canadian Journal of Surgery*, 23 (July 1980), 401-04.

In 1902 A. G. Nichols of McGill University first described an islet cell adenoma. Not until 1923 was the clinical syndrome of hyperinsulinism suspected. At
Toronto General Hospital in 1929 Dr. R. R. Graham resected the pancreas of a 54
year old woman, removing an islet cell carcinoma. The woman survived another
year. Hyperinsulinism had also caused hypoglycemia.

Holt, L. Emmett. "Primary Adenosarcoma of the Liver. Report of Case in a Child of Nine Months." *Archives of Pediatrics*, 71 (1954), 226-30.

The first case of a primary adenosarcoma of the liver was reported by Emmett Holt in Detroit, Michigan, in 1904, at the Sixteenth Annual Meeting of the American Pediatric Society. The child was a 9 month old male who was brought into the hospital with an extended abdomen, frequent vomiting, and discolored stool. Abdominal surgery revealed a large liver tumor, which could not be resected. A palliative procedure was used to relieve drainage pressures, but the child died two weeks later. An autopsy and pathological report revealed the adenosarcoma.

Hughes, E. S. R. "The Development of a Restorative Operation for Carcinoma of the Rectum." *Australian and New Zealand Journal of Surgery*, 51 (April 1981), 117-19.

(See Chapter 23: Hughes).

Imanaga, H. "Honoring Theodor Billroth by Attaining a Hundred Years Since His First Success in Gastric Cancer Resection." *Nippon Gans Chiryo Gakkai Shi*, 16 (June 20, 1981), 405-08.

(See Chapter 23: Brundschwig and Simandi).

Kirchner, John A. "A Historical and Histological View of Partial Laryngectomy." *Bulletin of the New York Academy of Medicine*, 62 (October 1986), 808-17.

(See Chapter 23: Kirchner).

Krolicki, T. A. "History of Cancer of the Rectum and Its Surgical Treatment." *Journal of the International College of Surgeons*, 25 (1956), 625-32.

(See Chapter 23: Gilbertsen; Chapter 23: Polglase; and Chapter 23: Hughes).

Morgan, C. N. "Carcinoma of the Rectum." *Annals of the Royal College of Surgeons of England*, 36 (1965), 73-97.

(See Chapter 23: Polglase and Chapter 23: Hughes).

Murakami, E., T. Nagatomo, and K. Hori. "Progress in Studies on Stomach Cancer in Japan." *Journal of Japanese Clinical Medicine*, 25 (July 1965), 1513-50.

Because of the high incidence of gastric cancer, the disease has had a prominent profile among Japanese oncologists. In the twentieth century the most important advances in the area of stomach cancer have been: 1) improved techniques for surgical resection of the lower esophagus, stomach, and duodenum; 2) the technology of fiber optics and development of a reliable, flexible gastroscope; and 3) epidemiological studies implicating diet and cooking methods in carcinogenesis.

Nakayama, K. "Progress in the Surgery of Oesophageal Carcinoma." *Nippon Kyobu Geka Gakkai Zasshi*, 23 (April 1975), 350-52.

(See Chapter 12: Gibbon).

Narula, I. M. S. "Historical Review of Carcinoma of the Gallbladder." *Indian Journal of the History of Medicine*, 16 (June 1971), 6-11.

In 1777 Maximillian de Stoll of Vienna published the first authentic record of carcinoma of the gallbladder. The next cases were reported by Halle in 1786 and Baille in 1794. Between 1800 and 1850 only 9 cases were reported in the literature, but that increased to 15 between 1850 and 1900. Since 1900 more than 4,000 cases of the disease have been reported. The etiology of gallbladder carcinoma has been a source of speculation. Cohnheim's theory of embryonic rests has been proposed, and several English researchers have argued for heredity. Benign neoplasms, like papillomas and adenomas, have been considered pre-malignant. Beginning with the animal research of Kazama in 1922, the association between gallstones and gallbladder carcinoma has been described many times.

Treatment of gallbladder carcinoma began in 1901 with the Mayo-Robson cholecystectomy and partial hepatectomy, with resection of the pylorus and the rectus muscle. Current opinion argues that adequate radical surgery for gallbladder carcinoma should include cholecystectomy, resection of the liver, meticulous dissection of the known lymph nodes, and resection of the involved ducts, neighboring organs, and abdominal wall.

Onuigbo, Wilson I. B. "Spontaneous Rupture of Hepatoma: Historical Perspectives." *Southern Medical Journal*, 78 (November 1985), 1335-36.

The author reviews several nineteenth century descriptions of ruptured hepatomas and the consistently fatal outcomes. He argues that physicians then knew of the vascularity of liver tumors and the likelihood of ruptures.

Polglase, A. L. "Rectal Excision for Cancer 1880 to 1980." *Medical Journal of Australia*, 10 (January 1981), 3-4.

(See Chapter 23: Polglase).

Polk, H. C. "Surgical Treatment for Carcinoma of the Colon and Rectum: Its Evolution in One University Hospital." *Archives of Surgery*, 91 (1965), 958-62.

(See Chapter 23: Polglase).

Rosenberg, Jerry C., Jack A. Roth, Allen S. Lichter, and David P. Kelsen. "Cancer of the Esophagus." In Vincent P. DeVita, Jr., Samuel Hellman, and Steven A. Rosenberg. *Cancer. Principles & Practice of Oncology.* 1985. Pp. 621-22.

Avenzoar, the Arab physician of the twelfth century, first described esophageal cancer. Nicholas Tulp of Amsterdam reported a carcinoma of the esophagus in the seventeenth century, as did Hermann Boerhaave and Gerhard van Swieten of The Netherlands in the eighteenth century. Surgical treatment of esophageal carcinomas waited until the nineteenth century. In 1877 Czerny resected a carcinoma of the cervical esophagus without reconnecting the esophagus. Franz Torek of New York City performed the first successful esophageal resection in 1913. In 1920 Hans Kirschner suggested an esophagogastrostomy to reconstruct the esophagus after an esophagectomy, and it was first performed in 1932 by T. Ohsawa in Japan. W. E. Adams and D. B. Phemister first performed it in the United States in 1938.

Because of high surgical mortality rates, physicians in the mid-twentieth century resorted heavily to radiotherapy in treating esophageal carcinoma. In the 1920s such treatment involved using radium bougies and external radiation in the 250-KeV range. The development of megavoltage equipment in the 1950s made radiotherapy the treatment of choice for esophageal carcinoma.

Rosenberg, P. J. "Total Laryngectomy and Cancer of the Larynx: A Historical Review." *Archives of Otolaryngology*, 94 (October 1971), 313-16.

(See Chapter 23: Schechter and Morfit).

Sindelar, William F. "Cancer of the Small Intestine. Historical Considerations." In Vincent T. DeVita, Jr., Samuel Hellman, and Steven A. Rosenberg. *Cancer. Principles & Practice of Oncology.* 1985. Pp. 771.

The medical recognition of cancer of the small intestine dates back to 1655, but the first clinical report of a duodenal carcinoma did not appear until 1746. Wesner described a leiomyosarcoma of the small intestine in 1883, and the first successful resection of a small intestinal tumor was reported by Fleiner in 1885.

Sindelar, William F., Timothy J. Kinsella, and Robert J. Mayer. "Cancer of the Pancreas. Historical Considerations." In Vincent P. DeVita, Jr., Samuel Hellman, and Steven A. Rosenberg. *Cancer. Principles & Practice of Oncology.* 1985. Pp. 691-92, 722-23.

The first reports of pancreatic carcinoma came from J. J. Bigsby in 1835, J. T. Mondiere in 1836, J. Da Costa in 1858, and L. Bard and A. Pic in 1888. Trendelberg first resected a pancreatic tumor in 1882, and in 1898 Codivilla resected a pancreatic carcinoma with duodenum involvement. W. S. Halsted performed a transduodenal resection of a malignant periampullary tumor in 1899. In 1935

A. O. Whipple described a two-stage surgical procedure consisting of a biliary diversion by bile duct ligation and cholecystogastronomy, followed by a limited resection of the duodenum and pancreas. By the 1940s Whipple and others were performing pancreaticoduodenal resections and gastric antrectomy. Total pancreatectomy was first performed by E. W. Rockey in 1943, but not until the 1970s did reduced surgical mortality rates make it a more common procedure.

Non-surgical treatment of pancreatic cancer began in 1922 when G. E. Richards began radiotherapy treatments with x-rays. In 1934 W. S. Handley developed the technique of radiation implants. In 1965 it was recognized that 5-fluorouracil was effective in reducing pancreatic carcinomas.

Sisson, G. A., J. C. Goldstein, and G. D. Becker. "Surgery of Limited Lesions of the Larynx (Past and Present)." *Otolaryngology Clinic of North America,* 3 (October 1970), 529-41.

(See Chapter 23: Schechter and Morfit).

Stell, P. M. "The First Laryngectomy for Carcinoma." *Archives of Otolaryngology,* 98 (November 1973), 293.

(See Chapter 23: Schechter and Morfit).

Supady, J. "Problematyka raka zolądka w pracach lekarzy polskich w koncu XIX i na początku XX wieku." *Wiadomosci Lekarskie,* 32 (April 15, 1979), 585-88.

By the end of the nineteenth century a group of Polish physicians like A. Mikulicz, who had trained under Theodor Billroth in Vienna, were making great strides in the surgical treatment of abdominal cancers. The most important development was their ability to perform resections of the larynx and esophagus, partial gastrectomies, and gastrojejunostomies.

Stolinsky, David C. "Trousseau's Phenomenon." *Blood,* 62 (December 1983), 1304.

In 1865 Armand Trousseau first pointed out the relationship between thromboembolic activity and cancer. He described migratory and non-migratory thrombophlebitis, in association with gastric cancer. In 1866, after noting phlebitis in his own left upper leg, Trousseau predicted his own death from cancer. He died of stomach cancer on January 1, 1867.

Trisolieri, V. N. "Storia dei carcinoidi del tenue con quadri anatomo-clinici e fisio-patologici." *Pagine di Storia della Medicina,* 13 (May-June 1969), 55-63.

(See Chapter 12: Sindelar).

Tsuchiya, R. "History of the Pancreatectomy—With Special Reference to Pancreatic Cancer." *Nippon Geka Gakkai Zasshi*, 86 (April 1985), 375-80.

(See Chapter 23: Zamora).

Watson, William L. and John T. Goodner. "Carcinoma of the Esophagus." *Journal of the International College of Surgeons*, 28 (December 1957), 715-23.

The study of the esophagus has been marked by three major contributions: 1) Adolf Kussmaul passed the first crude esophagoscope into a circus sword swallower in Frieberg, Germany, in 1868 and was able to observe the living esophagus; 2) Franz Torek, at the German Hospital in New York, performed the first successful subtotal thoracic esophagectomy for carcinoma in 1913 (the patient was free of disease until his death nine years later); and 3) the use of interstitial radium in the treatment of esophageal carcinoma by Dr. H. H. Janeway. He used the esophagoscope to implant radon seeds under direct vision. Esophageal cancer must be considered in three separate classifications: 1) the cervical portion of the esophagus gives rise to carcinomas which spread bilaterally to deep cervical lymph nodes and quickly metastasize; 2) tumors in the mid-thoracic portion of the esophagus are very difficult to treat because they often invade through the viscera before symptoms appear; because radiotherapy is very difficult; and because successful surgery requires a subtotal esophagectomy and a right colon retrosternal esophagoplasty; and 3) the distal portion of the esophagus gives rise to a carcinoma which often produces symptoms early and therefore is the most treatable through surgery; a left thoracoabdominal approach with wide surgical excision of the tumor is used, as is a pyloroplasty.

Weir, N. F. "Theodor Billroth: The First Laryngectomy for Cancer." *Journal of Laryngology and Otology*, 87 (December 1973), 1161-69.

(See Chapter 23: Schechter and Morfit).

Zamora, Jose L. "Cystic Neoplasms of the Pancreas. Evolution of a Concept." *American Journal of Surgery*, 149 (June 1985), 819-23.

Jean Cruveihlier first described a pancreatic cyst in 1816, and the first report of a pancreatic cystic tumor came in 1867. It was not until the end of the nineteenth century that physicians began to understand the nature of pancreatic disease, particularly the diverse origins of cystic lesions. In 1907 A. W. Mayo Robson and P. J. Cammidge divided pancreatic cysts into congenital, hydatidic, neoplastic, hemorrhagic, retention cysts, and pseudocysts. Their classification system is still used today. It was not until the 1970s that the two forms of neoplastic disease of the pancreas were classified: benign, microcystic adenoma and malignant, mucinous cystadenoma-cystadenocarcinoma.

In the seventeenth and eighteenth centuries the major treatment for abdominal cysts was puncture and external drainage. The first surgical resection of a solid pancreatic tumor was performed in 1882, and in 1894 Theodor Billroth performed the first total pancreatectomy. The discovery of insulin in 1922 made total pancreatectomy a reasonable treatment.

13 Gynecologic

Artner, Johanne, and A. Schaller. *Die Wertheimsche Radikaloperation; Anfange, Fortschrite, Ergebnisse, 1898-1968.* Vienna: 1968.

(See Chapter 13: Lopez de la Osa).

Berens, J. J. "Krukenberg Tumors of the Ovary." *American Journal of Surgery,* 81 (May 1951), 484.

(See Chapter 13: "Cancer Eponyms: Krukenberg Tumor").

"Cancer Eponyms: Krukenberg Tumor." *Cancer Bulletin,* 7 (January-February 1955), 5.

In 1896 Friedrich Ernst Krukenberg described five cases of ovarian tumor. Krukenberg was born on April 1, 1871, in Halle, Germany. He studied at Marburg. The tumors he identified were moderate in size, nodular, smooth, and without adhesions. They were characterized by signet ring cells surrounded by a fibrous stroma. At first Krukenberg thought they were primary sarcomas. Today it is believed the Krukenberg tumors are secondary growths and represent metastases from primary lesions in the gastrointestinal tract. The tumors are radioresistant and must be treated surgically through hysterectomy.

"Cancer Eponym: Rokitansky's Tumor." *Cancer Bulletin,* 14 (March-April 1962), 35.

Karl Rokitansky, a Viennese pathologist, in 1850 first described a rare, benign ovarian follicular cyst. In 1880 the British gynecologist Robert Lawson Tait credited Rokitansky with discovery of the ovarian cystoma. The disease was characterized by numerous translucent, thin-membraned cysts on the surface of the ovary.

Carmichael, Erskine. "Dr. Papanicolau and the Pap Smear." *The Alabama Journal of Medical Science*, 21 (January 1984), 101-04.

(See Chapter 2: PAPANICOLAU, GEORGES: Carmichael).

Candiani, G. B. "The Classification of Endometriosis: Historical Review and Present Status of the Art." *Acta European Fertility*, 17 (March-April 1986), 85-92.

The type of hyperplastic change in the endometrium, today called adenomatous hyperplasia, was first described by Thomas S. Cullen, a physician at Johns Hopkins University Medical School, in 1900. Ten years later I. C. Rubin of New York provided an excellent description of the cellular changes in the endometrium which lead to uterine cancer. By the 1930s and 1940s the work of people like S. R. Gusberg, A. T. Hertig, and S. C. Sommers had all confirmed the pre-malignant stage of endometrial carcinoma and the use of hysterectomy as a treatment to prevent development of the disease.

Identification of carcinoma *in situ* of the cervix also came from I. C. Rubin, even though a number of his contemporaries in Europe denied the possibility of identifying the beginning stages of cervical carcinoma. Working in Vienna early in the 1900s, Rubin established *in situ* carcinoma as a distinct pathological entity. In the 1920s Georges Papanicolaou and Aurel Babes independently developed early diagnosis of cervical carcinoma through cytological examination of vaginal smears.

Carrillo, Azcarate L. "Coloquio sobre endometriosis. I. Definici´on, historia, y sinonimia. Importancia actual de su conocimiento." *Cir Cir*, 36 (March-April 1968), 107-12.

(See Chapter 13: Candiani).

Cosbie, W. G. "Surgery for Ovarian Tumor." *Applied Therapeutics*, 9 (June 1967), 547.

In the 1870s an ovariotomy was still considered a major challenge to abdominal surgeons. Charles Clay of Manchester, England, had performed the first ovariotomy in 1842, but lack of reliable anesthetics and post-operative pain and distension left the procedure only a last resort option for ovarian tumor. The operative mortality rates did not drop until Robert Lawson Tait and others began returning the pedicle to the abdominal cavity after ligation. Today the abdominal incision would be governed by the need to remove the entire tumor intact, without causing a rupturing of fluids and possible peritonitis, and, in the case of malignant neoplasms, an abdominal metastasis.

Douglass, L. E. "A Further Comment on the Contributions of Aurel Babes to Cytology and Pathology." *Acta Cytologica*, 11 (1967), 217-24.

In 1928 Aurel A. Babes, a member of the faculty at the medical school of the University of Bucharest in Romania, suggested a relationship between cytological abnormalities in the vaginal smears of women and the likelihood of cervical or uterine cancer. Babes's discovery was announced almost simultaneously with the similar claim of Georges N. Papanicolaou of the Cornell Medical College.

"Eponym: Brenner's Tumor." *Cancer Bulletin*, 18 (September-October 1966), 89-90.

Fritz Brenner was born on December 16, 1877, in Osthofen, Germany, and raised in Frankfurt-am-Main. He received his medical degree from the University of Heidelberg. In 1907 he described what has since become known as Brenner's tumor: a rare ovarian tumor which is usually benign and occasionally functional in terms of hormone production and synthesis.

"Eponym: Wertheim Operation." *Cancer Bulletin*, 17 (March-April), 45.

(See Chapter 23: "Eponym: Wertheim Operation").

Fels, E. "Remarks on a Commentary on the Discovery of the Histogenesis of the Chorionepithelioma." *American Journal of Obstetrics and Gynecology*, 131 (July 15, 1978), 704-05.

(See Chapter 13: Ober and Fess).

Forster, Frank M. C. "A Case of Ovariotomy Instruments Sent by Thomas Spencer Wells to Richard Thomas Tracy." *Journal of Obstetrics and Gynecology of the British Commonwealth*, 72 (1965), 810-15.

(See Chapter 13: Forster).

Forster, Frank M. C. "Richard Thomas Tracy and His Part in the History of Ovariotomy." *Australian New Zealand Journal of Obstetrics and Gynecology*, 4 (1964), 128-38.

Richard Thomas Tracy was born in Limerick, Ireland, on September 19, 1826. He studied medicine in Dublin and in 1851 he emigrated to Australia, setting up a medical practice in Melbourne. In 1864 Tracy performed a successful ovariotomy. He subsequently performed dozens of ovariotomies and became widely known as a preeminent Australian surgeon. Richard Thomas Tracy died on November 7, 1874.

Gold, Michael. *A Conspiracy of Cells: One Woman's Immortal Legacy and The Medical Scandal it Caused.* Albany: 1986.

In 1950 researchers at Johns Hopkins University took cervical cells from Henrietta Lacks, who died of cervical carcinoma a year later. The scientists succeeded in getting her cancer cells to grow successfully *in vitro.* Scientists around the world requested samples of the cells, which were then widely distributed for research. Almost immediately the "HeLa" cell cultures contaminated other tissue cultures. In 1968 researchers determined that 24 of the 34 cell lines at the American Type Culture Collection were contaminated by HeLa cells. Walter Nelson-Rees, head of the Cell Culture Laboratory at the University of California at Berkeley, discovered in 1973 that some Russian tissue cultures were also contaminated, and he spent the next 8 years working to discover other contaminated cell cultures and the impact of the contamination on research results.

Gulbins, I. H. "Estudio crítico de la primera tésis Argentina sobre: Cancer del útero presentada por Francisco Cordoneda, ante la facultad de ciencias médicas de la Universidad Nacional de Buenos Aires, para optar al título de doctor en medicina, en el ano 1862." In *Congreso Nacional de Historia de la Medicina Argentina,* 2 (1970), 536-41.

In 1862 Francisco Cordoneda presented a doctoral thesis to the faculty of the medical school at the National University of Buenos Aires in Argentina. Cordeneda concentrated on the problem of cancer of the cervix and uterus, arguing that cervical carcinoma was confined to married women and almost never seen in Roman Catholic nuns, which made it a lifestyle disease associated with sexual habits. He also talked about the disease's tendency to invade surrounding tissues and spread to distant areas.

Hasegawa, T. "Development of the Studies on Trophoblastic Neoplasia in Japan." In *Trophoblastic Neoplasia: Its Basic and Clinical Aspects.* Tokyo: 1971. Pp. 6-95.

(See Chapter 13: Li.)

Held, E. R. *Die Abdominale Erweiterie Hysterektomie; Geschichte, Grundlagen, Technik, und Ergebnisse.* Basel: 1966.

(See Chapter: Lopez de la Osa).

Herbst, Arthur L., Howard Ulfelder, and David C. Poskanzer. "Adenocarcinoma of the Vagina: Association of Maternal Stilbesterol Therapy with Tumor Appearances in Young Women." *New England Journal of Medicine*, 284 (1971), 878-81.

After World War II gynecologists began administering diethylstilbestrol to women with a history of miscarriages in order to allow them to carry their babies to full term. The therapy was successful and the drug, an estrogen hormone, came into common use. But in 1969 Arthur Herbst and Robert Scully, a gynecologist and pathologist respectively, noticed an unusually high rate of adenocarcinoma of the vagina in adolescent girls. Howard Ulfelder, another gynecologist, suggested an epidemiological study, which David Poskanzer then conducted. The 1971 study showed an undeniable correlation between administration of diethylstilbestrol to pregnant women and the subsequent development of vaginal adenocarcinoma in their daughters. The hormone was without question carcinogenic to human beings during gestation.

Hertig, Arthur T. "Early Concepts of Dysplasia and Carcinoma *In Situ* (A Backward Glance at a Forward Process)." *Obstetrical and Gynecological Survey*, 34 (November 1979), 795-803.

The relationship between carcinoma *in situ* of the cervix and a full-blown invasive carcinoma was first hinted at in 1886 by Williams in England, and other pathologists like Cullen (1900), Rubin (1910), and Novak (1929) were aware of the disturbing changes which could occur in the cellular structure of the cervix. Still, pathologists did not recognize the preinvasive stages of cervical cancer as a biologic entity until the 1930s. In 1933 Schiller introduced the iodine test for non-glycogenated squamous epithelium. During the 1930s at the Free Hospital for Women in Boston, Frank A. Pemberton, George V. Smith, and Paul A. Younge clarified the relationship between carcinoma in situ and invasive carcinoma. Younge coined the term "carcinoma *in situ*."

Kazanowska, W., P. Knapp, and K. Kubalowa. "Wkład ginekologow polskich w walce z nowotworomi zenskiego narzadu plciowego." *Ginekologow Polski*, 57 (September 1986), 626-30.

(See Chapter 13: Lopez de la Osa).

Kessler, Irving I. "Cervical Cancer Epidemiology in Historical Perspective." *Journal of Reproductive Medicine*, 12 (May 1974), 173-85.

(See Chapter 5: Kessler).

Kjellgren, O. "The Development of Gynecological Oncology in Scandinavia During the Last 50 Years." *Acta Obstetrica et Gynecologie Scandinavica*, 120 (1984), 27-34.

The most important developments during the last fifty years in gynecological oncology have been the following: the cytological studies of Georges Papanicolaou and the development of the vaginal smear to detect early carcinoma *in situ*; the development megavoltage external beam radiotherapy for the treatment of uterine and endometrial cancers; the revival of the Wertheim surgical procedure for abdominal hysterectomy; and the development of methotrexate therapy for choriocarcinomas.

Kyank, H., and R. Schwarz. "Ergebnisse der Behandlung des Zervixkarzinoms an der Universtats-Frauenklinik Rostock von 1959 bis 1972." *Zentralblatt für Gynakologie*, 102 (1980), 481-85.

(See Chapter 13: Lopez de la Osa).

Li, Min Chiu. "The Historical Background of Successful Chemotherapy for Advanced Gestational Trophoblastic Tumors." *American Journal of Gynecology and Obstetrics*, 135 (September 15, 1979), 266-72.

(See Chapter 25: Li).

Lopez de la Osa, Garces L. "Estudio histórico de la evolución del tratamiento del carcinomen de cuello uterino." *Revista de España Oncologiae*, 28 (1981), 569-90.

Uterine cancer was a recognizable disease entity as far back as the time of the ancient Greeks, but the first surgery for the disease, a vaginal hysterectomy, was performed by Langenback in 1813. In the 1790s Heinrich Wrisberg and Friedich Osiander of Germany had suggested surgical removal of the uterus as a treatment for carcinoma, and Langenback had been the first to act on their proposal. Throughout most of the nineteenth century surgeons used a vaginal approach, but it was unsatisfactory because of their inability to perform an *en bloc* excision and reach the regional lymph nodes, where metastatic tumors were common. The surgical research of people like William Halsted and John Clark at Johns Hopkins in the 1880s was accumulating undeniable evidence that *en bloc* excision with suitable margins of healthy tissue was the only way of preventing local recurrences.

The first abdominal hysterectomy was performed by Wilhelm Freund in 1878, and in 1895 Emil Ries, a French student of Freund's, suggested simultaneous dissection of the pelvic lymph nodes. In 1898 Ernst Wertheim of Vienna perfected the Ries procedure, removing the uterus, tubes, ovaries, parametria, much of the vagina, paravaginal tissue, and pelvic lymph nodes up to the aorta. Wertheim reduced the surgical mortality rate to 20 percent, compared to the 80 to 90 percent of his predecessors.

But even a 20 percent surgical mortality rate was too high, and as radio-therapy, particularly radium implants, developed early in the twentieth century, the Wertheim procedure was largely abandoned. Radiotherapy, however, left high recurrence rates, and after World War II, Joe Vincent Meigs of the Massachusetts General Hospital in Boston revived the Wertheim procedure, adding bilateral lymph node dissection. New blood replacement techniques and sulpha drugs helped Meigs reduce the surgical mortality to one percent, and once again surgery became the treatment of choice. Mortality rates from cervical and uterine cancer were also reduced after World War II because of widespread use of the Pap smear.

Naylor, B. "The History of Exfoliate Cancer Cytology." *University of Michigan Medical Bulletin*, 26 (1960), 289-96.

(See Chapter 13: Douglass and Chapter 2: PAPANICOLAU, GEORGES: Carmichael).

Negru, I. "Momente remarcabile din trecutul luptei importriva cancerului in Romania." *Viata Medicina*, 28 (September 1980), 213-15.

(See Chapter 13: Douglass).

Norris, J. C. "Krukenberg Tumors." *Southern Medical Journal*, 47 (February 1954), 116.

(See Chapter 13: "Cancer Eponyms: Krukenberg Tumor").

Ober, William B. "History of the Brenner Tumor of the Ovary." *Pathology Annual*, 14 (1979), 107-24.

(See Chapter 13: "Eponym: Brenner's Tumor").

Ober, William B., "Trophoblastic Disease: A Retrospective View." *Human Reproduction*, 1 (December 1986), 553-57.

(See Chapter 25: Li and Chapter 13: Ober and Fass).

Ober, William B. and Richard O. Fass. "The Early History of Choriocarcinoma." *Journal of the History of Medicine and Allied Sciences*, 16 (January 1961), 49-63.

Choriocarcinoma, or cancer of the placenta in pregnant women, was not segregated until 1895, when Max Sanger in Germany argued that the tumor was a non-epithelial neoplasm, or what he called a sarcoma. The first unequivocal report of a choriocarcinoma came from English physician William Wilton in 1840 and later in Vienna in 1877 by pathologist Hans Chiari. Felix Marchand, a pathologist at Leipzig, argued that the tumors were epithelial in origin and he coined the term chorioepithelioma in 1898. By 1903 Marchand's theories had been widely disseminated and accepted by the scientific community. Eventually choriocarcinoma would become one of the most curable of cancers because it is so vulnerable to methotrexate therapy.

Olsson, J. E., and H. Reichard. "Mannen Bakom Syndromet: Pierre Ménétrier. Tumörpatolog och Mikrobiolog med Tidig Insikt om Precancerösa Förändringar." *Lakartidningen*, 81 (October 1981), 3705-06.

Pierre Ménétrier, an early and prominent French pathologist and microbiologist, believed that cytological studies could reveal pre-cancerous lesions in certain tissues, such as cervical tissues and expectorated lung tissues.

Onuigbo, Wilson I. B. "Historical Notes on Cancer in Married Couples." *The Netherlands Journal of Surgery*, 36 (1984), 112-15.

As far back as 1842 William Budd of the British Medical Society noticed a connection between penis cancer in men and cervical or uterine cancer in their wives. Throughout the nineteenth century others speculated that the reason for the connection was that cancer had a parasitical origin that could be sexually transmitted. Today interest centers on the question of viral transmission and the reality of cervical cancer being essentially a venereal disease.

Pantoja, Enrique, Alexander G. Gabriels, and Thomas A. Caputo. "Melanoma of the Female Genitalia. Historical Commentary." *New York State Journal of Medicine*, 77 (February 1977), 248-51.

(See Chapter 18: Pantoja, Gabriels, and Caputo).

Pantoja, Enrique, R. W. Axtmayer, et al. "Ovarian Dermoids and Their Complications. Comprehensive Historical Review." *Obstetrics and Gynecology Survey*, 30 (January 1975), 1-20.

Ovarian dermoids are rare ovarian cysts containing a variety of immature, embryonic cells capable of malignant transformation, especially if they consist of embryonic nerve tissues. The histogenesis of ovarian dermoids was not really understood until the mid-twentieth century, although their treatment has been the same as for other other ovarian lesions—surgical excision.

Pantoja, Enrique, R. W. Axtmayer, and Rodríguez-Ibañez, I. "Procidentia Uteri and Its Mythical Protection Against Cervical Cancer. Historical Review." *Boletín de la Asociación de Medicina de Puerto Rico*, 68 (October 1976), 252-56.

Ever since the Middle Ages physicians believed that the uterus was the seat of health, both mental and physical, in women, and that changes in the position of the uterus could explain the onset of a variety of illnesses. One common ailment of women, especially those who had given birth, was procedentia uterus, in which the uterus sags down toward the cervix and vagina. As late as the nineteenth century physicians were convinced that procedentia uterus protected women against cervical cancer. Not until systematic studies on the incidence of cervical cancer were completed in the early twentieth century did the myth of protection die out among physicians.

Pejovic, M. H., and M. Thuaire. "Etiologie des cancers du col de l'uterus. Le point sur 150 ans de recherche." *Journal de gynecologie, obstetrice, biologie, et reproduction,* 15 (1986), 37-43.

In the nineteenth and early twentieth centuries physicians frequently connected cervical cancer with sexual habits, since nuns and Jewish women had such low rates, and they also attributed the disease to multiparity and the trauma of childbirth to the uterus and cervix. But in 1931 Smith noted a higher incidence of cervical cancer in poor women. Late in the 1940s epidemiological research demonstrated that socioeconomic status was relevant and that single women had lower rates of the disease than married and widowed women. In 1962 Rotkin showed that low socioeconomic status and early first coitus were closely connected to cervical cancer. Contemporary data clearly implicates a sexual factor in the etiology of cervical carcinoma.

Pratt, Joseph H. "Ephraim McDowell. The First Five Cases of Ovariotomy, 1809 to 1818." *Mayo Clinic Proceedings,* 52 (February 1977), 125-28.

Ephraim McDowell, a Kentucky surgeon, is credited with the first performance of an ovariotomy. He performed the first ovariotomy in 1809 and did many more during the course of his career. The first patient lived for thirty years after the surgery, which involved the removal of a large, ovarian tumor, probably a benign cyst. His surgeries were all performed before the age of antisepsis, yet he practiced careful surgical techniques and washing of the wounds in hot water.

Querleu, Denis. "Pregnancy and Adenocarcinoma." *Obstetrics & Gynecology,* 53 (June 1979), 767-68.

The first cases of adenocarcinoma in the urethra of pregnant women were reported in French and British medical journals in the 1930s.

Rather, L. J. "Ambroise Paré, The Countess Margaret, Multiple Births, and the Hydatidiform Mole." *Bulletin of the New York Academy of Medicine,* 47 (May 1971), 508-15.

Ambroise Paré, the famous sixteenth century French physician, reported in 1579 that the Countess Margaret of Cracow, Poland, had given birth to 36 live infants on January 20, 1269. In his written works, Paré also describes a "mole of the uterus," which is probably a hydatidiform mole.

Ries, J. "Zur Entwicklung der Gynäkologischen Strahlen-Therapie; 50 Jahre Er-
fahrungen an der 1. Frauenklinik der Universität Munchen." *Munchener
Medizinische Wochenschrift*, 109 (6 January 1967), 3-9.

In the last half century four developments altered the practice of gynecological
oncology and affected clinical treatment at the Women's Clinic of the University
of Munich. They are: Margaret Cleaves's use of radium for treating carcinoma of
the cervix and subsequent developments in radiotherapy; I. C. Rubin's development of the notion of carcinoma *in situ* in 1910; Georges N. Papanicolaou's vaginal
cytology test in the 1920s and 1930s; Joe Meigs's revival in the late 1930s of Ernst
Wertheim's abdominal hysterectomy for cancer of the uterus; and Min Li's and
Roy Hertz's use of methotrexate as a chemotherapeutic cure for choriocarcinoma
in the 1950s.

Roman, C. "A Propos du syndrome de Demon-Meigs. Une Observation qui
pourrait être la première mondiale." *Gynecologie Pratiquée*, 15 (1964), 185-
88.

Joe Meigs, the prominent gynecological surgeon in the first half of the twentieth century, first described an association of ascites and hydrothorax with ovarian
fibromas, noting that any woman with ascites and pleural effusion should be examined for ovarian neoplasms.

"Sarcoma Botryoides in Children." *Cancer Bulletin*, 12 (May-June 1960), 49-50.

(See Chapter 19: "Sarcoma Botryoides in Children").

Shingleton, Hugh M. "Cervical Treatment: A Treatment Evolves." *Gynecologic
Oncology*, 25 (1986), 261-70.

The morbid anatomy of cervical cancer was well known in the nineteenth century; Matthew Baillie's atlas of 1793 clearly illustrates the disease. Prior to 1850
treatment of cervical cancer was confined to use of a hot-iron cautery to destroy
the disease. During the 1850s an instrument called the "ecraseur" was used to
remove pedunculated masses and to perform cervical amputations. Late in the
nineteenth century the electrocautery came into to use to treat cervical lesions. By
that time J. Marion Sims and a few other gynecologists were surgically removing
the cervix and then packing the raw cavity wound with such caustics as sulphate
of iron and zinc chloride. The cure of cervical cancer, however, did not begin to
develop until the 1890s, when Roentgen discovered x-rays, the Curies discovered
radium, and John G. Clark and Ernst Wertheim developed a new surgical approach for cervical cancer. In the twentieth century the great advancements were
invention of the colposcopy by Von Hinselman, cytology by Papanicalaou and
Traut, and new surgical innovations by Bonney, Meigs, Brunschwig, and others.

Silva, K. "Historical Landmarks in Trophoblastic Aberrations and Neoplasms." *Ceylon Medical Journal,* 14 (December 1969), 178-84.

(See Chapter 13: Li and Chapter 13: Ober and Fass).

Sjovold, T. "A Pregnant Woman from the Middle Ages with Exostosis Multiplex." *OSSA,* 1 (1974), 3-23.

Skeletal remains of a young, pregnant female who lived approximately in the twelfth century show a series of abnormal lesions in the bones, indicating the presence of metastatic breast carcinoma, metastatic choriocarcinoma, or multiple myeloma.

Stallworthy, John. "Progress in Gynecologic Oncology. A Personal Retrospective View." *Gynecologic Oncology,* 8 (1979), 253-64.

In 1809 Ephraim McDowell of Kentucky performed the first surgical removal of a large ovarian tumor. Between 1857 and 1880 Dr. Spencer Wells of the Samaritan Hospital for Women in London performed more than 1,000 ovariotomies, and because of his work to prevent surgical infections, he reduced mortality rates in the procedure from 49 to 20 percent. In 1897 Wertheim in Vienna performed the first radical hysterectomy for cervical cancer on a living patient. Through autopsies he had studied the pathology of the disease and its drainage sites. In 1898 Pierre and Marie Curie discovered the radioactivity of pitchblende and isolated radium, and in 1910 the Radiumhemmet in Stockholm began its famous radiotherapy program for gynecologic cancer. Because of all these developments, and many more, we can now prevent or cure 80 percent of the cancers which a century ago were terminal.

Stallworthy, John. "Surgery of Endometrial Cancer in the Bonney Tradition." *Annals of the Royal College of Surgeons of England,* 48 (May 1971), 293-305.

William Francis Victor Bonney (1872-1953) was a brilliant gynecological surgeon in England who pursued the Wertheim procedure even when radiotherapy seemed to be displacing it in the 1920s and 1930s. He also played an important role in the revival of the procedure in the 1940s. Because of Bonney's extensive experience in surgery for endometrial carcinoma, he came to a number of conclusions about the disease and its treatment:

1. The "field at risk" with endometrial cancer is similar to that of cervical cancer, although the percentage of metastasis distribution is different. It includes, in order of occurrence, the whole uterus (endometrium and endocervix) 10 percent, pelvic nodes 14 percent, adnexa 5 percent, and vagina 2 percent.

2. In Stage 1 tumors a five year survival rate of over 80 percent can be obtained by total hysterectomy with bilateral salpingo-oophorectomy combined with pre-operative radiotherapy, or packing and suturing of the cervix, or both.

3. The risk of pelvic node metastases is minimal when the primary tumor is superficial but is 30 to 40 percent with deep myometrial penetration.

4. Poor differentiation and anaplasia of the primary tumor increase the danger of dissemination both within the field of risk and beyond the pelvis.

Steinfeld, Alan D. and Henry C. McDuff. "An Ancient Report of a Dermoid Cyst of the Vagina." *Surgery, Gynecology & Obstetrics*, 150 (January 1980), 95-96.

Reports of a sacrococcygeal teratoma appear in Babylonian cuneiform 4,000 years ago. In the Tohoroth section of the Talmud, a description of a vaginal dermoid cyst is found. Because sexual relations were forbidden during menstruation, unusual bleeding required physical examinations in order for the rabbi to counsel married couples on their sexual relations.

Strouhal, Eugen. "Ein Verkalktes Myoma Uteri aus der Spaten Romerzeit in Agyptisch-Nubien." *Mitteilungen der Anthropologischen Gesellschaft in Wien*, 107 (1977), 215-21.

Anthropologists discovered what appeared to be a uterine carcinoma in the remains of an Egyptian female from the ancient period. The mummification process afforded to royalty and nobility preserved soft tissues, permitting the diagnosis.

Tschakert, H. "Funfjahresheilungsergebnisse bei der Strahlentherapie von 4347 Collum-Uteri-Karzinom im Zeitraum von 1928 bis 1977. Historischer Uberblick über einen Berichyszeitraum eines Halben Jahrunderts." *Strahlentherapie Onkologie*, 162 (November 1986), 680-85.

Early in the 1900s the Wertheim surgical procedure for uterine and cervical carcinoma was largely abandoned because of new developments in radiotherapy. During the 1920s radium implants were used, with both intracavity and interstitial approaches, and by the 1930s the development of the 200 kilovolts external beam therapy was widely used. The use of fractionated doses of radiation exposure was also fine-tuned. Megavoltage external beam therapy came of age in the 1950s and 1960s when developments in high-energy physics permitted construction of new machines.

Ulfelder, Howard. "Cancer of the Female Genital Tract. Historical Survey." *Oncology: Proceedings of the Tenth International Cancer Congress*, IV (1970), 199-203.

The starting point in the history of modern gynecologic oncology is the middle of the nineteenth century when the studies of Rudolf Virchow and other European pathologists first demonstrated the nature of microscopic cancer spread. The most important contribution in the twentieth century to therapeutic pelvic oncology is the recognition that early diagnosis would lead to high cure rates, and the development of cytological techniques, like those of Georges Papanicolaou, permitting early diagnosis. Another important contribution to pelvic oncology was the notion of *en bloc* therapy, either surgically or radiotherapeutically, which reduced both local recurrences and metastases by securing margins of normal tissue around the tumor.

Usandizaga, Miguel. "Evolución historica del tratamiento operatorio del cancer del cuello uterino." *Acta Obstetrica y Gynecología Hispano-Lusitana,* 20 (May 1972), 201-22.

(See Chapter 13: Lopez de la Osa).

Usandizaga, Miguel. "Introduccion historica al estudio de la mola vesicular y del corioepitelioma." *Acta Obstetrica y Gynecologica Hispano-Lusitana,* 20 (June 1972), 225-35.

(See Chapter 13: Ober and Fass).

Vacha, Karel. "Vyvoj onkolokicko-gynekologicke prevence v Ceskoslovenska za poslednich 50 Let." *Ceskoslovensku Gynekologicky,* 33 (November 1968), 692-703.

During the last fifty years the major development in preventing cancer and reducing mortality for gynecological cancer in Czechoslovakia has been early diagnosis, the increasingly widespread use of the Pap smear, and aggressive combinations of surgical resection and radiotherapy.

Woodruff, J. Donald. "History of Ovarian Neoplasia: Facts and Fancy." *Obstetrics and Gynecology Annual,* 5 (1976), 331-44.

The first successful ovariotomy was performed by Ephraim McDowell of Kentucky in 1809. Between 1809 and 1851 there are records of another 219 ovariotomies in the United States, with a surgical mortality rate of more than 25 percent. The most comprehensive study of ovarian cancer in the nineteenth century was done by Spencer Wells, an English physician, in 1872, but generally early physicians had no idea about the etiology of the disease. In the early twentieth century, animal experimentation indicated that ovarian tumors are often hormone dependent and that performance of the hypophysectomy will generally protect animals from the disease. After World War II new cancer treatments have been developed, but no single or multiple chemotherapy modality has brought on a cure of ovarian cancer, at least not in the way that success has been achieved in the chemotherapy of trophoblastic disease, leukemia, and lymphoma. Also, if tumors are accurately graded and staged, radiotherapy has not really improved five-year survival rates. Consequently, *en bloc* surgical resection of the tumor remains the only treatment capable of achieving a long-term cure.

Zander, Johanne. "100 Jahre Gynäkologische Krebstherapie." *Geburtshilfe Frauen-heilkd*, 38 (September 1978), 711-15.

(See Chapter 13: Lopez dela Osa).

Zuckerman, C. "Anataciones acerca de la historia del conocimiento del cancer del útero in Mexico." *Prensa Medicina Argentina*, 52 (1965), 548-49.

(See Chapter 13: Lopez de la Osa).

Zuech, S. "L'evoluzione della terapía del carcinoma dell' útero nella storia." *Minerva Medicina*, 59 (10 November 1968), 4800-22.

(See Chapter 13: Lopez de la Osa).

14 Head and Neck

Ayer, E., and D. Montandon. "Pierre Franco (1506-1580) and the Treatment of a Cheek Ulcer." *Chirurgica plastica*, 5 (1980), 289-93.

Pierre Franco, a sixteenth century French surgeon, was one of the earliest practitioners of plastic surgery for treatment of skin lesions because he advocated surgical excision of tumors on the face and, when possible, repair of the surgical wound with suturing and skin from the patient himself. His primitive but forward-looking techniques represented the embryonic beginnings of the surgical discipline of plastic surgery.

Baden, Ernest. "Terminology of the Ameloblastoma: History and Current Usage." *Journal of Oral Surgery, Anesthesia, and Hospital Dental Service*, 23 (1965), 40

Since the middle of the nineteenth century the ameloblastoma, a rare odontogenic tumor, has attracted considerable attention among researchers. It is a benign lesion with the capacity to do widespread local damage, and the only treatment is wide surgical excision. Over the years the tumor has been described as an odontoma, epithelioma adamantin, cystosarcoma, follicular cystoid, adamantinoma, and, according to Churchill in 1895, an ameloblastoma. The ameloblastoma is an odontogenic tumor of ectodermal origin, along with the enameloma, adenoamelblastoma, melanoameloblastoma, and malignant ameloblastoma. The author suggests renaming the tumor an odontogenic epithelioma, which he feels is a more accurate pathological title for the lesion, given its histological characteristics.

Bryce, D. P. "The Conacher Memorial Lecture: '100 Years of Effort'." *Laryngoscope*, 85 (February 1975), 241-53.

(See Chapter 23: Schechter and Morfit).

Cruciani, A. "Sul granuloma della polpa dentaria. (Rassegna cronologica della letteratura e contributo clinico)." *Annali di Stomatologia*, 16 (January 1967), 51-68.

(See Chapter 14: Baden).

"The Development of Head and Neck Surgery." *Cancer Bulletin*, 5 (May-June 1953), 68-69.

Celsus (100 AD), a Roman physician, first described surgical excision of lip and facial carcinomas. In Arabia, Avicenna (980-1037) performed surgical procedures for removal of the tongue. Until the eighteenth century there were no new techniques. Aseptic modern surgery began in the nineteenth century. In 1842 Crawford Long used ether as an anesthetic for removing a "vascular tumor" of the neck. Pioneers in head and neck surgery included Auguste B. Berard (excision of the partoid gland); Nicholas Senn (resection of the mandible and maxilla); Henry T. Butlin (removal of the tongue and lymph nodes); and John Bland-Sutton (bronchiogenic carcinoma).

Duke-Elder, S. "The History of the Treatment of Intraocular Tumours." *Bibliography of Ophthalmology*, 75 (1968), 2-6.

The classic treatment for intraocular tumors, which usually are choroidal melanomas and retinoblastomas, has been immediate surgical enucleation. But alternative treatments have emerged in recent years. In 1952 G. Meyer-Schwickerath reported the successful use of photocoagulation on small, intraocular melanomas. Although melanomas are not particularly radiosensitive, eliminating much use of external beam therapy, suturing a radiation source into the sclera at the base of the lesion has been used since R. F. Moore's first attempt in 1930, when he placed gold radon seeds into the oral cavity of a melanoma patient. In 1966 H. B. Stallard used radon seeds and later a Co-60 placque sutured to the area of a retinoblastoma.

Dunphy, Edwin B. "The Story of Retinoblastoma." *Transactions of the American Academy of Ophthalmology and Otolaryngology*, 68 (1964), 249-64.

Retinoblastoma had many early names, including "soft cancer," "fungus hematodes," and "encephaloid cancer." The first microscopic description of the lesion came from Langenback in 1836. He placed the origin of the tumor cells at the inner granular layer of the retina. Rudolf Virchow called the tumor "glioma of the retina" in 1864. Verhoeff coined the term "retinoblastoma" in 1922. In 1941 Parkhill and Benedict described three basic types of the lesion: 1) the retinoblastoma with highly undifferentiated cells resembling the neuroblastoma; 2) the neuroepithelioma with partially differentiated cells similar to primitive spongioblastomas; and 3) the astrocytoma with astrocyte cells similar to gliomas of the brain.

By the 1850s surgical enucleation of the eye was the recommended treatment for retinoblastoma. Herman Knapp of the United States was the surgeon who perfected the early technique, which included removal of the optic nerve, since the tumor tended to spread along that pathway. H. L. Hilgarten of Austin, Texas, became the first physician to use radiotherapy on the tumor when he successfully applied fractionated x-ray treatments to a child's retinoblastoma and achieved total remission. Subsequent research revealed that the tumor was highly radiosensitive. Chemotherapy for treatment of retinoblastoma came in 1946 when Gillette and Bodenstein learned that triethylenemelamine, a nitrogen mustard, was effective against the lesion.

Dymarskii, L. Iu. "O nekotorykh istoricheskich korniakh sovremennykh deontologicheskikh postulatov v onkologii." *Voprosy Onkologii*, 32 (1986), 67-73.

(See Chapter 14: Baden).

"Eponym: Rathke's Pouch Tumor." *Cancer Bulletin*, 18 (March-April 1966), 32-33.

(See Chapter 10: "Eponym: Rathke's Pouch Tumor").

Fournier, George, et al. "Symbol of Boston's Museum of Science Has Eye Tumor." *New England Journal of Medicine*, 308 (March 31, 1983), 782-83.

Veterinary surgeons removed an eye tumor and performed a sector iridectomy on "Spooky," an owl at the Boston Museum of Science.

Gerlings, P. G. "Laryngeal Carcinoma—Some Considertions with Reference to the Illness of Emperor Frederick III." *The Eye, Ear, Nose and Throat Monthly*, 47 (November 1968), 566-71.

(See Chapter 3: FREDERICK III: Lin).

Gierek, T., G. Namyslowski, and E. Kondracka. "Nowotwory złośliwe ucha leczone w i Klinice ORL Śląskiej Akademii Medycznej w okresie od 1967 to 1977 r." *Otolaryngologia Polska*, 34 (1980), 11-16.

The article focuses on the surgical and radiotherapeutic treatment of malignant tumors of the ear at the ORL Clinic of the Silesian Medical Academy between 1967 and 1977 and the success they achieved in reducing local recurrence rates because of the combined therapy.

Glasscock, Michael E. "History of the Diagnosis and Treatment of Acoustic Neuroma." *Archives of Otolaryngology*, 88 (December 1968), 578-85.

The first post-mortem examination of this benign but deadly lesion was by
Sandifort in Leyden, Germany, in 1777, but not until late in the 1800s was the
localization of an acoustic neuroma made on the basis of clinical symptoms before
death. Surgical removal of the tumor had a mortality rate of 80 percent. Harvey
Cushing began performing subtotal resections and reduced the surgical mortality
rate to 20 percent. In 1934 Dandy began using the unilateral suboccipital exposure in total resections of acoustic neuromas, but the incidence of increased cranial
nerve deficit was appalling. The modern era of treatment began in 1961. New
developments in audiometric techniques and radiology allowed for earlier diagnosis, and William House and John B. Doyle developed a surgical approach going
through the middle fossa to the internal auditory canal, which permitted more
definitive treatment of the disease by providing for more success in achieving a
better surgical margin of healthy tissue around the tumor.

Haneveld, G. T. "An Early Nineteenth Century Case of Ameloblastoma of the
Jaw." *Archiv Chirugia Neederland*, 29 (1977), 9-17.

(See Chapter 14: Baden).

Hoogland, G. A. "Some Historical Remarks on Acoustic Neuroma." *Advances in
Otorhinolaryngology*, 34 (1984), 3-7.

(See Chapter 14: Glasscock).

Horwitz, Norman H. "Sir Geoffrey Jefferson on Invasive Pituitary Adenomas."
Journal of Neurosurgery, 42 (February 1975), 244.

(See Chapter 10: Horwitz).

Hutt, M. S. R. "Historical Introduction, Burkitt's Lymphoma, Nasopharyngeal
Carcinoma, and Kaposi's Sarcoma." *Transactions of the Royal Society of
Tropical Medicine and Hygiene*, 75 (No. 6), 761-65.

(See Chapter 17: Hutt).

Jacques, Darrell A. "The Fraternity of Strangers." *The American Journal of
Surgery*, 148 (October 1984), 426-27.

In his presidential address to the Society of Head and Neck Surgeons, Darrell
Jacques looks back at the history of cancer of the head and neck and deals with
current concerns: whether cancers of the upper aerodigestive tract are similar
enough so they can be grouped together to provide more statistically significant
data; how to determine safe resection margins around tumors; whether multimodal
therapy improves survival rates; when should mandibular replacement take place;

what is the true incidence of radiation complications; can modified or functional neck dissection replace standard radical neck dissection; and how far can surgeons and radiotherapists go in reducing tissue loss in surgical procedures by employing radiotherapy without increasing the risk of local recurrences. Post-operative quality of life for head and neck surgical patients must be an important consideration for all surgical oncologists in determining treatment modalities.

Jonecko, A. "Wkład uczonych polskich do badań nad branchiogennymi odchyleniami rozwojowymi szyi na przełomie XIX i XX wieku." *Polski Przeglad Chirurgiczny*, 51 (September 1979), 921-26.

The author deals with the incidence and treatment of lung cancer in the nineteenth and twentieth centuries, particularly the use of lobectomies and pneumonectomies after the 1930s.

Kasperski, A. "Występowanie raka krtani u chorych na obszarze byłego województwa bydgoskiego w latach 1955-1975 z uwzględnieniem niektórych czynników epidemiologicznych." *Otolaryngologia Polska*, 34 (1980), 125-26.

(See Chapter 5: Kasperski).

Linnik, L. F. "Pervaia operatsiia udaleniia opukholi raduzhnoi obolochki putem korneoskieral'noi trepanatsii." *Vestnik Oftalmalogii*, 80 (March-April 1967), 87-88.

(See Chapter 14: Duke-Elder).

Maynard, John. "Historical and Pathological Curiosities of Parotid Disease." *Guy's Hospital Report*, 121 (1972), 45-49.

Until recently physicians ignored or misunderstood the nature and function of the parotid glands. A medieval sculpture left a stone gargoyle on the west facade of the Trocadero Museum in Paris, and the statue showed evidence of a large tumor of the left parotid region. In the nineteenth century the Chinese artist Lam-Qua painted a number of portraits of individuals suffering from parotid tumors. Johannes von Mikulicz-Radecki (1850-1905), a Vienna surgeon, described parotid tumors, and they subsequently became known as Mikulicz disease, although they were probably a collection of tuberculosis, lymphoma, leukemia, sarcoid, adenolymphoma, and Sjogren's disease. Real understanding of malignant parotid tumors did not occur until 1965 when David Patey established the Cancer Research Campaign Salivary Gland Panel in London. They then saw enough patients over the years to establish statistical patterns and reliable grading systems for tumors.

McInnis, W. E., W. Egan, and J. B. Aust. "The Management of Cancer of the Larynx in a Prominent Patient, or Did Morell Mackenzie Really Cause World War I?" *American Journal of Surgery*, 132 (October 1976), 515-22.

(See Chapter 3: FREDERICK III: Lin).

Meyer-Schwickerath, G. "Die Geschichte der Photokoagulation und die Behandlung der Intraocularen Tumoren mit Dieser Methode." *Klinik Oczena*, 83
   (1981), 59-61.

Meyer-Schwickerath pioneered the use of photocoagulation for treatment of
small, malignant melanomas of the choroid through the use of a xenon arc therapy. The xenon arc was used to encircle the tumor and obliterate the choroidal
vasculature supply to the lesion, sometimes preventing the use of enucleation for
tumor treatment.

Michel, J. "Recherches historiques sur la découverte des maladies des sinus, le
   XIX siècle." *Journal de francais otorhinolaryngologie*, 28 (November 1979),
   577-90.

Nasopharyngeal and sinus carcinomas have been recognized since ancient times.
In 1837 the French physician Durand-Fardel described a case of nasopharyngeal
cancer, as did L. Michaux in 1845. In 1904 Laval described three cases: nasopharyngeal carcinoma, a maxillary sinus carcinoma, and a metastatic thyroid
carcinoma which had spread into the throat and nasopharynx. Another French
surgeon—Flour—identified in 1873 a nasopharyngeal carcinoma which had ob-
structed the the posterior orifice of the right nasal fossa.

Michel, J. "Recherches historiques sur la découverte des maladies des sinus." *Annales des otorlaryngologie, chirurgie de cervicofaciale*, 94 (December 1977),
   753-69.

(See Chapter 14: Michel).

Monteil, R. A., and J. F. Knoche. "Etude de l'evolution du terme odontome
   depuis sa creation jusqua'au concept anatomo-patholgique actuel." *Actu-
   alites Odonto-Stomatologique*, 132 (1980), 583-95.

(See Chapter 14: Baden).

Morgan, G. "The History and Natural History of Malignant Melanomata of the
   Uvea." *Transactions of the Ophthalmology Society*, 93 (1973), 71-78.

(See Chapter 14: Duke-Elder).

Muir, C. S. "Nasopharyngeal Cancer—A Historical Vignette." *CA-A Cancer
   Journal for Clinicians*, 33 (May/June 1983), 180-85.

Skulls from ancient Egyptians indicate that nasopharyngeal carcinoma is a
disease which has existed for thousands of years. The first confirmed case of nasopharyngeal carcinoma was described by L. Michaux in 1845. J. Maisonneuve
described another case in 1859, as did R. Fluor in 1873. Early treatments for

the disease included a variety of caustic applications as well as surgical excision, the use of the cold snare and the curette, galvanic ignipuncture, and lymph node dissection. Scientists in the early twentieth century generally attributed the disease to tobacco use and environmental pollution. In 1930 K. H. Digby indicated that nasopharyngeal carcinoma was far more common in China than in the west. Subsequent epidemiological studies indicate that the disease is also common in ethnic Chinese communities located in other parts of the world.

Muratori, G. "I tumori delle ghiandole salivari." *Dentisti Cadmos*, 49 (May 1981), 73-74.

(See Chapter 14: Maynard).

Muratori, G. "Odontoiarria del passato. I tumori delle labbra e della mucosa orale." *Dentisti Cadmos*, 49 (May 1981), 71-72.

The major developments in treatment of squamous cell carcinomas of the lip, tongue, and oral cavity have been surgical excision combined with megavoltage radiotherapy, which has dramatically reduced the incidence of local recurrences as well as the need for wide surgical excisions and tissue losses. Also, epidemiological studies have indicated the role tobacco products play in the etiology of oral cavity tumors.

Muratori, G. "Odontoiartria del passato. I tumori odontogeni." *Dentisti Cadmos*, 49 (April 1981), 65-67.

(See Chapter 14: Baden).

Olszewski, E., W. Jaszcz, and W. Popek. "Pierwszy opis raka brodawkowatego krtani." *Otolaryngologia Polska*, 34 (1980), 11-16.

The article reports the first description in Polish of a carcinoma of the larynx.

Shapiro, S. L. "Radiotherapy for Laryngeal Cancer." *The Eye, Ear, Nose, and Throat Monthly*, 48 (March 1969), 174-78.

(See Chapter 24: Shapiro).

Steckler, Robert M., Milton T. Edgerton, and William Gogel. "Andy Gump." *American Journal of Surgery*, 128 (October 1974), 545-47.

On August 28, 1915, physicians at The Johns Hopkins University Medical School operated on David Hoag, performing a resection of the anterior arch of the mandible and floor of the mouth, leaving the patient permanently without a lower jaw. The patient returned home to Canandaigua, New York. It was also the home of Sidney Smith, a cartoonist who, using Hoag as his model, developed the popular character of Andy Gump.

Stockwell, Richard M. "Irradiation Related Thyroid Cancer. History and Current Recommendations." *Connecticut Medicine*, 43 (February 1979), 63-67.

In 1907 A. Friedlander first reported successfully treating a thyroid carcinoma with x-rays. Radiotherapy gained popularity over the next few decades as a treatment superior to surgical excision. But in 1950 Duffy and Fitzgerald reported high rates of thyroid cancer in individuals who had been treated with radiation therapy earlier in their lives at the Sloan-Kettering Institute in New York. Subsequent studies comparing thousands of individuals receiving radiotherapy with their non-treated siblings completely documented the association between irradiation and thyroid neoplasia, and magnified the importance of reducing dosages, whenever possible, in treating younger patients suffering from the leukemias and lymphomas.

Strouhal, Eugen. "Ancient Egyptian Case of Carcinoma." *Bulletin of the New York Academy of Medicine*, 54 (March 1978), 290-302.

The skull was excavated in 1901 and represented the remains of a 35 to 45 year old female from ancient Egypt. The skull suffered from extensive destruction by a nasopharyngeal carcinoma.

Suarez, Nieto C. "Evolución historica en el diagnóstico y tratamiento de los neurinomos del acústico." *Acta Otorinolaryngolico Ibero America*, 24 (1973), 48-88.

(See Chapter 14: Glasscock).

Suraiya, J. N. "Medicine in Ancient India with Special Reference to Cancer." *Indian Journal of Cancer*, 10 (December 1973), 391-402.

(See Chapter 1: Suraiya).

von Haam, Emmerich. "The Historical Background of Oral Cytology." *Acta Cytologica*, 9 (1965), 270-72.

(See Chapter 22: von Haam).

Vozza, J. V. "Historiographical Commentary Concerning the Knowledge of the Acoustic Tumours." *Revue de Laryngologie*, 86 (1965), 253-61.

(See Chapter 14: Glasscock).

Vozza, J. V., and G. J. Marcone. "La enfermedad de Lagleyze-Von Hippel-Landau (Insistiendo en una cuestion de prioridad)." *Archivos de Oftalmologia de Buenos Aires*, 41 (May 1966), 91-96.

Eugen von Hippel, an ophthalmalogist in Halle, Germany, published several careful descriptions of retinal angiomatosis between 1895 and 1918. In 1926 Lindau noted that hemangioblastomata of the cerebellum was present in many patients. Lagelyze later noted the hypernephromata and polycystic lesions in the kidney and pancreas of many patients.

Wells, Calvin. "Ancient Egyptian Pathology." *Journal of Laryngology and Otolaryngology*, 77 (1963), 261-65.

The skull was excavated from an archeaological site in Egypt and came from a 30 to 35 year old male who lived approximately 3,000 B.C. The skull showed evidence of a primary tumor of the soft tissues which had destroyed much of the face and upper jaw, with widespread cranial metastases. Most likely the lesion was a nasopharyngeal carcinoma.

15 Heart and Lung

Bartecchi, Carl E. "Primary Cardiac Tumors: Historically Elusive Lesions." *Southern Medical Journal*, 75 (October 1982), 1249-50.

The first recorded case of primary cardiac neoplasms was offered by the Italian physician Columbus in 1559, but Thomas Hodgkin offered the first sophisticated description in 1845. In 1837 I. Bricheteau offered an excellent clinical description of a primary cardiac tumor, but his work was ignored. It was not until 1934 that the first clinical diagnosis of a cardiac tumor was made. A. R. Barnes, D. C. Beaver, and A. M. Snell described it in the *American Heart Journal*.

Bednarski, Z. "Wladyslaw florkiewicz—autor pierwszych w Polsce opisow pierwotnego raka płuc i promienicy." *Wiadomosci Lekarskie*, 38 (June 15, 1985), 891-95.

Wladyslaw Florkiewicz provided the first description in Polish of a primary lung carcinoma.

Brewer, Lyman A. "Historical Notes on Lung Cancer Before and After Graham's Successful Pneumonectomy in 1933." *The American Journal of Surgery*, 143 (June 1982), 650-59.

Early in the sixteenth century Agricola and Van Swietan described lung carcinomas as resembling brain tissue, and they used the terms "encephaloid" and "cerebriform" to describe the lesion. In 1819 Laènnec differentiated lung cancer from tuberculosis, and Storer offered the report of the disease in the United States in 1851. In 1862 Rudolf Virchow offered the first histological description of the disease. In 1866 Flint identified lung carcinoma microscopically, and in 1882 Ehrlich found cancer cells in the pleural fluid. In 1887 Kronig developed a technique for needle aspiration of the lung as a positive diagnostic method. The discovery of the roentgen ray in 1895 and Killian's development of bronchoscopy in 1897 greatly facilitated noninvasive diagnosis of the disease.

Surgical treatment of lung cancer has gone through four stages: 1) the period of "fortuitous" pulmonary resection between 1496 and 1895; 2) the period of animal experimentation between 1880 and 1900; 3) the beginning of the modern era between 1900 and 1928, when Meltzer and Auer developed intratracheal anesthesia and surgeons provided for surgical control of the hilar stump in lobectomies; and 4) the modern era from 1928 to the present, characterized by Brunn's successful lobectomies using interlocking catgut sutures to secure the hilar stump and a drainage catheter, and by Graham's 1933 one-stage pneumonectomy. By the 1950s surgeons were learning that lobectomies were as successful as pneumonectomies in improving survival rates, although some surgeons were performing radical pneumonectomies characterized by intrapericardial ligature and extensive lymph node resection.

New diagnostic techniques in the second half of the twentieth century included the scalene biopsy, fiberoptic segmental bronchial biopsy, transthoracic needle biopsy, refinement of the Papanicolaou stains of the sputum, transcervical mediastinoscopy, anterior thoracic mediastinotomy, gallium and technetium scans, and computer axial tomograms.

Brewer, Lyman A. "The First Pneumonectomy: Historical Notes." *Journal of Cardiovascular Surgery*, 88 (November 1984), Suppl., 810-26.

Evarts A. Graham of Washington University performed the first single stage removal of an entire lung on April 5, 1933, for treatment of a squamous cell carcinoma. The patient lived for 30 years. It was a surgical milestone built on a long history of scientific progress. In 1821 Milton Anthony first opened the thorax and removed diseased, tuberculor lung tissue. Widespread experimental pneumonectomies were performed on animals between 1880 and 1930. In 1909 S. J. Meltzer used intratracheal anesthesia to counteract the forces of pneumothorax during thoracotomy. In 1928 H. Brunn began the era of pulmonary resection by securing the hilar stump of the lobe with massive interlocking sutures. In the first pneumonectomy Graham clamped the main pulmonary artery, used massive transfixion ligatures in the hilus, removed the lung, and left behind seven radon seeds of 1.5 millicuries each into the stump to destroy any localized tumor.

Brock, Russell. "Thoracic Surgery and the Long-Term Results of Operation for Bronchial Carcinoma." *Annals of the Royal College of Surgeons of England*, (October 1964), 195-213.

(See Chapter 23: Brock).

"Cancer Eponyms: Pancoast's Tumor." *Cancer Bulletin*, 7 (July-August 1955), 67.

(See Chapter 2: PANCOAST, HENRY KHUNRATH: "Cancer Eponyms: Pancoast's Tumor").

"Early Pulmonary Surgery." *Cancer Bulletin*, 11 (November-December 1959), 114-15.

(See Chapter 23: "Early Pulmonary Surgery").

Graham, Evarts. "The First Pneumonectomy." *Cancer Bulletin*, 2 (January-February 1949), 2-4.

(See Chapter 15: Brewer).

Herbsman, Horace. "Early History of Pulmonary Surgery." *Journal of the History of Medicine*, 13 (July 1958), 329-48.

(See Chapter 23: "Early Pulmonary Surgery").

Krawczyk, K. "Rak płuc wśród chorych leczonych w oddziałach chorób płuc krakowskiego szpitala specjalistycznego im. Dr Anki w latach 1956-1977." *Pneumonologia Polska*, 47 (August-September 1979), 573-80.

The article deals with the treatment of lung and bronchial carcinomas in the Department of Pulmonary Illness at the Krakow Special Hospital between 1956 and 1977.

Molinieri, J. "Estudio crítico de la primera tésis Argentina sobre: Comentarios clínicos sobre algunos casos de tumores de pulmón, por Francisco Emparanza, ano 1897." *Congreso Nacional de Historia de la Medicina Argentina*, 2 (1970), 76-81.

In 1897 Francisco Emparanza presented his doctoral thesis at the National University of Buenos Aires, where he summarized the current state of knowledge concerning the etiology and treatment of lung cancer. He argued that the old comparisons between lung cancer tissue and brain tissue were no longer useful, because even though they might resemble one another in terms of morbid anatomy, they were quite different histologically. Emparanza also argued that surgical removal of the tumors was the only hope of ever dealing with them successfully, even though the problem of lung collapse made pulmonary surgery a dangerous proposition at best. Finally, he described the clinical results of a variety of individual cases of metastatic lung carcinomas.

Nissen, Rudolph. "Historical Development of Pulmonary Surgery." *American Journal of Surgery*, 89 (January 1955), 9-15.

(See Chapter 14: Brewer).

Olakowski, T., H. Rudzinska, and H. Gadomska. "Epidemiologia raka płuca w polsce do roku 1977." *Pneumonologia Polska*, 47 (August-September 1979), 553-64.

(See Chapter 5: Olakowski, Rudzinska, and Gadomska).

Onuigbo, Wilson I. B. "Lung Cancer in the Nineteenth Century." *Medical History*, 3 (1959), 69-77.

The first diagnosis of a lung carcinoma was in 1819, but physicians had a very difficult time distinguishing between tuberculosis and lung cancer. Not until the last decade of the nineteenth century, when x-rays and bronchoscopy became available, could tumors be clinically described in a living patient. Lymph node metastasis was carefully described by Fox in 1891, and in 1895 Coats described retrograde metastasis to distant abdominal nodes. In 1899 Russell held that bronchial carcinoma frequently led to brain metastases. During the nineteenth century there was no treatment for lung carcinoma.

Onuigbo, Wilson I. B. "Some Nineteenth Century Ideas on Links between Tuberculosis and Cancerous Diseases of the Lung." *British Journal of Diseases of the Chest*, 69 (1975), 207-10.

It was not until the 1870s that physicians began to distinguish carefully between pulmonary tuberculosis and lung cancer. Early in the 1800s many believed that cancer evolved out of tuberculosis because the diseases had a similar naked-eye appearance. Most nineteenth century physicians also believed that both diseases had an infective etiology.

Onuigbo, Wilson I. B. "Patterns of Metastasis in Lung Cancer: A Review." *Cancer Research*, 21 (October 1961), 1077-85.

(See Chapter 8: Onuigbo).

"Pancoast's Tumor." *Cancer Bulletin*, 16 (September-October 1964), 72.

(See Chapter 2: PANCOAST, HENRY KHUNRATH: "Cancer Eponyms: Pancoast's Tumor").

Onuigbo, Wilson I. B. "The Diagnosis of Lung Cancer in the 19th Century." *British Journal of Diseases of the Chest*, 65 (April 1971), 119-24.

The first comprehensive report on lung cancer was Laènnec's work in 1815, where he said the disease resembled brain tissue. His name for lung cancer tissue, therefore, was "encephaloides." French physicians thereafter expressed great interest in the disease and a variety of clinical descriptions were forthcoming. One of the earliest British physicians interested in lung cancer was William Stokes, who wrote about diseases of the chest in 1837. In 1838 Hare described the clinical picture when lung cancer invades the cervical sympathetic ganglia and brachial plexus. By the 1840s physicians had distinguished between lung cancer and inflammatory lesions through use of a stethoscope. They also were aware of the disease's capacity to metastasize. In 1844 Burrows described the compression of the superior vena cava by involvement of mediastinal lymph nodes.

By the second half of the nineteenth century the whole notion of cellular pathology had changed views of the disease. The term "encephaloid" was gradually dropped as useless. Metastasis came to be more clearly understood when similar cellular deposits could be found scattered throughout the body. In 1861 the French surgeon E. Aviolat published his book on lung cancer. The emergence of the physical examination of the chest as a routine diagnostic procedure contributed greatly to increased interest in lung cancer, as did increasing lung cancer rates in developed areas. In 1882 Birch-Hirschfeld wrote that primary lung carcinoma was an outgrowth of the epithelial mucosa of the bronchi or of the mucous glands and that it spread through the lymphatic channels and along the mucosal surface into the lumen of the alveoli. Enormous diagnostic progress was launched in 1895 with the development of the x-ray by Wilhelm Roentgen, and by Hampeln's demonstration in 1887 that lung cancer could be diagnosed clinically from expectorated tissue. Subsequent cytological studies refined diagnostic techniques.

Pearson, F. G. "Lung Cancer. The Past Twenty-Five Years." *Chest*, 89 (April 1986), 200S-05S.

Progress in the surgical management of lung cancer has been slow, but there have been important advances in the past twenty-five years. At the University of Toronto, because of improvements in staging and patient selection, the number of patients with unresectable tumors has dropped from 25 percent to 5 percent. Operative mortality has declined from 10 percent to 3 percent. The five-year survival rate of patients operated on has increased from 23 percent to 40 percent, although the improvement is largely the result of patient selection rather than improvements in surgical technique.

Perret, L. "Retrospektiva synpunkter pa lungkancer." *Finska Lakaresallskapets Handlingar*, 108 (1964), 94-100.

(See Chapter 15: Nissen and Chapter 15: Vincent).

Pruitt, Raymond D. "William Osler and His Gulstonian Lectures on Malignant Endocarditis." *Mayo Clinic Proceedings*, 57 (January 1982), 4-9.

William Osler, a medical professor at McGill University and pathologist at the Montreal General Hospital, delivered the Gulsonian Lectures in London in 1885. His subject was "malignant endocarditis," a dangerous lesion of bacterial origins which affected the heart.

Rosenblatt, Milton B. and James R. Lisa. "Diagnostic Progress in Lung Cancer: Historical Perspectives." *Journal of the American Geriatric Society*, 16 (August 1968), 919-29.

(See Chapter 22: Rosenblatt).

Shimkin, Michael B. "Pneumonectomy and Lobectomy in Bronchogenic Carcinoma." *Journal of Thoracic and Cardiovascular Surgery*, 44 (1962), 503-19.

(See Chapter 23: Shimkin).

Spath, F. "Das Cardiakarzinom. Zum Gedachtnis Viktor v. Hackers." *Wiener Klinische Wochenschrift*, 76 (31 January 1964), 77-79.

(See Chapter 15: Bartecchi).

Steinfeld, Jesse L. "Smoking and Lung Cancer. A Milestone in Awareness." *Journal of the American Medical Association*, 253 (May 24-31, 1985), 2995-97.

(See Chapter 4: Steinfeld).

Vincent, Ronald G. "Lung Cancer—an Overview." In Williams, T. E., Jr., H. E. Wilson, and D. S. Yohn. *Perspectives in Lung Cancer*. 1977.

The story of lung cancer begins in 1420 with the opening of the cobalt and nickle mines in Schneeberg, Austria. In 1521 Agricola described a respiratory disease which claimed the lives of half the miners working there. Härting and Hesse confirmed the disease in 1879 as pulmonary carcinoma. G. B. Morgagni first described lung carcinoma in 1761, but it was not until 1904 that Sehrt published the first comprehensive study of 177 cases. I. A. M. Adler published the first comprehensive monograph in 1912 describing 374 cases of the disease. In 1908 surgeons began performing thoracotomies and partial pulmonary excisions. Between 1926 and 1933 a number of lobectomies were performed with some success, and in 1933 Evarts Graham performed the first single stage pneumonectomy in a lung cancer patient.

The connection between lung cancer and smoking began in 1932 when Cook fractionated two tons of pitch and identified dibenzanthracene as a carcinogenic hydrocarbon. Ochsner and Debakey in 1939 reviewed 86 pneumonectomies and postulated that increased smoking, especially the practice of inhaling, explained the absolute and relative increases in lung cancer rates. In the late 1940s and 1950s a series of monumental epidemiological studies led to the 1962 report of the Royal College of Surgeons and the 1964 report of the Surgeon General of the United States that smoking and lung carcinoma were unequivocably connected. Finally, in 1967, Kreyberg developed a histopathological classification system for pulmonary carcinomas.

Wynder, Ernst L. "A Corner on History. Microepidemiology (Evarts A. Graham and David Karnofsky)." *Preventive Medicine*, 2 (November 1973), 465-71.

  (See Chapter 4: Wynder).

Wynder, Ernst L. "Some Reflections on Smoking and Lung Cancer." *Journal of Thoracic and Cardiovascular Surgery*, 88 (November 1984), Suppl., 854-57.

  (See Chapter 4: Wynder).

16 Leukemia

Bennett, John M. "Myelomonocytic Leukemias: A Historical Review and Perspective." *Cancer*, 27 (May 1971), 1218-20.

Because of John Bennett and Rudolf Virchow, both chronic granulocytic leukemia and chronic lymphocytic leukemia were well established as pathologic entities by the latter half of the nineteenth century. Acute leukemia as a separate entity was first recognized as early as 1857 by Friedreich. Ehrlich, utilizing panoptic stains, elaborated for the first time the cellular details of different leukocytes and recognized various cell types in acute leukemia. He also traced the origin of the granular cells back to a precursor cell—the "myelocyte." Naegeli used the term "myeloblast" to describe cells in the bone marrow that resembled "large lymphocites" and the stage was set finally at the beginning of the twentieth century for the pathologic and clinical evaluation of the acute leukemias. One of the first observations that red cell precursors might be involved in the leukemic process was made by Hirschfeld in 1914. At the same time, Schilliry reported a new form of leukemia in which the monocyte was the malignant cell. The distinction between acute myeloblastic and acute lymphocytic leukemia was not fully appreciated until John Auer described the presence of thin cytoplasmic rods in cases of acute leukemia in 1915.

Bessis, Marcel, and Jean Bernard. "Remissions After Exchange Transfusions in Acute Leukemia. On the Possible Antileukemic Properties of Normal Blood— Historical Notes and Recent Reflections." *Blood Cells*, 9 (1983), 75-82.

In 1947 acute leukemia was always rapidly fatal. Few patients survived more than eight weeks after diagnosis. The technique of exchange transfusion was introduced in 1947 to treat adults for massive hemolysis after abortion to prevent kidney failure. Exchange transfusions as a treatment for acute lymphocytic leukemia in children was launched in Paris by Marcel Bessis and Jean Bernard in

1947. The children were suffering from all the classic symptoms: high temperature, gingival lesions, and the typical blood picture of low RBC, absent platelets, 86,000 WBC, 98 percent lymphoblasts, and bone marrow containing 99 percent blasts. The first transfusions were tolerated well and brought on immediate clinical improvement. Remissions lasted from three weeks to fourteen weeks.

"Chloroma ... Aran's Green Cancer." *Cancer Bulletin,* 13 (January-February 1961), 5.

Chloroma is a neoplasm of localized, green-pigmented tumors in children with acute leukemia. The English physician A. A. King first used the term chloroma in 1853, but it was first described systematically by Francois-Amlicar Aran (1817-1861) in 1854.

Dameshek, W. and F. Gunz. *Leukemia.* New York: 1964.

In this systematic treatment of leukemia, the authors trace the evolution of scientific understanding of the disease. John Hughes Bennett of Glasgow and Rudolf Virchow of Germany simultaneously provided case reports of leukemia in 1845. Both men noted enlarged spleens and the presence of large amounts of "pus" in the blood, which Virchow later identified as white corpuscles. Virchow introduced the term "leukemia" into the scientific literature in 1856 and by 1870 had identified two types of leukemia: myelocytic and lymphocytic. In 1857 N. Friedreich identified acute leukemia, and in 1893 H. Kundrat first described lymphosarcoma.

Evans, Audrey E. "Leukemia: Historical Development of Cancer Therapy." *Frontiers of Radiation Therapy and Oncology* , 16 (1982), 18-29.

In 1905 Dessauer proposed that leukemia was a systemic disease and should be treated by total body irradiation. During the 1940s the major breakthrough came in 1948 when Sidney Farber of the Children's Hospital in Boston achieved temporary remission of a few months in ten of sixteen children suffering from leukemia. He used therapy with the folic acid antagonist aminopterin. Early in the 1950s came the discovery and clinical use of the purine antagonists. Later in the 1950s, methotrexate was used in conjunction with prednisone and together they accounted for longer remissions. By 1960 the median survival time in acute lymphocytic leukemia cases was up from four to ten months. In the 1960s new treatment regimens of multiple doses and cyclical therapy were clinically tried to reduce cell populations and prevent the development of resistant cells. Low dose radiation was also aimed at sanctuary sites for leukemia cells in the liver, kidney, and central nervous system. Bone marrow transplantation incorporating total body irradiation also came of age. During the 1970s the first cases of clinical cures of acute lymphocytic leukemia began to appear, and by the late 1970s the five-year survival rate had reached 50 percent of all patients.

Fleming, Alan F. "HTLV from Africa to Japan." *Lancet*, 1 (4 February 1984), 279.

(See Chapter 16: Gallo, Sliski, and Wong-Stall).

Furth, Jacob. "An Historical Sketch of Experimental Leukemia." In Marvin A. Rich. *Experimental Leukemia.* New York: 1968. Pp. 1-11.

Extensive research on viral leukemia began with V. Ellerman's 1908 discovery of a filterable agent in chickens capable of producing "systemic" leukemia as well as solid tumors of lymphoid cells. In 1911 Peyton Rous isolated the chicken sarcoma virus. In 1926 and 1927 E. P. Snidjers and Tio T. Gie transplanted malignant lymphomas through fifty-eight passages of guinea pigs. In 1930 C. H. Krebs demonstrated that radiation exposure led to a higher incidence of leukemia. The chemical carcinogenesis of leukemia was shown with benzol (Lignac, 1932), trypan blue (Gillman, 1949), and polycyclic aromatic hydrocarbons (1956).

Gallo, Robert, Ann Sliski, and Flossie Wong-Stall. "Origin of Human T-Cell Leukemia-Lymphoma Virus." *Lancet*, 2 (22 October 1983), 962-63.

Human T-Cell Leukemia Virus (HTLV) entered a wide range of Old World primates from an unidentified source. A similar strain of virus is involved in divergent animal species. Black Africans have widespread rates of HTLV because of the presence of Old World primates in Africa. HTLV in the Caribbean, United States, and South America came from slave transportation. Japanese HTLV is confined to the coastal regions of Kyushu and Shikoku, probably from sixteenth century Portuguese traders who had picked up HTLV in Africa and brought it to Japan.

Gavosto, F. "Evoluzione storica delle leucemie umane." *Minerva Médica*, 60 (August 11, 1969), 2993-99.

(See Chapter 16: Seufert, Walter and Wolf D. Seufert).

Gross, R. "Rudolf Virchow, 1821-1902. Leukamie. Lungenembolie." *Internist*, 10 (March 1969), 79-82.

(See Chapter 16: Seufert, Walter and Wolf D. Seufert).

Hino, Shigeo, Kenichiro Kinoshita, and Tsutomu Kitamura. "HTLV and the Propagation of Christianity in Nagasaki." *Lancet*, 2 (2 September 1984), 572-73.

They agree with Gallo (Chapter 16: Gallo, Sliski, and Wong-Stall) that HTLV was brought into Japan by the Portuguese in the sixteenth century. The virus is endemic in southwest Japan, and Adult T-Cell Leukemia/Lymphoma (ATLL) develops in HTLV carriers. HTLV is not a very communicable virus. From the middle of the seventeenth century Japan's isolationist policy meant that Nagasaki was the only port open to western culture. In the past ten years 150 ATLL patients have registered in Nagasaki. The cases occur more frequently in Roman Catholic parts of the population, consistent with the presence of Portuguese missionaries and traders 400 years ago.

Janicki, K. "Charakterystyka zachorowalności na białaczki w regionie Krakowskim w latach 1961-1968 w świetle oceny prawdopodobieństwa według rozkładu poissona. Doniesienie I: Analiza rozkładu czestoscibialaczek w 18 powiatowych jednostkach administracyjnych, przy założeniu równomiernego rozrzutu w całym regionie krakowskim." *Folia Médica Cracoviensia*, 21 (1979), 275-94.

The article provides an assessment of the occurrence of leukemia in Krakow and distribution and frequency of leukemia in eighteen Polish administrative districts.

Johnson, F. Leonard. "Marrow Transplantation in the Treatment of Acute Childhood Leukemia. Historical Development and Current Approaches." *The American Journal of Pediatric Hematology/Oncology*, 3 (Winter 1981), 389-95.

In 1891 two French physicians, Brown-Sequard and d'Arsonaval, attempted bone marrow transplantation in a leukemia case by administering a small dose of marrow orally, but the first injection of marrow directly into the medullary cavity did not occur until 1939. Bone marrow transplants were used in the 1940s for aplastic anemia cases. By that time Osgood had developed the technique for administering the marrow intravenously. What physicians could not do, however, was how to prevent rejection of the transplanted marrow. But in 1948 Jacobsen observed that irradiating the medullary cavity in mice produced bone marrow aplasia but no anemia because the spleen assumed the role of erythrocyte production. In 1951 Lorenz demonstrated that the intravenous or intraperitoneal injections of syngeneic and allogeneic marrow suspensions were also effective in protecting irradiated mice and guinea pigs. In 1966 D. E. Pegg showed that the rejection of the donated marrow could usually be prevented by the destruction of a rat's immunocompetent marrow with the administration of a dose of 1000 rads of total body irradiation. These animal experiments led the way for human therapeutic marrow transplantations. Scientists realized that one method of treating acute leukemia would be to administer 1000 rads of total body irradiation, which hopefully would kill all the leukemia cells as well as the patient's marrow cells, and then rescue the patient's immunological system through a marrow transplant.

The next problem encountered was a high mortality rate from graft- vs. -host disease (GVHD). Patients often died of opportunistic infections after the irradiation and transplants since their immune systems had been so totally, if temporarily, compromised. The death rate was so high that the transplants stopped in the early 1960s. What changed the picture dramatically, however, in the mid-1960s was the discovery by J. Dausset and F. T. Rappaport of the histocompatibility complex in human beings. The step of matching the bone marrow donor with the marrow recipient for histocompatibility substantially reduced GVHD. So the three major steps leading to bone marrow transplants for acute leukemia patients were: 1) safe intravenous infusion of large amounts of marrow; 2) prevention of host rejection by total body irradiation; and 3) decrease of fatal graft-vs.-host disease by using donors matched at the major histocompatibility complex. Bone marrow transplants for acute leukemia recommenced in 1969.

Kass, Lawrence, and Bertram Schnitzer. "Acute Erythremic Myelosis," In *Refractory Anemia*. 1975. Pp. 3-9.

Acute erythremic myelosis is a rare disorder characterized by fever, striking proliferation of neoplastic erythroid precursors, hepatosplenomegaly, and neoplastic reticulum cells in the bone marrow. Events leading to the initial description of acute erythremic myelosis in 1923 by Giovanni DiGuglielmo had their origin in the early descriptions of pernicious anemia and the morphologic features of the megaloblast. Biermer in 1872 and then Ehrlich in 1880 first described pernicious anemia. In 1907 Luzzatto described two cases of severe "megaloblastic anemia without corresponding hematologic findings." Copelli described in 1912 a case of "erythroblastic hyperplasia" in a 60 year old male. After his first report in 1923, DiGuglielmo spent the rest of his career studying the disease, and by 1958 he had distinguished several different varieties of acute erythremic myelosis: 1) a pseudopernicious anemia type; 2) a pseudoerythroblastomatous type; 3) a pseudoneoplastic type; 4) an erythremic or hypoerythremic type; 5) a type with initial anaplastic phase; and 6) mixed varieties including acute erythroleukemia, acute erythromegakaryocytemia, and acute erythroleukomegakaryocytemia. In 1956 Rosenbaum described a case of malignant erythroblastoma.

Kass, Lawrence, and Bertram Schnitzer. "Erythroleukemia." In *Refractory Anemia*. 1975. Pp. 82-84.

Erythroleukemia is characterized by uncontrolled proliferation of neoplastic-appearing erythroid precursors, myeloblasts, neoplastic granulocytic precursors in the bone marrow, retinal hemorrhages, and hepatosplenomegaly. Von Luebe described the first case of erythroleukemia in 1900. Other early descriptions of the disease came from Parks-Weber in 1904 and Treadgold in 1913. In 1917 Giovanni DiGuglielmo coined the term erythroleukemia to describe the disease.

Kass, Lawrence, and Bertram Schnitzer. "Refractory Sideroblastic Anemia." In *Refractory Anemia*. 1975. Pp. 113-115.

Refractory sideroblastic anemia is characterized by normoblastic or macronormoblastic erythroid hyperplasia of the bone marrow and normocytic, normochronic refractory anemia, and occasionally macrocytic anemia and hepatosplenomegaly. In 1936 Israels and Wilkinson used the name "achrestic" for a group of illnesses with hypercellular bone marrow and anemia unresponsive to therapy. They observed high levels of stainable iron in the bone marrow. Then in 1956 Bjorkman described four cases of "chronic refractory anemia with sideroblastic bone marrow." In 1971 J. P. Kushner described seventeen cases of refractory sideroblastic anemia in which he observed hypochromia and basophilic stippling of erythrocytes, macrocytosis, monocytosis, normoblastic erythroid hyperplasia, and high levels of free erythrocyte protoporphyrin.

Kirk, Judy, et al. "Outcome for Acute Lymphoblastic Leukemia Since 1975: A Comparison of Two Treatment Protocols." *Oncology*, 10 (Summer 1988), 93-98.

In the mid-1970s the most prominent treatment protocol for children with acute lymphoblastic leukemia was a radiotherapy-chemotherapy regimen developed by the Memorial Sloan-Kettering Cancer Center in New York. It had been used for non-Hodgkin's lymphoma but was revised for acute lymphoblastic leukemia patients by adding a 2,400 rad cranial radiotherapy administered during the second month of treatment. Chemotherapy consisted of induction of cyclophosphamide (CPA), vincristine (VCR), prednisolone (PNL), and daunomycin (DNR), followed by cranial prophylaxis with four doses of intreathecal methotrexate (IT MTX) and oral 6-thioguanine (TG) during radiotherapy. Consolidation consisted of cytosine arabinoside (Ara-C), TG, 1-asparaginase (1-asp), and lomustine (CCNU). Maintenance was continued until a time three to four years from diagnosis, with cycles of TG and CPA, hydroxyurea and DNR, MTX and CCNU, Ara-C and VCR, and IT MTX given every ten weeks. More than 50 percent of the patients had an event-free survival for more than five years.

Early in the 1980s the German Berlin-Frankfurt-Munster (BFM) treatment altered the Memorial Sloan-Kettering protocol. They reduced the cranial radiotherapy to 1,800 rads for all except high-risk patients and shortened the duration of the treatment, hoping to reduce long-term toxicity. The BFM treatment had a similar induction of VCR, PNL, DNR, and 1-asp. The cranial radiotherapy was given in conjunction with Ara-C, 6-mercaptopurine (6MP), high dose CPA, and four doses of IT MTX. An interim maintenance of oral 6MP and MTX was given before an innovative reinduction phase, which was modified according to risk of relapse, so that patients with a high risk of relapse were given more intensive chemotherapy. The results indicated a 69 percent, event-free survival rate.

Lehndorff, H. "Leukemia One Hundred Years Ago." *Archives of Pediatrics*, 72 (January 1955), 26-30.

In 1845 Rudolf Virchow discovered "white blood" as a pathologic entity, and in 1854 Dr. Jules Vogel of the University of Giessen in Germany wrote an article entitled "The Symptomatology of Leukemia" in which he described the disease as "an extreme increase of the colorless cells and a decrease of the red cells simultaneously." At the time the disease was looked upon as a peculiar, incomprehensible disease and always fatal.

"Polycythemia Vera." *Cancer Bulletin*, 13 (July-August 1961), 77-78.

In 1892 Louis Henri Vaquez first described polycythemia vera, and in 1903 William Osler defined it as excessive red cell masses in the blood which lead eventually to thrombosis and hemorrhaging. It usually affects older males.

Seufert, Walter and Wolf D. Seufert. "The Recognition of Leukemia as a Systemic Disease." *Journal of the History of Medicine and Allied Sciences*, 37 (January 1982), 34-50.

In 1845 Rudolf Virchow concluded that leukemia was a pathologic entity by itself and not a symptomatic suppuration of the blood. He came to this conclusion four years before John Hughes Bennett of Edinburgh, the physician most often credited with discovering leukemia. Virchow parted with his original belief that an accumulation of pus made the blood appear yellowish white. Virchow defined leukemia as a massive increase in white blood cells, not as an extensive pyemia. By 1849 he had identified two forms of leukemia—splenic and lymphatic. In 1870 Ernst Neumann made the bone marrow connection with the physiology of leukemia. He called it myelogenous leukemia. In 1887 Paul Ehrlich concluded that leukemia was a primary disease of the hematopoietic system—that more and more cells are produced and released into the bloodstream.

"Some Historical Aspects of Leukemia." *Cancer Bulletin*, 17 (November- December 1965), 105.

The first accurate description of a patient with leukemia was made by Velpeau in 1827, who observed pus in the blood of a sick adult male. In 1845 John Hughes Bennett of Scotland and Rudolf Virchow of Germany both published descriptions of leukemia patients, although Virchow was most correct in describing the illness as a "white blood disease." In 1856 Virchow published another paper accurately identifying white corpuscles as a normal blood product and as abnormally present in leukemia. By 1870 two types of chronic leukemia were known.

Stavem, Per. "Acute Hypergranular Promyelocytic Leukaemia. Priority of Discovery." *Scandinavian Journal of Hematology*, 20 (March 1978), 287-88.

He argues that Leif Hillestad (1957) first coined the term acute promyelocytic leukemia, not Jean Bernard (1973). The term acute hypergranular promyelocytic leukemia is used because of the high numbers of Auer rods in faggots and the heavy granulation.

Storti, E. "The History of Leukemia Therapy." *Haematologica*, 63 (February 1978), 74-85.

In 1845 John Hughes Bennett of Scotland and Rudolf Virchow of Germany simultaneously described leukemia for the first time. Both of them were intrigued by the excess of colorless blood cells and the enlarged spleen. In 1852 Bennett further reported on 37 cases, and in 1856 Virchow coined the term "leukemia." He also noted that there were two types of the disease, one characterized by the enlarged spleen and the other by enlarged lymph nodes. Eventually these were recognized as myelocytic leukemia and lymphocytic leukemia. Acute leukemia was first described by N. Friedreich in 1857, and in 1893 K. Kundrat first recognized lymphosarcoma.

Treatment of the disease, however, lagged badly until the post-World War II years. Until then, leukemia was virtually a death sentence. Potassium arsenite (Fowler's solution) had been used before the war to treat myelocytic leukemia. During World War II modern chemotherapy was born when researchers noted the antineoplastic properties of nitrogen mustard. The nitrogen mustard therapies eventually included chlorambusil for chronic lymphocytic leukemia and busulfan for chronic granulytic leukemia. In 1946-47 Sidney Farber noted the effect of folic acid on children with acute leukemia, and that led in the 1950s and 1960s to the development of the antifolic acid drugs—pterolyglumatic acid and methotrexate. In the 1960s experiments with the periwinkle plant led to the development of vincristine and vinblastine, both treatments for acute leukemia.

Stransky, Eugene. "Contributions to the History of Chloroleukemia." *Episteme*, 4 (January-March 1970), 69-71.

Twenty years before Virchow and Bennett described acute leukemia in 1845, physicians and particularly ophthalmologists had already described chloroleukemia. They observed exophthalmus and swellings on the skull and a universally fatal outcome. At first they attributed it to some type of sarcoma. The American ophthalmologist Allan Burns described the first case of chloroleukemia in 1820, while a host of others had added their observations by the mid-1830s. King, an English ophthalmologist, coined the term "chloroma" to describe the tumor in 1854. He used the term because of the greenish color of the tumor. Gradually, through the use of autopsies and blood examinations of the enormous proliferation of white blood cells, pathologists by the 1880s had identified the disease as a form of lymphatic leukemia. Turck reported the first case of "myleoid chloroma" in 1903. After 1924 all cases of chloroleukemia were labeled "acute myelogenous leukemia."

Stransky, Eugene. "Contributions to the History of Leukemia." *Episteme*, 4 (July-September 1970), 241-316.

The history of leukemia generally falls into four chronological periods. They are:

1. Between 1845 and 1880 leukemia was identified as a pathological entity. Almost simultaneously John Bennett in Edinburgh and Rudolf Virchow published papers in 1845 describing the first real cases of leukemia. Over the next three decades both men fought over the priority of discovery. Only the most primitive staining methods were used for histologic examination, but physicians did gain an appreciation for the importance of bone marrow in the etiology of leukemia.

2. Between 1880 and 1900 new changes occurred in the scientific understanding of leukemia. In 1880 Paul Ehrlich introduced new staining procedures which greatly enhanced histologic studies of leukemia cells. During this period acute leukemia was distinguished from chronic leukemia and myeloblasts from lymphoblasts.

3. Between 1901 and 1930 more progress was made. The peroxydase was introduced in 1909 for the differentiation of myelogenous and lymphatic cells. The first case of monocytic leukemia was published in 1913, and during the 1920s monocytic, basophilic, eosinophilic, plasma-cell and megakaryocytic leukemias, erythremic myelosis, and erythroleukemia were first described. The last two leukemias were not really accepted as pathologic entities until the 1950s.

Stransky, Eugene. "On the History of 'Pseudoleukemia'." *Episteme*, 4 (January-March 1970), 3-18.

In 1865 Julius Cohnheim coined the term "pseudoleukemia" to describe what was believed to be a well-defined disease entity characterized by symptoms of leukemia, like severe anemia, hepatosplenomegaly, generalized lymphodenopathy, fever, and fatal outcome, but without the elevated white blood cell count of leukemia. In the late nineteenth century a host of researchers went on to describe such diseases as "acute pseudoleukemia," "chronic pseudoleukemia," "lineal pseudoleukemia," "lymphatic pseudoleukemia," "myeloid pseudoleukemia," and "medullary pseudoleukemia." But beginning with the research of Wilhelm Turk in 1899 and Hans Hirschfield in 1911, the term "pseudoleukemia" gradually fell into disuse as scientists recognized that the earlier accounts of "pseudoleukemias" were either leukemia without elevated leucocyte counts, Hodgkin's disease, lymphosarcoma, or tuberculosis lymphadenitis.

Supady, J. "Poglady na temat białaczki w pracach lekarzy polskich na przełomie XIX i XX wieku." *Wiadomosci Lekarskie*, 32 (October 1, 1979), 1415-19.

By 1900 most Polish physicians had come to agree with the theories of Rudolf Virchow and Paul Ehrlich that leukemia was a primary disease of the hematopoietic system.

Thorburn, A. Lennox. "Alfred Francois Donne 1801-1878, Discoverer of Tri-
chomonas Vaginalis and Leukemia." *British Journal of Venereal Diseases*,
50 (October 1974), 377-80.

Alfred Francois Donne was born September 13, 1801, at Noyon, France. He
received his medical degree from the Sorbonne in 1831 and worked at the Charité
Hopital in Paris. In 1836 through microscopic studies he discovered the proto-
zoan trichomones vaginalis. In 1843 and 1844 he reported excess white cells in
the blood of leukemia patients. Donne died on March 7, 1878, by which time his
stature as a prominent pathologist was well-established.

17 Lymphoma

Barduagni, A. "I tumori del sistema reticolo-istiocitario." *Medica Secoli*, 3 (December 1966), 3-12.

(See Chapter 17: Rywlin).

Bergsagel, Daniel E., and Walter Rider. "Plasma Cell Neoplasms. History." In Vincent P. DeVita, Jr., Samuel Hellman, and Steven A. Rosenberg. *Cancer. Principles & Practice of Oncology.* 1985. Pp. 1753-54.

Although John Dalrymple, Henry Bence Jones, and William MacIntyre first described the clinical features of the disease between 1846 and 1850, the term "multiple myeloma" was coined in 1873 by Johann Rustizky. The elevated serum protein and increased erythrocyte sedimentation rate in multiple myeloma patients was reported by Ellinger in 1899, and in 1900 Wright described the close relationship between myeloma cells and plasma cells. That diagnosis, however, was not experimentally proven until the 1930s when marrow aspiration and studies of serum proteins by ultracentrifugation and electrophoresis began. Treatment was impossible until 1947 when urethane was shown to have positive chemotherapeutic effects. In 1958 the drug Sarcolysin produced significant improvement. In the 1970s the beneficial effects of cyclophosphamide and adrenocortical steroids became apparent.

Brooks, Sheilagh and Jerome Melbye. "Skeletal Lesions of Pre-Columbian Multiple Myeloma." *Paleopathology*, 1 (1967), 23-29.

(See Chapter 9: Brooks and Melbye).

Burkitt, Denis P. "Classics in Oncology. A Sarcoma Involving the Jaws in African Children." *CA-A Cancer Journal for Clinicians,* 22 (November-December 1972), 345-55.

(See Chapter 17: Glemser).

Burkitt, Denis P. "The Discovery of Burkitt's Lymphoma." *Cancer,* 51 (May 15, 1983), 1777-86.

The author provides an autobiographical essay recalling his work for the British government in Central Africa in the 1940s and 1950s and his identification of the disease which has subsequently become known as Burkitt's lymphoma. (See Chapter 17: Glemser).

"Cancer Eponyms: Hodgkin's Disease." *Cancer Bulletin,* 7 (March-April 1955), 29.

Thomas Hodgkin, a Quaker, was born at Tottenham, England, in 1798. He graduated from Edinburgh University in 1823 and then studied in Paris. Hodgkin became head of morbid anatomy at Guy's Hospital in London in 1827, and in 1832 he published an article describing the lymphoma which now bears his name. He died in 1868. Sir Samuel Wiks first used the term "Hodgkin's Disease" in 1865. In 1878 Greenfield provided the first careful description of the multinucleated giant cells; in 1892, Goldmann described the frequent occurrence of eosinophils; and in 1898 Sternberg noted the "pseudoleukemic" properties. In 1902 Dorothy Reed described the diagnostic giant cells now referred to as Dorothy Reed or Reed-Sternberg cells.

Clamp, John R. "Some Aspects of the First Recorded Case of Multiple Myeloma." *Lancet,* No. 7530 (23 December 1967), 1354-56.

In a series of papers published between 1846 and 1850, John Dalrymple, Henry Bence Jones, and William MacIntyre described all the essential features of multiple myeloma. The patient was a man named Thomas Alexander McBean. They described the clinical aspect of the disease, the presence and properties of Bence-Jones protein in the patient's urine, and, after post-mortem examination, the tumors of the ribs, sternum, and the cervical, lumbar, and thoracic vertebrae, concluding that the disorder was a malignant disease of the bone. It was the first cancer in which a specific biochemical agent was identified—the Bence-Jones protein.

Dawson, Peter J. "The Original Illustrations of Hodgkin's Disease." *Archives of Internal Medicine*, 121 (March 1968), 288-90.

In 1828 Dr. Robert Carswell of the Hospital St. Louis in Paris made several anatomical drawings. Thomas Hodgkin saw the drawings and noticed "the enlarged spleen, loaded with large tubercles ..." He used the drawings in his own initial presentations on the lymphoma which now bears his name. Robert Carswell (1793- 1857) was an artist and anatomist.

Epstein, M. A. "Historical Background: Burkitt's Lymphoma and Epstein-Barr Virus." *IARC Scientific Publications*, No. 60, 17-27.

Denis Burkitt first described the disease in 1958 and soon argued that it was endemic to a tropical region across Central Africa, suggesting some biological agent in its etiology. Epstein had been working with chicken tumor viruses and surmised that a climate-dependent arthropod vector might be spreading an oncogenic virus. In 1964 we isolated a herpes virus in the lymphoid cells. Eventually we realized it was a new virus active *in vitro* only on interaction with human and certain sub-human primate B lymphocytes. It became known as the Epstein-Barr virus (after co-researcher Yvonne Barr). The Epstein-Barr Virus transforms normal human B cells into continuous growing cell lines carrying the viral DNA and showing features of malignant transformation. Epstein-Barr Virus is an essential link in a series of several interlocking steps toward malignant transformation. We have also seen an Epstein-Barr virus link in nasopharyngeal carcinoma.

Gellar, Stephen A. "Comments on the Anniversary of the Description of Hodgkin's Disease." *Journal of the National Medical Association*, 76 (1984), 815-17.

In 1832 Thomas Hodgkin issued a paper showing the interrelationship between lymph nodes and the spleen in normal function and in disease. He helped establish the concept of the lymphoreticular system. Hodgkin recognized the neoplastic nature of the seven lymphoma cases he described. In 1865 Dr. Samuel Wiks at Guy's Hospital first used the term "Hodgkin's Disease" to describe lymphatic cancer.

Glemser, Bernard. *Mr. Burkitt and Africa.* New York: 1970.

In 1958, while doing field work in Africa, Dr. Denis Burkitt identified a lymphoma primarily afflicting children. The disease most commonly appeared as a rapidly growing tumor of the jaw. Burkitt concluded that there was a relationship between temperature and humidity, suggesting that an insect might be carrying the disease. Subsequent research indicated the presence of the Epstein-Barr virus. Along with Dr. Joseph H. Burchenal of the Sloan-Kettering Institute for Cancer Research in New York City, Burkitt developed a highly effective chemotherapy treatment involving antifolates. The disease has become known as "Burkitt's Lymphoma."

Gyenes, G. "Adatok a magyarországi Hodgkin-kor kutatáshoz." *Orvosi Hetilap*,
120 (November 18, 1979), 2812-14.

The article briefly correlates the success in treating Hodgkin's disease with
the development of multiple-site and preventive radiotherapy and multiple series
of chemotherapy treatments.

Hutt, M. S. R. "Historical Introduction, Burkitt's Lymphoma, Nasopharyngeal
Carcinoma, and Kaposi's Sarcoma." *Transactions of the Royal Society of
Tropical Medicine and Hygiene*, 75 (No. 6), 761-65.

Contrary to conventional wisdom, cancer is not rare in the tropics. In 1958
Burkitt identified the malignant lymphoma that bears his name. Today we know
that the Epstein-Barr virus is strongly indicated in the process of neoplastic
change. The disease is connected with the endemic malaria belt of Africa and
New Guinea. Heavy infection with malaria suppresses the immune system, en-
hances proliferation of lymphocytes, and may make people more susceptible to
the oncogenic effects of the Epstein-Barr virus. The Epstein-Barr virus is also
implicated in nasopharyngeal carcinoma—squamous cell carcinoma arising in the
mucous membranes of the nasopharynx. Epidemiologists have known for years, as
have paleopathologists, that the incidence of nasopharyngeal carcinoma is much
higher in South Asia and East Asia than in other regions of the world. Finally,
Kaposi's sarcoma occurs in men in central Africa. In the United States all patients
with Kaposi's sarcoma have antibodies to the cytomegalic viruscytomegalic virus.

Hutt, M. S. R. "Introduction and Historical Background." In Denis P. Burkitt
and D. H. Wright. *Burkitt's Lymphoma*. Edinburgh: 1970.

(See Chapter 17: Glemser).

Jackson, H. and F. Parker. *Hodgkin's Disease and Allied Disorders*. New York:
1947.

(See Chapter 17: Gellar).

Kaplan, H. S. "Historical Aspects." In *Hodgkin's Disease*. Cambridge, Mass.:
1972. Pp. 1-14.

(See Chapter 17: Gellar).

Morse, Dan, R. C. Dailey, and Jennings Bunn. "Prehistoric Multiple Myeloma."
Bulletin of the New York Academy of Medicine, 50 (April 1974), 447-58.

(See Chapter 9: Morse and Bunn).

Nuland, Sherman B. "The Lymphatic Contiguity of Hodgkin's Disease: A Historical Study." *Bulletin of the New York Academy of Medicine*, 57 (November 1981), 776-86.

Early in the 1960s Henry Kaplan, a researcher at Stanford University, using lymphangiographic mapping techniques, demonstrated that the spread of Hodgkin's disease was not random and unpredictable but in an orderly manner from one lymph node chain to the next adjacent lymphatic area. By using supervoltage radiation to sterilize diseased areas and their contiguous nodal chains, physicians were able to achieve dramatic improvement in survival rates.

Marcello Malpighi in 1668 first described the enlarged spleen of a Hodgkin's victim. Thomas Hodgkin in 1832 noted that the enlargement of the spleen occurred after enlargement of the lymph nodes. Dr. Samuel Wiks of Guy's Hospital in London noted the spread of disease from the lymphatic system to the spleen. In 1903 Francis Williams first tried Roentgen treatment of Hodgkin's disease with good results. The real breakthrough came when Gilbert and Vera Peters of Toronto treated 250 patients between 1924 and 1942 with radiation of tumor sites and adjacent lymph nodes. They achieved a 51 percent 5-year survival rate and a 35 percent 10-year survival rate. Their work set the stage for the more aggressive radiotherapy modalities which were launched in the 1960s and 1970s.

Ober, W. B. "Hodgkin's Disease: Historical Notes." *New York State Medical Journal*, 77 (January 1977), 126-33.

(See Chapter 17: Kaplan).

Peters, M. Vera. "Historical Perspective in Hodgkin's Disease." *Oncology: Proceedings of the Tenth International Cancer Congress*, IV (1970), 483-93.

The most exciting era in the treatment of Hodgkin's disease came after 1965 when lymphography was developed on a routine basis. Pathologists began using new histological criteria based on the publication of Lukes and Butler in 1966. Dramatic improvements in survival rates were achieved in the 1970s when combined chemotherapy replaced single drug therapy, laparotomy improved techniques for finding occult disease, and more aggressive radiotherapy was used for early stage disease. As a result of combined therapies, survival rates have steadily improved.

Rather, L. J. "Who Discovered the Pathognomonic Giant Cell of Hodgkin's Disease?" *Bulletin of the New York Academic of Medicine*, 48 (August 1972), 943-50.

What actually happened in regard to the discovery of the pathognomonic cell of Hodgkin's disease was that many investigators, beginning in the 1860s, recognized and described one or more varieties of large cells in patients with a disease characterized by enlargement of the lymph nodes and spleen in the absence of a leukemic blood picture, a disease usually referred back to Hodgkin's report in 1832. Virchow in Germany and Cornil and Ranvier in France described a large cell with only a few nuclei and another, the true giant cell of Virchow, containing ten or twenty or more nuclei. In Great Britain Murchison and Tuckwell described the smaller of the two kinds of cell in 1870, and in the same year Bristowe and Pick gave an excellent description of that cell in tissues from Tuckwell's patient, calling attention to the prominent nucleoli probably for the first time. Two years later Langhans noted both kinds of cells and distinguished the larger, the so-called true giant cell, from another highly multinucleated cell seen in tubercles (now called Langhan's cell). The presence of peculiar large cells in the involved tissue was by now common knowledge.

Later in the 1970s the reports of Greenfield, Coupland, and Turner appeared. In 1892 Goldmann, using Ehrlich's staining procedures, described the nucleolar acidophilia of the smaller "giant" cells (whose presence he took for granted). Good descriptions of the smaller cell were also given by Hausse in 1890 and Glockner in 1895. In 1898 Sternberg, using the new staining procedures, gave his outstanding description of the cell now regarded as pathognomonic of Hodgkin's disease. In 1902 came Dorothy Reed's equally good description and superior illustrations of that cell. The elevation of the Sternberg-Reed cell to its present status of *sina qua non* took place only a few decades ago.

Ritchie, William A. and Stafford Warren. "The Occurrence of Multiple Bony Lesions Suggesting Myelomas in the Skeleton of a Pre-Columbian Indian." *American Journal of Roentgenology*, 28 (1932), 622-28.

(See Chapter 9: Ritchie and Warren).

Rywlin, Arkadi M. "Non-Hodgkin's Malignant Lymphomas. Brief Historical Review and Simple Unifying Classification." *The American Journal of Dermatopathology*, 2 (Spring 1980), 17-24.

The designation "malignant lymphoma" is given to a group of tumors which arise primarily in the lymph nodes. The term also includes Burkitt's lymphoma, mycosis fungoides, and multiple myeloma—cancers which are composed of lymphoid or lymphocyte-derived plasma cells. Hodgkin's disease has been classified on a histological basis according to the following types: 1) lymphocytic predominance, 2) nodular sclerosis, 3) mixed cellularity, and 4) lymphocytic depletion. But classifying the non-Hodgkin's lymphomas has been very difficult. In 1864 Rudolf Virchow coined the term "lymphosarcoma" to describe primary tumors arising in the lymph nodes, while he used the term "lymphoma" for both inflammatory and neoplastic growths in the lymph nodes. By the 1880s the term "lymphoblastoma" was in wide use to describe all neoplasms. In the early years of the twentieth century, pathologists like James Ewing and Charles Oberling separated out the lymphosarcomas, so that by the 1940s the generally accepted classification for what are today's non-Hodgkin's lymphomas was lymphosarcoma for the small cell malignant lymphoma, reticulum cell sarcoma for the large cell malignant lymphoma, and giant follicle lymphoblastoma for follicular lymphomas.

In the 1950s Rappaport introduced what became a new standard classification system. He argued that no lymphomas arise from germinal center cells and all malignant lymphomas may exhibit a nodular or diffuse growth pattern. Rappaport did not recognize "giant follicle lymphoblastoma" and renamed reticulum cell sarcoma as "histiocytic lymphoma." Malignant lymphomas made up of smaller cells were subdivided into well-differentiated and poorly differentiated types. In recent years new knowledge about B-lymphocytes, T-lymphocytes, and monocytes has sophisticated the classification system for non-Hodgkin's lymphomas. The author proposes a new classification based on the following assumptions: 1) that neoplastic cells be named after the normal cells they most resemble; 2) that the germinal center is truly a germinal center as well as a reaction center; 3) that lymphoid cells can be subdivided by size and cytologic characteristics into small, intermediate, and large types; and 4) that precise correlations of cytology and function are not possible yet.

Sandison, A. T. "Kanam Mandible's Tumor." *Lancet*, 1, No. 7901 (February 1, 1975), 279.

The author doubts that the growth in the skull found in Kenya by Richard Leakey was due to Burkitt's lymphoma. He argues instead that it is the result of trauma or a low-grade inflammation, not a malignancy. (See Chapter 17: Stathopoulos).

Stathopoulas, G. "Kanam Mandible's Tumour." *Lancet*, 1, No. 7894 (January 18, 1975), 165.

In 1932 Richard Leakey excavated the Kanam mandible in Kenya. The young adult lived between 500,000 and 1,000,000 years ago, and his mandible had an asymmetrical fullness on the left side, which some anthropologists diagnosed as an osteosarcoma. The author suggests it might have been caused by Burkitt's lymphoma.

Sreuli, Rolf A. and John E. Ultmann. "Non-Hodgkin's Lymphomas: Historical Perspective and Future Prospects." *Seminars in Oncology*, 7 (September 1980), 223-33.

The interest in lymphomas began in 1832 when Thomas Hodgkin described the clinical features and the postmortem findings of seven cases of tumors involving "the absorbent glands and the spleen." In 1865 Samuel Wiks published a second series of fifteen patients with the same disease and named the condition Hodgkin's disease. A half century later John Dreschfeld distinguished lymphosarcoma from Hodgkin's disease. It was not until the early part of the century that James Ewing's histologic description of lymphosarcoma received wide acceptance. Ewing described two types of lymphosarcoma, the malignant lymphosarcoma containing rather small cells and the large round cell lymphosarcoma or reticulum cell sarcoma. N. E. Brill in 1925 described for the first time follicular lymphomas as a distinct group and recognized the radiosensitivity of these tumors. This disease has since come to be known as "giant follicle hyperplasia," "follicular lymphoblastoma," or "Brill-Symmers disease." Finally, in 1958 Denis Burkitt described a unique lymphoma in African children which had unusual epidemiological manifestations and a connection to the Epstein-Barr virus.

In terms of pathological classification, Rappaport in 1956 abandoned the older methods of classifying lymphomas on the basis of cell structure and proposed five groups of lymphomas: 1) lymphocytic, well-differentiated lymphoma; 2) lymphocytic, poorly differentiated lymphoma; 3) mixed cell (histiocytic-lymphocytic) lymphoma; 4) histiocytic lymphoma; and 5) undifferentiated lymphoma. In the 1970s and 1980s new classification systems incorporated the knowledge that the follicular center is the site of B cell transformation and the inclusion of two additional cell types—the U cell (undefined cell) and the true histiocyte.

Today the Ann Arbor Classification System used for Hodgkin's disease is also used for the non-Hodgkin's lymphomas, but the system is unsatisfactory because they are a very heterogeneous set of diseases. In terms of clinical staging technology, one of the most important improvements came in 1952 with the Kinmonth extremity lymphangiography, which provided for a noninvasive assessment of iliac and paraortic lymph nodes. Other roentgenologic and isotopic procedures, such as pulmonary tomography, skeletal scintigraphy, gallium scanning, liver/spleen scanning, and computer axial tomography have further improved clinical staging techniques. The introduction of laparotomy with splenectomy and liver biopsy in recent years have improved clinical staging even more.

Treatment of lymphomas has undergone dramatic improvements in the last generation. W. A. Pusey first used x-ray therapy on malignant lymphomas in 1902, and in 1903 N. Senn reported dramatic improvements in Hodgkin's disease patients. Because the dosages were so low, however, remissions were only temporary. In the 1930s R. Gilbert began advocating extension of the radiation fields from areas of known disease to areas likely to become involved. In 1950 M. V. Peters published her classic study on the curative potential of radiation therapy in Hodgkin's disease. Radiotherapeutic management of non-Hodgkin's lymphomas is more difficult because of the wide variety of histologic types, although radiation treatments of patients with non-Hodgkin's lymphoma and histiocytic lymphoma have been highly effective.

Chemotherapeutic treatments have also been dramatically effective. During World War II a derivative of mustard gas (tris-beta-chloroethylamine hydrochloride) was used for the first time on leukemia and lymphoma patients, and temporary remissions were achieved. Other alkylating drugs were added in the late 1940s and early 1950s. Sidney Farber developed the folic acid antagonists in the early 1950s, and 5-fluorouracil appeared in the early 1960s. The vinca alkaloids were introduced by Noble in 1958, and daunorubicin and doxorubicin were developed in Italy and France in the early 1960s. Alkalyting agents, vincristine, and prednisone have represented the backbone of combination chemotherapy programs for malignant lymphomas in the late 1960s and 1970s.

Williams, G. D., W. A. Ritchie, and P. F. Titterington. "Multiple Bony Lesions Suggesting Myeloma in a Pre-Columbian Indian Aged 10 Years." *American Journal of Roentgenology*, 46 (1941), 351-55.

(See Chapter 9: Williams, Ritchie, and Titterington).

Ziegler, J. L. "Early Studies of Burkitt's Tumor in Africa." *American Journal of Pediatric Hematology and Oncology*, 8 (Spring 1986), 63-65.

(See Chapter 17: Glemser).

18 Skin

Baruchin, A. M., and H. Zirkin. "From the Times of Mar-Samuel to Those of Marjolin." *Burns Including Thermal Injuries*, 12 (October 1985), 68-70.

Mar-Samuel was director of a school for higher learning in Nehardea in Babylon whose medical teachings appear in the Jewish Gemara. His medical counsel tried to help Jewish leaders distinguish between types of lesions, so they would know the difference between infections, leprosy, burns, and Marjolin's ulcer, a squamous cell carcinoma arising from the skin of a severely burned area. If the lesion was leprosy, community leaders were required to declare the victim "unclean." Mar-Samuel's description of tumors arising in burned tissue is the earliest description of Marjolin's ulcer.

Bennett, John P. "From Noli-Me-Tangere to Rodent Ulcer: The Recognition of Basal Cell Carcinoma." *British Journal of Plastic Surgery*, 27 (April 1974), 144-54.

"Noli-me-tangere" ("touch me not") was the term applied to slowly spreading lesions of the skin in the Middle Ages. Physicians assumed that the lesions were incurable, because neither surgery nor caustics seemed to permanently remove the disease. In 1755 Jacques Daviel spoke to the Royal Society of London and suggested that certain varieties of "noli-me-tangere" in the peri-orbital region could be cured by wide surgical excision. Daviel's claim that the patient had suffered from a facial lesion for 23 years indicates that the tumor was probably a basal cell carcinoma. Had it been a squamous cell carcinoma or a melanoma, metastases would most likely have developed and caused death. The Irish surgeon Arthur Jacob described basal cell carcinomas in 1827. Subsequent reports were offered by Benjamin Travers (1829), William Mackenzie (1830), and John Warren Collins (1837). The first major critical assessment of the disease was published by Jonathan Hutchinson in 1860, when he described 42 cases of "rodent ulcer." The disease had now become a recognizable clinical entity distinct from lupus or venereal lesions. Physicians also realized that "rodent ulcer" did not usually involve the lymphatic system and was not life threatening. The classic description of the disease was offered by Charles Moore in his 1867 book "Rodent Cancer." By the late nineteenth century the disease was widely recognized as a superficial but potentially destructive disease of local tissues. The histogenesis of the lesion was disputed however. Moore and Warren believed it to be a variety of epithelioma; Thiersch, a carcinoma of the sebaceous glands; Thin (1880), a carcinoma of the sweat glands; Sangster (1882) and Hume (1884), a carcinoma of the hair follicles. As for treatment, Daviel called for wide surgical excision in 1755, but the treatment of choice was the use of caustics, especially arsenical compounds and zinc sulphate. Eventually Mohs (1956) developed a highly effective form of chemosurgery on histologically controlled basal cell carcinomas. Rodent ulcer was first treated by radiation in Sweden in 1899. The rise of plastic surgery coincided with the understanding of basal cell carcinoma and provided for surgical repair of excision wounds, as did the development of the Moh's technique.

Blum, Harold F. "General History and Outline of the Concept." *National Cancer Institute Monographs*, 50 (Decrmber 1978), 211-12.

(See Chapter 4: Blum).

Braun, M. "Classics in Oncology: Idiopathic Multiple Pigmented Sarcoma of the Skin by Kaposi." *Cancer; Diagnosis, Treatment, Research*, 32 (November-December, 1982), 340-47.

(See Chapter 19: Braun).

Braverman, Irwin M. "Commentary: Migratory Necrolytic Erythema." *Archives of Dermatology*, 118 (October 1982), 796-98.

(See Chapter 8: Braverman).

"Cancer Eponyms: Bowen's Disease." *Cancer Bulletin*, 7 (November-December 1957), 104.

John Templeton Bowen was born in Boston in 1857. He took a medical degree at Harvard and taught dermatology there all his life. Bowen was also associated with the Massachusetts General Hospital from 1887 to his death in 1940. In 1912 and 1915 he wrote papers on the disease which now bears his name—a squamous cell carcinoma *in situ* which metastasizes very slowly.

"Cancer Eponyms: Kaposi's Sarcoma." *Cancer Bulletin*, 9 (January-February 1957), 5.

(See Chapter 2: KAPOSI, MORITZ: Bluefarb, S. M.).

"Cancer Eponyms: Marjolin's Ulcer." *Cancer Bulletin*, 8 (July-August 1956), 69.

(See Chapter 2: MARJOLIN, JEAN-NICHOLAS: Steffen).

Clemmensen, Ole. "Hutchinson's Freckle." *The American Journal of Dermatology*, 4 (October 1982), 425-28.

Because of his accurate clinical descriptions taken from cancer patients in the 1890s, Jonathan Hutchinson is credited with the first scientific description of melanoma of the face. He recognized the heavily pigmented lesions as cancerous.

Crouch, H. E. "History of Basal Cell Carcinoma and Its Treatment." *Journal of the Royal Society of Medicine*, 76 (April 1983), 302-06.

(See Chapter 18: Bennett and Chapter 18: Swanson).

Cruikshank, A. H. and E. Gaskell. "Jean-Nicolas Marjolin: Destined to be Forgotten?" *Medical History*, 7 (1963), 383-84.

They argue that Marjolin did not describe malignant "degeneration" in burn ulcers and that the erroneous ascription of the phenomena came into being from the mistakes of Robert W. Smith (1850) who labeled cancerous ulcers appearing in scars as the "warty ulcers of Marjolin." Marjolin never described the lesions as cancerous, even though Smith and John Fordyce (1914) said he did. Marjolin actually described a cancroidal ulcer.

Davis, Neville C. "William Norris, M. D.: A Pioneer in the Study of Melanoma." *Medical Journal of Australia*, 1 (January 26, 1980), 52-54.

(See Chapter 2: NORRIS, WILLIAM: Davis).

Eller, J. J. and W. D. Eller. *Tumors of the Skin*. Philadelphia: 1951.

The disease known today as Marjolin's Ulcer was first described in 1828 by Jean-Nicholas Marjolin of L'Hotel Dieu in France. In 1839 Dupuytren reported treating a similar lesion with sulphuric acid. In 1860 Hertaux wrote a brochure about "Marjolin's Ulcer." Broca in 1862 observed an epithelioma in an ulcerated scar 51 years after the burn. In 1881 Neve reported 2,000 cases of kangri cancer from burns by the portable basket fires used in Kashmir, India. These were usually squamous cell carcinomas.

Garofalo, F. "L'epitelioma cutaneo attraverso i secoli." *Atti* (1964), 488-95.

(See Chapter 18: Bennett and Chapter 18: Swanson).

Greenwood, Ronald D. "19th Century Medicine in Indiana." *Indiana Medicine*, 77 (June 1984), 476.

In 1869 Dr. J. S. Bobbs, a surgeon at the Indiana Central Medical College, performed the surgical excision of a large facial hemangioma in a 7 month old infant.

Greenwood, Ronald D. "Surgical Treatment for Facial Hemangiomas." *Alabama Medicine*, 54 (August 1984), 27.

In 1834 Herbert Mayo of the Middlesex Hospital in England treated a large facial hemangioma in a 5 year old boy by tying off the common cartoid artery and limiting the lesion's blood supply.

Hart, Gary D. "Trichoepithelioma and the Kings of Ancient Parthia." *Canadian Medical Association Journal*, 94 (March 12, 1966), 547-49.

Trichoepithelioma is a benign lesion of squamous cell origin usually occurring on the forehead. Many coins from ancient Parthia portray a facial lesion on the reigning monarch's head. Between 123 B.C. and 222 A.D. each of the kings in a familial succession had the lesion, indicating a genetic component in the disease.

Haynes, Harley A., Kevin W. Mead, and Robert M. Goldwyn. "Historical Background of Skin Cancer." In Vincent P. DeVita, Jr., Samuel Hellman, and Steven A. Rosenberg. *Cancer. Principles & Practice of Oncology.* 1985. Pp. 1343-44.

(See Chapter 4: Haynes, Mead, and Goldwyn).

Hiles, R. W. "Malignant Melanoma." *Journal of the Royal College of Surgeons of Edinburgh*, 18 (November 1973), 368-372.

Primary malignant melanoma often metastasizes by the lymphatic route but it is only lesions on the head, neck and limbs that have a clearly restricted nodal lymphatic exit from the region. When discussing the problems of management of lymph nodes it is essential to distinguish between lesions draining primarily to a single group of nodes and those arising on the trunk. The prognosis following removal of cervical and inguinal nodes invaded from head and neck or leg melanoma is very much better than that following removal of any of the six groups which may be implicated in trunk primaries. Historically, the demonstration of lymphatic spread of malignant melanoma by Sampson Handley (1907) led to an *en bloc* excision of the primary lesion, the regional nodes and a continuous strip of skin and subcutaneous tissue between the two. Today we know that the best treatment for melanoma is surgical excision of the primary tumor as early as possible. Regional lymph nodes should be removed only when they are definitely clinically involved or when they remain doubtfully enlarged for more than four weeks. Follow-up must be carefully and frequently carried out for at least 10 years.

Holubar, Karl. "Angioendotheliomatosis Proliferans Systemisata (Tappeiner-Pfleger Disease)." *American Journal of Dermatopathology*, 6 (December 1984), 537-39.

In 1959 Josef Tappeiner and Lilly Pfleger of the University of Vienna first identified what became known as Tappeiner-Pfleger Disease, or angioendotheliomatosis proliferans systemisata. It is a malignant, multifocal lesion of the vascular endothelium. It is fatal in 6 to 24 months.

Howell, James B. and Amir H. Mehregan. "Story of the Pitts. A Historic Vignette." *Archives of Dermatology*, 102 (December 1970), 583-85.

J. Pollitzer of Vienna first described the nevoid basal cell carcinoma (NBCC) syndrome in 1905. NBCC is characterized by highly destructive, pigmented, multiple basal cell cancers and has a genetic component. W. H. Ward of Australia in 1960 offered the next major description of the disease. Ward also described dental follicular cysts and skeletal abnormalities as part of the NBCC syndrome.

Hunter, John A. and Karl Holubar, eds. "In Praise of Alexander Breslow." *American Journal of Dermatopathology*, 6 (Summer 1984), Suppl. 1, 151-57.

Alexander Breslow was a pathologist at the George Washington University School of Medicine and responsible for assessing the prognosis of malignant melanoma by measuring the thickness of the lesion. His realization that "wide and deep" excision for primary lesions of thin malignant melanomas (1 centimeter instead of the standard 5 centimeters) saved thousands of patients from mutilating surgery.

Hutt, M. S. R. "Historical Introduction, Burkitt's Lymphoma, Nasopharyngeal Carcinoma, and Kaposi's Sarcoma." *Transactions of the Royal Society of Tropical Medicine and Hygiene*, 75 (No. 6), 761-65.

(See Chapter 17: Hutt).

Ichikawa, A. "Discovery of the Effect of Bleomycin on Squamous Cell Carcinoma and the Development of Its Research." *Journal of the Japanese Medical Association*, 62 (15 July 1969), 153-58.

(See Chapter 25: Ichikawa).

Jackson, Robert. "Early Clinical Descriptions of Skin Cancer." *Canadian Medical Association Journal,* 109 (November 1973), 906-08.

The first report of squamous cell carcinoma was given by Percivall Pott in 1775 when he recognized scrotum tumors in chimney sweeps. He recommended early, wide surgical excision as the only treatment. William Norris provided the first written description of metastatic malignant melanoma in 1820. In 1827 Arthur Jacob reported the first basal cell carcinoma, which he called "rodent ulcer." Finally, the first report of keratoacanthoma was completed by Jonathan Hutchinson in 1889.

Jackson, Robert. "Medicine and History. How Caustics Were Used to Treat Skin Cancer." *The Journal of Dermatologic Surgery and Oncology,* 5 (December 1979), 949-50.

(See Chapter 25: Jackson).

King, D. Friday. "Chronic Atypical Epithelial Proliferation of Bowen: A Historical and Biographical Note." *American Journal of Dermatopathology,* 6 (February 1984), 35-38.

In 1912 John Templeton Bowen first described the precancerous cutaneous condition which now bears his name. It is a squamous cell carcinoma *in situ* of the skin.

Marmelzat, Willard L. "Daviel on the 'Noli-me-tangere.' A Lost Chapter in the History of Cutaneous Cancer of the Face." *Journal of the History of Medicine,* 4 (Spring 1949), 188-95.

Jacques Daviel (1696-1762) was the first physician to extract the lens in the treatment of cataracts. He was an eye specialist practicing in Paris. In treating what was probably basal cell carcinomas, Daviel argued that nothing less than total surgical removal would effect a cure. He urged patients to avoid caustics. Although he was wrong in his assumption that such cancers originated in the periosteum or perichondrium, he was right in insisting on total excision as the preferred treatment.

Marmelzat, Willard L. "The First Case of Malignant Melanoma Formally Reported in America (1837), Case of Melanosis by Isaac Parrish, M. D." *Journal of Dermatology and Surgical Oncology,* 3 (January/February 1977), 30-31.

In 1837 Isaac Parrish, a physician at Wills' Hospital in Philadelphia, examined a 43 year old woman with a large, dark growth on her big toe and swollen lymph glands. Within weeks she was dead, and in a subsequent autopsy, Parrish found metastatic lesions of what he called "melanosis" in the lymphatic tissues of the groin, both lungs, and the abdominal cavity. His published description of the case is the first account in the United States of a malignant melanoma.

Marmelzat, Willard L. " 'Noli-me-tangere' circa 1754: Jacques Daviel's Forgotten Contribution to Skin Cancer." *Archives of Dermatology*, 90 (1964), 280-83.

(See Chapter 18: Marmelzat, Willard L. "Daviel on the 'Noli-me-tangere.' ").

Morgan, G. "The History and Natural History of Malignant Melanomata of the Uvea." *Transactions of the Ophthalmology Society*, 93 (1973), 71-78.

(See Chapter 14: Duke-Elder).

Onuigbo, Wilson I. B. "Secondary Skin Cancer in Nineteenth-Century Britain." *British Journal of Dermatology*, 94 (1976), 457-63.

As early as 1805 British physicians recognized metastatic lesions of primary tumors occurring in the skin, but they had no idea of the mechanism which brought the lesions to distant sites. Astley Cooper in the 1840s argued that secondary deposits of breast cancer must be transferred to their locations by the lymphatic system. In 1883 D. W. Finlay argued that secondary lesions of gastric carcinoma are carried to their new locations by the bloodstream. Nineteenth century surgeons realized that patient prognosis after the appearance of secondary skin lesions was quite poor, but they nevertheless recommended surgical excision of the new tumors.

Pantoja, Enrique, Alexander G. Gavbriels, and Thomas A. Caputo. "Melanoma of Female Genitalia. Historical Commentary." *New York State Journal of Medicine*, 77 (February 1977), 248-51.

Melanoma of the female genitalia was first recognized by Laènnec in 1806, and over the years he thoroughly studied the disease, described pulmonary metastases, and distinguished it from pigment-free encephaloid. He named it melanosis, and it was not until late in the nineteenth century, after the pathological studies of people like Virchow, Hooper, Cooper, and Pemberton, that the term melanoma came into general use. Schwann offered the first microscopic description of the lesion's cellular structure in 1847. In 1917 B. Bloch of the University of Zurich demonstrated that the naturally-occurring amino acid dioxyphenylalanine (DOPA) was converted by certain basal cells of the epidermis into melanin. The DOPA reaction then became a way of identifying cells capable of producing melanin. It was in 1949 that A. C. Allen described the altered appearance of the melanoblasts at the dermoepidermal junction and their subsequent infiltration of the various layers of the epidermis in the form atypical clear cells as heralding the inception of a malignant melanoma. The earliest recorded case of a vulvar melanoma was reported by Cullen and Carswell, two Scottish physicians, in 1824. Generally, because of social conditions and moral values, careful examinations of the female genitalia were not performed by physicians, so the disease often went unrecognized. The first case of vaginal melanoma was reported by Parona in 1887. As late as the 1970s, physicians often miss vulvovaginal melanomas on pelvic examinations and pathologists misinterpret them histologically.

Pillsbury, Donald M. "General Eisenhower's 'Melanoma'." *Journal of the American Society of Dermatology*, 4 (May 1981), 631-32.

(See Chapter 3: Pillsbury).

Ronchese, F. "Kaposi's Sarcoma: An Overlooked Essay of 1882." *Archives of Dermatology*, 77 (1958), 542-45.

(See Chapter 19: Ronchese).

Ronchese, F. and A. B. Kern. "Kaposi's Sarcoma." *Postgraduate Medicine*, 14 (August 1953), 101.

(See Chapter 19: Ronchese and Kern).

Silvers, David N. and James D. Gorham. "Observations on a Melanoma by William Norris, M.D., a Country Practitioner of the Early 19th Century." *The American Journal of Dermatology*, 4 (October 1982), 421-24.

In 1820 Dr. William Norris, an English physician, treated a 59 year old man with a mole located just above the pubis. The mole had a "brownish hue" and soon turned into a tumor with small nodules around it. Norris excised the tumor but it returned six weeks later. Eventually the patient died. Because the patient's father had died of a similar disease thirty years before, Norris speculated in his written report that the tumor had a hereditary basis. In 1857 Norris wrote "Eight Cases of Melanoma with Pathological and Therapeutical Remarks on that Disease." Although recognition of Norris's contribution did not come until long after his death, it was the first instance of a malignant melanoma reported in English literature.

"Speigler's Tumors." *Cancer Bulletin*, 13 (July-August 1961), 70, 74.

Edward Speigler (1860-1908), a dermatologist in Vienna, in 1899 published an article describing benign, basal cell epitheliomas arising in the scalp as multiple, individual nodules. They are disfiguring but not life-threatening. The disease became known as Speigler's Tumor.

Steffen, Charles. "Jean-Nicolas Marjolin." *The American Journal of Dermatopathology*, 6 (April 1984), 163-65.

(See Chapter 2: Steffen).

Steffen, Charles. "Marjolin's Ulcer: Report of Two Cases and Evidence that Marjolin Did Not Describe Cancer Arising in Scars of Burns." *American Journal of Dermatopathology*, 6 (April 1984), 187-93.

(See Chapter 18: Cruikshank and Gaskell).

Swanson, Neil A. "The Evolution of Mohs' Surgery: Introduction." *Journal of Dermatologic Surgery and Oncology*, 8 (August 1982), 650.

Dr. Frederic Mohs developed the technique for surgical removal of basal cell carcinoma early in the 1950s. The tumor is excised in thin, saucer-shaped layers, and each layer is prepared for horizontal sectioning of mapped and color-coded tissue so as to enable the surgeon to examine microscopically the entire base as well as the epidermal wound edge of the removed tissue.

Taylor, William B. "Mohs' Chemosurgery, Fixed Tissue Technique." *Journal of Dermatologic Surgery and Oncology*, 8 (August 1982), 650-51.

Mohs' chemosurgery for basal cell carcinoma was instituted in 1952 at the University of Michigan. From 1958 to 1980 Dr. Neil Swanson directed the program. Early in the nineteenth century a Dr. Canquoin in Paris had used zinc chloride paste. Such paste applications without microscopic follow-up were used until the 1950s when Mohs' fixed-tissue technique replaced it.

Tromovitch, Theodore A. "Mohs' Surgery, Fresh-Tissue Technique." *Journal of Dermatologic Surgery and Oncology*, 8 (August 1982), 651-53.

The author had performed Mohs' surgery between 1963 and 1966 using the fixed tissue technique but he was not comfortable with the amount of pain the procedure caused patients. Gradually, between 1966 and 1980, he switched to the fresh-tissue technique, and today 95 percent of chemosurgery for basic cell carcinoma involves the fresh-tissue approach rather than the use of zinc chloride paste.

Urteaga, Oscar and George T. Pack. "On the Antiquity of Melanoma." *Cancer*, 19 (1966), 607-10.

Hippocrates first mentioned melanoma in the fifth century, B.C. Several references to "fatal black tumors with metastases and black fluid in the body" appear in European literature during the seventeenth and eighteenth centuries. Robert Carswell first used the term "melanoma" in 1838. Anthropologists have found metastatic melanomas in the bodies of Peruvian Incan mummies.

Walsh, M. Y., and H. Bharucha. "Malignant Melanoma Over a Fifty-Year Period: A Histological Evaluation." *Ulster Medical Journal,* 55 (October 1986), 118-23.

Melanoma was recognized anciently by Hippocrates as a "black cancer," but Laènnec provided the first modern report of a melanoma in 1806. William Norris, an English surgeon, offered the first description of metastatic melanoma in 1820. In 1838 Robert Carswell first used the term "melanoma" to describe the lesion. The most dramatic change in the understanding of the histogenesis of melanoma has occurred since the 1940s. In 1949 A. C. Allen reported on changes in the appearance of melanoblasts at the dermo-epidermal junction. When these atypical cells invade the layers of the epidermis, it is the beginning of a malignant melanoma. The epidermal change takes place just before the invasion of the dermis by the malignant cells, proving that melanoma originates in this junctional activity. Common moles, which are completely intradermal and without a junctional component, do not serve as the source of melanoma. The incidence of primary cutaneous malignant melanoma is increasing in the developed countries. In a study at the Queen's University of Belfast, oncologists found that between 1930 and 1955 only 10 percent of melanomas presented were at a stage where adequate local excision could provide hope for a cure. By 1980 only 20 percent were of the less infiltrating stage with a hope of a surgical cure.

White, C. J. "John Templeton Bowen, M. D." *Archives of Dermatology,* 43 (February 1941), 386.

(See Chapter 18: "Cancer Eponyms: Bowen's Disease").

Wischhusen, H., N. Heiling, and E. Ehler. "Ueber die Cambucca des Paracelsus. (Aus Einer Doktorabelt J. L. Ehlers aud dem Jahre 1756." *Dermatologische Monatsschrift,* 160 (June 1974), 497-502.

J. L. Ehlers, an eighteenth century German surgeon, came to the conclusion that malignant skin lesions were not products of an excess of black bile but were instead localized tumors which could be cured through wide surgical excision. Ehlers was a follower of the Paracelsian theories which would soon sweep away the ancient humoral theories which had dominated medical thought since the time of the Greeks.

Wood, James O. "Woman With a Horn." *Huntington Library Quarterly,* 29 (May 1966), 295-300.

In 1588 a Welsh woman named Margaret Vergh Gryffith was living in London and suffering from a four-inch "horn" tumor growing on her forehead. Contemporaries associated the growth as a sign of adultery, proof that God punished unchastity. It was probably a rare bone tumor, usually benign and painless, but her repeated attempts to remove it surgically were unsuccessful and exacerbated the condition.

Wood, James O. "A Horned Woman." *Isis*, 58 (Summer 1967), 239-40.

(See Chapter 18: Wood).

Zubiri, A. "Dermatología y cancer." *Actas Dermosifiliografia*, 67 (September-October 1976), 637-39.

(See Chapter 18: Haynes, Mead, and Goldwyn).

19 Soft-Tissue Sarcomas

Braun, M. "Classics in Oncology: Idiopathic Multiple Pigmented Sarcoma of the Skin by Kaposi." *Cancer; Diagnosis, Treatment, Research*, 32 (November-December, 1982), 340-47.

In 1872 Moritz Kaposi, a dermatologist in Vienna, Austria, wrote an essay, "Idiopathic Multiple Pigment Sarcoma of the Skin," describing the disease which later became known as Kaposi's sarcoma, a spindle cell neoplasm originating in connective tissue and appearing most frequently in adult males. The lesions for the most part appear on the skin, especially in the extremities, but in its advanced stage, Kaposi's sarcoma metastasizes to internal organs, particularly the lungs.

"Cancer Eponym: Abrikosov's Tumor." *Cancer Bulletin*, 12 (September-October 1960), 92.

Aleksei Ivanovich Abrikosov (1875-1855) was educated at Moscow University and later taught there as a physician and professor of pathology. In 1926 he wrote an article for *Virchow's Archiv* describing what he called "myoblastoma myomas." Today the granular cell myoblastoma is referred to as Abrikosov's tumor.

Davison, Roderick C. "Rhabdomyosarcoma of the Middle Ear." *The Laryngoscope*, 76 (1966), 1889-1920.

Weber first mentioned a rhabdomyosarcoma in 1854 in *Virchow's Archiv*. It is a muscle sarcoma. Other reports appeared throughout the late 1800s. The first case of the tumor in the middle ear was reported by Soderberg in 1933. The tumor is resistant to radiotherapy and chemotherapy, and the only hope for a cure is wide surgical excision.

Peltier, Leonard F. "Historical Note on Bone and Soft-Tissue Sarcoma." *Journal of Surgical Oncology*, 30 (December 1985), 201-05.

Although bone and soft-tissue tumors were not unknown to the older surgical authorities, it was not until the beginning of the nineteenth century that such lesions were clearly distinguished from other diseases. Alexis Boyer (1757-1833) first used the term osteosarcoma to describe bone tumors, and in 1818 Astley Cooper (1768-1841) separated bone tumors into two groups—intramedullary and extramedullary. The French pathologist J. C. A. Recamier (1774-1852) was the first to distinguish between primary and metastatic bone lesions. Rudolf Virchow (1821-1902) first separated the sarcomas from other cancers and defined them as a variety of tumors originating in non-epithelial and non-hematagenous tissues. Virchow identified six major types of sarcomas: fibrosarcoma, myxosarcoma, gliosarcoma, melanosarcoma, chondrosarcoma, and osteosarcoma.

Treatment of bone and soft-tissue tumors has always involved wide-excision and, if necessary, amputation. For a time in the 1940s the surgeon Albert B. Ferguson claimed higher survival rates in osteogenic sarcoma cases by using preoperative radiotherapy and wide excision of the tumor, resorting to amputation only after local recurrence. The delay introduced a bias in favor of slowly growing, less aggressive tumors and against rapidly growing tumors that metastasized early. His theories proved to be shortlived and counterproductive. By the 1950s surgeons had returned to radical, early ablation as the best form of surgical treatment. That pathologists now could now distinguish between varieties of bone and soft-tissue sarcomas allowed for less radical surgical procedures when possible. For soft-tissue sarcomas the development of megavoltage radiotherapy in the 1950s allowed for wide excision followed by radiation treatments, which sometimes eliminated the need for amputation. In the 1960s and 1970s new chemotherapy treatments increased survival rates for osteogenic sarcomas.

"Primary Retriperitoneal Sarcoma—Lobstein's Cancer." *Cancer Bulletin*, 12 (November-December 1960), 114-15.

John Georg Christian Lobstein was born May 8, 1777, in Giessen, Germany. He served as a professor of medicine at the University of Strasbourg and died on March 7, 1835. In 1829 he first described soft-tissue sarcomas arising in the retroperitoneal space. Today we know that those lesions are most commonly rhabdomyosarcomas, lymphosarcomas, liposarcomas, fibrosarcomas, leiomyosarcomas, and synovial sarcomas.

Ronchese, F. "Kaposi's Sarcoma: An Overlooked Essay of 1882." *Archives of Dermatology*, 77 (1958), 542-45.

In 1882 Tomasso De Amicis, an Italian physician, wrote a monograph describing twelve cases of Kaposi's sarcoma and providing photographs of patients suffering from the lesion. The disease is particularly prominent in African males and in men living in the Mediterranean area, although its etiology is unknown.

Ronchese, F. and A. B. Kern. "Kaposi's Sarcoma." *Postgraduate Medicine*, 14 (August 1953), 101.

Kaposi's sarcoma is a cutaneous tumor first appearing on the distal area of the lower extremities. Symmetric pitting edema of the extremities is common. Tumors may appear anywhere in the body and scientists do not know whether it is the result of metastasis or multiple primary tumor foci. The lesions are far more common in males than in females and seem to have an epidemiological bias in favor of Africa and the Mediterranean regions, where the incidence is the highest in the world.

"Sarcoma Botryoides in Children." *Cancer Bulletin*, 12 (May-June 1960), 49-50.

M. P. Guersant first described sarcoma botryoides in 1854, and cervical lesions were first reported by Weber in 1867. Sarcoma botryoides most commonly occurs in female children. The tumors most commonly are found in the vagina, bladder, urethra, and uterine cervix. The rumor is rare, multifocal, and rapidly growing.

Sears, Henry F. "Soft Tissue Sarcoma: A Historical Overview." *Seminars in Oncology*, 8 (June 1981), 129-32.

Sarcomas, malignant tumors originating in connective tissues, account for only one percent of all reported neoplasms. The wide morphological range of sarcomas reflects the complexity of the mesenchymal tissue from which they stem. It was not until the eighteenth century that technology and medicine advanced sufficiently to make relevant investigations of sarcomas possible. The development of the achromatic microscope, thin tissue sectioning techniques, and the recognition of different germ layers of embryonic development made differentiation possible. Rudolf Virchow first described a lipoma lyxomatodes with lung metastases in the 1850s, and by the 1860s he had accurately described and classified the major types of soft-tissue sarcomas. It was not until the 1970s, however, that histological analysis had become sophisticated enough to make consistent, reliable diagnoses of the diseases.

Smith, Maria Wilkins and Lester S. King. "Description of Another Dreadful and Unusual Disease Drawn Up by Hermann Boerhaave." *Journal of the History of Medicine and Allied Sciences*, 23 (October 1968), 331-48.

Dr. Hermann Boerhaave, a physician practicing medicine in Leyden, Holland, early in the eighteenth century, reported the disease and death of a patient from a lung metastasis of what was probably a myxoliposarcoma or poorly differentiated mesenchymal tumor.

Volberding, Paul A. "Kaposi's Sarcoma and the Acquired Immune Deficiency Syndrome." *The Medical Clinic of North America*, 70 (May 1986), 665-76.

Kaposi's sarcoma was an uncommon disease before 1981, with its incidence usually confined to elderly men of African and Mediterranean descent. It was also known to appear in renal graft cases as a form of exogenous immune suppression. But in 1981 Kaposi's sarcoma became the first clear sign that a new disease had appeared when young male homosexuals in the United States and Western Europe began coming down with high rates of the disease. Its etiology is still unknown, except for its indirect relationship to the AIDS virus. Also, Kaposi's sarcoma is much more likely to occur in male homosexuals with AIDS than among male or female heterosexuals with AIDS.

20 Urinary Tract

"Adrenalectomy." *Cancer Bulletin*, 5 (September-October 1953), 116-17.

In 1945 Charles Huggins and W. W. Scott reported the first bilateral adrenalectomy for prostate carcinoma. Most patients with prostate cancer and those with distant metastases can benefit from hormonal therapy, including castration and adrenalectomy, because the tumors are hormone-sensitive and likely to regress once they are starved of the appropriate hormones.

"Cancer Eponyms: Grawitz's Tumor." *Cancer Bulletin*, 9 (March-April 1957), 30.

(See Chapter 2: GRAWITZ, PAUL: "Cancer Eponyms: Grawitz's Tumor").

Depalma, D. A. "Tumores renales: Aspectos históricos." *Seminario en Medicina*, 154 (19 January 1979), 94-97.

In 1883 Paul Grawitz first argued that renal tumors arose from the adrenal rests. Under microscopic examination, the tissue resembled adrenal tissues. The term he coined for the disease was hypernephroma. Paul Sudek in 1893 argued that the tumors were of renal tubular origin, and Otto Stoerk confirmed that opinion with his research in 1908. By the 1940s the term renal adenoma was used for tumors less than 2 centimeters in size, while renal adenocarcinoma described tumors larger than 2 centimeters. The recommended treatment for renal tumors was surgical removal of the diseased kidney, adrenal gland, surrounding perinephric fat, Gerota's fascia, and renal lymph nodes. Radiotherapy was proven effective in 1935 by the research of C. A. Walters. Chemotherapy has been of little use against metastatic renal lesions.

Finkelstein, Jerry Z. "Introduction: Historical Review of Wilms' Tumor." In Carl Pochedly and Denis R. Miller. *Wilms' Tumor*. 1975. Pp. 1-9.

Although there were earlier suggestions of the disease, the first clinical description of Wilms' tumor was offered by F. Van der Byl in 1856. English surgeons performed the first nephrectomies for Wilms' tumor in 1877. By the 1870s excellent descriptions, both clinical and pathological, of Wilms' tumor had been offered by William Osler, Julius Cohnheim, amd Vincenz Czerny. It was an embryonal sarcoma of the kidney. Surgical removal was the only available treatment until 1915 when Alfred Friedlander of Cincinnati began treating the disease with x-ray therapy. It was not until the 1950s that the first chemotherapeutic agents for Wilms' tumor were reported, when Sidney Farber described the effectiveness of actinomycin D in producing tumor regression. Vincristine was added to the therapy in the mid-1960s.

Greene, Frederick L. "A Review of the Historical Development and Results of the Chemotherapy of Wilms' Tumor." *Southern Medical Journal*, 63 (December 1970), 1405-08.

Wilms' tumor is an embryonal renal adenomyosarcoma and constitutes up to 25 percent of all malignancies in children, second only to leukemia. The first reference to the tumor was in 1814 when Thomas Rance described "Fungus Haematodes of the Kidnies." In 1877 the British surgeon L. Jessup performed the first successful nephrectomy for a malignant renal tumor in a child. Max Wilms described the tumor carefully in 1899 and earned the eponymic honors. By the 1920s German physicians were using radiotherapy before surgery to treat the disease. In 1940 researchers isolated the drug actinomycin, and actinomycin D has proven the most effective in treating Wilms' tumor. The drug acts by binding the guanine moiety of deoxyribonucleic acid and thereby preventing the formation of the enzyme, ribonucleic acid polymerase. As a result, ribonucleic acid and protein synthesis are suppressed and cellular damage occurs. In the 1960s researchers began using vinblastine and vincristine, along with actinomycin D, in conjunction with surgery and radiotherapy.

Hafermann, M. "External Radiotherapy." *Urology*, 17 (April 1981), 15.

Until the 1950s, the kilovoltage delivery system for external irradiation was inadequate to treat deep-seated prostate carcinomas. The advent of megavoltage external beam radiation therapy in the 1950s allowed delivery of cancercidal doses to deep tissues without exceeding the radiation tolerance of the skin and other surface tissues. The first trials began in the 1950s, and by the early 1960s external beam radiotherapy had become an important new tool in the fight against prostrate cancer.

Jacobs, Edwin M., Franco M. Muggia, and Marcel Rozencweig. "Chemotherapy of Testicular Cancer: From Palliation to Curative Adjuvant Therapy." *Seminars in Oncology*, 6 (March 1979), 3-12.

In the 1950s the success of the antimetabolites on leukemias and lymphomas launched a vigorous search for curative chemotherapy drugs. The success of methotrexate therapy on gestational choriocarcinomas in the late 1950s inspired even more activity. In the case of testicular cancer, single agent chemotherapy was launched in the early 1960s, and researchers discovered that the alkylating agents had some effect in testicular seminomas and the cytotoxic antibiotics induced some regressions in embryonal cell testicular carcinomas. Eventually it became clear that actinomycin D, mithramycin, adriamycin, bleomycin, vinblastine, and Cis-diamminedichloroplatinum all had tumor fighting capabilities. When it became clear, however, that single drug therapy could not achieve permanent remissions, only palliation, researchers turned to combination drug therapy. By the 1970s the use of combination drug therapies was making testicular carcinomas some of the most curable of malignant lesions.

Jensen, O. M., and A. Larsen. "Blaerecancer i Danmark 1943-1977. Kraefstatistik." *Ugeskrift for Laeger*, 144 (November 15, 1982), 3458-60.

During the past 30 years the incidences of bladder cancer has increased in Denmark, probably because of increased chemical exposure. Tumor pathologists have also been more successful at staging bladder cancer in terms of whether it has penetrated the muscle wall of the bladder, reached adjacent lymph nodes, or metastasized to distant sites. Public health officials have made a particular attempt to improve working conditions in areas where individuals are exposed to carcinogenic metals and dyes so that the incidence of bladder cancer can be reduced.

Jewett, Hugh J. "The Historical Development of the Staging of Bladder Tumors: Personal Reminiscences." *Urological Survey*, 27 (April 1977), 37-40.

Under the direction of Hugh H. Young of the Johns Hopkins University Medical School, Hugh Jewett began a research project in 1942 to provide some classification system for bladder tumors. The original staging system they developed was based on the existence of submucosal invasion (A), muscular invasion (B), and perivesical extension (C). After determining the clinical significance of such a segregation after cystectomy, he found that no class C patients survived 3 years. The B classification, however, had to be subdivided into B1 (superficial muscular invasion) and B2 (deep muscular invasion).

In June 1949 Dukes and Masina developed another approach. Stage 1A represented a tumor confined to the mucous membrane and submucosa only, while Stage 1B indicated spread to the bladder muscle. Stage 2 represented tumors which had spread to the perivesical fat and adjacent tissues. Stage 3 was characterized by regional lymph node involvement, while Stage 4 had distant metastases present. The American Joint Committee for Cancer Staging began in 1959 to convert the staging systems to the International TNM System by adding the histological grade of the tumor. That work was completed in 1967.

Murphy, Gerald P. "Bladder Neoplasms." *Journal of the American Medical Association,* 250 (September 9, 1983), 1326.

Until 1874 urologic surgeons relied on either blind transurethral manipulation or lateral perineal incisions for removal of bladder tumors. In 1874 Billroth employed suprapubic incisions and removed a bladder tumor under direct visual contact. But in 1910 Edwin Beer of Mount Sinai Hospital developed the first successful transurethral removal of a bladder tumor under direct vision. A high frequency current from a Oudin resonator was attached to an ordinary x-ray machine. Underwater endoscopic fulguration and destruction of the tumor was achieved. In 1917 H. H. Young and Howard Kelly of Baltimore pioneered endoscopic radium seed insertion.

"Note sur un cas de cancer au penis." *Union médicale du Canada,* 72 (1943), 188-89.

In 1874 Dr. J. O. Mousseau, a French Canadian physician, surgically excised a squamous cell carcinoma from the penis of an adult male. The immediate surgery was successful but the tumor eventually recurred locally in the urethra, bladder, and regional lymph nodes, ulcerated and hemorrhaged, and caused the patient's death just over a year later.

Perez, Carlos A., William R. Fair, Daniel C. Ihde, and Ferdinand Labrie. "Cancer of the Prostate." In Vincent P. DeVita, Jr., Samuel Hellman, and Steven A. Rosenberg. *Cancer. Principles & Practice of Oncology.* 1985. Pp. 929.

The role of prostate tumors in causing bladder outlet obstruction was first described by Antonio Ferri in Naples in 1530. Eight years later Vesalius provided the first anatomical drawings of the prostate. In 1649 Riolan described a prostate tumor, and in 1794 Baillie first reported prostatic carcinoma. The English anatomist John Hunter demonstrated in 1786 that removing the testicles from young male animals prevented the growth of the prostate, and in the 1940s Charles Huggins showed that regression of prostate carcinomas could be induced by endocrine controls.

Price, James M. "Etiology of Bladder Cancer." In James E. Maltry. ed. *Benign and Malignant Tumors of the Urinary Bladder.* Flushing, N.Y.: 1971. Pp. 189-216.

In 1895 Ludwig Rehn, a German surgeon, reported an unusually high incidence of bladder cancer among aniline dye workers. Reports from other industrialized countries with similar industries soon confirmed Rehn's suspicions that aniline dye was carcinogenic. Those conclusions were experimentally confirmed in 1938 when W. C. Hueper induced bladder cancer in dogs after repeated injections of 2-naphthylamine. Hueper believed bladder cancer was induced by substances in the urine which irritated the interior lining of the bladder. R. S. Ferguson, another oncologist of the 1930s, believed the tumors were produced by unknown products of aniline metabolism, which were delivered to the bladder wall by blood vessels and produced edema, hemorrhages, and benign papillomas. Eventually the benign papillomas were transformed into carcinomas. Subsequent research revealed that Hueper's view of the etiology of bladder cancer was the correct one.

Pyrah, L. N. "John Hunter and After: Renal Calculi and Cancer of the Bladder." *Annals of the Royal College of Surgeons of England,* 45 (July 1969), 1-22.

John Hunter, the famous eighteenth century British surgeon, observed bladder neoplasms in autopsies, but he did not recognize the exact nature of the lesion. The German urologist Rehn in 1895 observed a high incidence of bladder cancers in chemical plant workers. Subsequent research by W. C. Hueper (1938) and G. M. Bonser (1943) demonstrated that the carcinogenic substances in bladder cancer were 1-naphthylamine, 2-naphthylamine, the dye-stuffs auramine and magenta, benzidine, and 4-aminodiphenyl. The bladder tumors are actually produced by the body's metabolite of the chemical, rather than the chemical itself, because the neoplasms appear along the excretion route rather than the ingestion route. The concentration of the metabolite in the bladder, where it is in continuous contact with the transitional epithelium of the bladder, causes those tumors to develop.

Rohl, Lars. "Max Wilms (1867-1918)." *Investigations in Urology,* 4 (1966), 194-96.

In 1814 T. F. Rance described a case of what later became known as Wilms' tumor, and in 1870s there were several descriptions of the lesion, although the nomenclature differed because the pathologists disagreed on the tissue's histology. In 1899 Max Wilms correctly argued that the tumors originated in embryonic mesoderm, and the tumor became known as Wilms' tumor.

Scott, William W. "Historical Overview of the Treatment of Prostate Cancer."
The Prostate, 4 (1983), 435-40.

There have been four major developments in the history of the treatment of
prostatic cancer. In 1904 Hugh H. Young of Johns Hopkins University performed
the first radical prostatectomy. It was known as the radical perineal prostatectomy. In 1945 Terrence Millin pioneered the retropubic prostatectomy. Second,
radiation therapy for prostate cancer began before 1920 with the use of radium.
In the 1960s J. A. Del Regato led the way in external megavoltage therapy of
prostate cancer. Third, in the early 1930s, Charles Huggins discovered the efficacy of hormonal therapy through castration and estrogen dosage. Finally, Dr.
Gerald Murphy of the National Prostate Cancer Project in the 1970s and 1980s
developed several chemotherapeutic protocols using cyclophosphamide, estramus-
tine, 5-fluorouracil, semustine, dacarbazine, and streptozotocin.

Shelley, Harry S. "The Enlarged Prostate. A Brief History of Its Treatment."
The Journal of the History of Medicine and Allied Sciences, 24 (October
1969), 452-73.

Although Morgagni described prostatic enlargement in the mid-1750s, with
involvement of the seminal vesicles, the first genuine description of a prostatic
carcinoma was given by George Langstaff of London in 1817. In 1847 Benjamin
Brodie described prostatic carcinoma and metastasis to the vertebra. Theodor
Billroth performed the first perineal prostatectomy for carcinoma of the prostate
in 1867, but the patient died of metastatic disease a year later. Hugh Young of
Johns Hopkins developed his radical perineal prostatectomy in 1904. The operation involved removal of the entire prostate gland, the seminal vesicles, and a small
cuff of bladder, with the bladder then sutured to the cut end of the urethra. That
became the surgery of choice until the 1940s when Terrence Millin developed his
retropubic approach. In 1956 Brice Vallett of the United States began employing
the transsacral prostatectomy. Another important development in the treatment
of prostate cancer was Charles Huggins's realization in the early 1940s that some
prostatic carcinomas were androgen dependent. Castration or estrogen therapy
could retard growth and relieve the pain caused by metastases to the bones.

Sproul, Edith E. "Acid Phosphatase and Prostate Cancer: Historical Overview."
The Prostate, 1 (1980), 411-13.

The author recalls her collaboration with Alexander Gutman and Ethel Benedict at the Presbyterian Hospital in New York during the 1930s when they demonstrated striking elevations of acid phosphatase at the site of prostatic cancer metastases in bone. The research showed that blood levels of acid phosphatase could be
correlated with progress of the disease. And since acid phosphatase levels in the
prostate rise with maturity and vary with hormonal status, it became clear that
cancer cells could be functionally mature, not embryonic, which was the prevailing
belief of the time.

Tkocz, Izabella and Franz Bierring. "A Medieval Case of Metastasizing Carcinoma with Multiple Osteosclerotic Bone Lesions." *American Journal of Physical Anthropology*, 65 (December 1984), 373-80.

(See Chapter 9: Tkocz and Bierring).

Waldron, H. A. "On the History of Scrotal Cancer." *Annals of the Royal College of Surgeons of England*, 65 (November 1983), 420-22.

Since Percivall Pott's description of scrotal cancer in 1775, there have been three major occupational groups in which the risk of contracting the disease has been unusually great. English chimney sweeps had high rates of the disease, which was usually preceded by the development of hyperkeratic lesions on the scrotum. By the early 1800s surgeons recommended wide excision as the only treatment. The second group of men suffering from the disease were brown coal and parrafin workers who contracted scrotal cancer after long exposure to the tar from gas works, blast furnaces, and coke ovens. The association between the occupation and the lesion was first suggested by von Volkmann in 1873. The third occupational group with a high propensity for scrotal cancer was mineral oil workers: shale oil workers, mule spinners, and engineering workers. The association between these workers in the cotton industry and the disease was well established by the 1920s.

Waldron, H. A. "On the History of Scrotal Cancer." *British Journal of Indian Medicine*, 40 (November 1983), 390-401.

(See Chapter 20: Waldron).

Zorgniotti, Adrian W. "Bladder Cancer in the Pre-Cystoscopic Era." *Progress in Clinical and Biological Research*, 162A (1984), 1-9.

French urology began with the work of Jean Civiale (1792-1867) who revolutionized the treatment of bladder stones with lithotrity. But even before Civiale, another French surgeon, Francois Chopart (1743-1795), had differentiated between low-grade and high-grade tumors of the bladder. Before the invention of the cystoscope in 1879, bladder cancer was diagnosed by the presence of painless hematuria, frequent urination, the passage of tumor fragments in the urine, a cadaveric odor in the urine, and general cachexia. Late in the nineteenth century Henry Thompson in England had developed a small perineal incision to allow a physician to insert the index finger and palpate the bladder. The only treatment for bladder cancer throughout most of the nineteenth century was the use of opium to control pain until death. The problem with surgery was its technology and the serious threat to patient survival posed by the operation. Not until 1895 did Clado develop a method for wide excision and cauterization of bladder carcinomas, using a suprapubic approach.

21 Endocrine Tumors

"Adrenalectomy." *Cancer Bulletin,* 5 (September-October 1953), 116-17.

(See Chapter 20: "Adrenalectomy").

Besson, A., R. Chabloz, and F. Saegesser. "Pheochromocytomes sporadiques, familiaux ou associes a une neurocristopathie. 27 Observations dont 26 chirurgicales (1926 a 1985)." *Schweizerische Rundshau für Medizin Praxis,* 74 (November 12, 1985), 1267-82.

(See Chapter 21: Brennan and Macdonald).

Brennan, Murray F., and John S. Macdonald. "Cancer of the Endocrine System." In Vincent DeVita, Jr., Samuel Hellman, and Steven A. Rosenberg. *Cancer. Principles & Practice of Oncology.* 1985. Pp. 1179-1241.

Hyperthyroidism was described by Parry in 1786, Graves in 1835, and Von Basedow in 1840. In 1850 Curling first described myxedema in 1850, as did Gull in 1875. Reverdin performed a thyroidectomy in 1882 but noticed the subsequent development of myxedema. Murray and Howitz began treating myxedema with thyroid extract in 1890, and Kendall isolated the hormone thyroxine in 1914. The first successful thyroidectomy was performed by the Moor physician Albucasis in Spain in 950 A.D., but the real pioneer in the surgery was Theodor Kocher of Berne, Switzerland. He performed thousands of thyroid operations, and to avoid myxedema he pioneered the subtotal thyroidectomy. Kocher received the Nobel Prize in 1909. Thyroxin was first synthesized by Harrington and Barger in 1927, and thiouracil, the first anti-thyroid drug, appeared in 1943.

The adrenal gland was first described by Bartolomeu Eustacchio in 1563, but the function of the adrenal remained shrouded in mystery until the twentieth century. In 1927 F. A. Hartman suggested that the general function of the adrenal gland was production of a hormone, and in 1927 he demonstrated that adrenal extracts sustained life in animals without adrenal glands. In 1899 William Osler first described what became known as Cushing's syndrome, and the adrenal tumor was confirmed by Parkes-Weber in 1913.

The Zollinger-Ellison Syndrome fulminant ulcer disease, gastric hyperacidity, and a gastrin-producing islet cell tumor. It was first described by Robert Zollinger and Edwin Ellison in 1955.

In 1899 Mering and Minkowski discovered that total pancreatectomy in dogs resulted in fatal diabetes. Laguesse suggested in 1911 that the islet might be the source of pancreatic secretions. The internal secretion of the pancreas was described by F. G. Banting and C. H. Best in 1922 at the University of Toronto. The first case of carcinoma of the islets of Langerhans, or insulinoma, was published in 1927. The pancreatic endocrine neoplasm known as a glucagonoma, composed of pancreatic alpha cells, was first discovered in 1942. In 1958 J. V. Verner and A. B. Morrison first reported what became known as WDHA syndrome—the watery diarrhea, hypokalemia, and achlorhydria of an islet-cell tumor. The first case of pancreatic somatostatinoma was reported in 1977.

Multiple Endocrine Neoplasia Syndrome I (MEN-1) involves the parathyroid, pituitary, and pancreatic islet cells. Adrenal and thyroid adenomas are rarely found. The first report of MEN-1 was presented by Erdheim in 1903. The patient had a pituitary tumor with multiple gland parathyroid disease. Cushing reported in 1927 a patient with an eosinophilic adenoma of the pituitary, two parathyroid adenomas, and a pancreatic islet tumor. In 1953 Underdahl presented eight patients with muliple adenomas involving pituitary islet cells and the parathyroid glands. Werner in 1954 postulated a genetic origin to the neoplasm. MEN-2 is a medullary carcinoma of the thyroid gland. MEN-2 was first reported by Hazard in 1959, but in 1961 John Sipple of the State University of New York at Syracuse described an association of pheochromocytoma and thyroid cancer. E. D. Williams of London Hospital in 1965 associated medullary carcinoma with a family history and bilateral pheochromocytoma.

Collins, W. F. "Hypophysectomy: Historical and Personal Perspective." *Clinical Neurosurgery*, 21 (1974), 68-78.

(See Chapter 26: "Some Aspects of Hormonal Therapy").

"Cushing's Syndrome." *Cancer Bulletin*, 15 (May-June 1963), 45.

Harvey Cushing, the famed Harvard neurosurgeon, first described in 1932 the disease which now bears his name—hyperadrenocorticism caused by excess secretion from the pituitary gland. It is caused by an adenoma, carcinoma, bilateral hyperplasia, or unilateral hyperplasia. The clinical symptoms of Cushing's syndrome are protein depletion, shrinking of muscle mass, osteoporosis, hypertension, and peripheral edema.

Emmanuel, I. G. "Symposium on Pituitary Tumours: Historical Aspects of Radiotherapy, Present Treatment and Results." *Clinical Radiology*, 17 (1966), 154-60.

(See Chapter 10: Emmanuel).

German, William J., and Stevenson Flanigan. "Pituitary Adenomas: A Follow-Up Study of the Cushing Series." *Clinical Neurosurgery*, 10 (1964), 72-81.

(See Chapter 10: German and Flanigan).

Harrison, R. Cameron and F. Miks. "Canadian Contributions Towards the Comprehension of Hyperinsulinism: The First Successful Excision of an Insulinoma." *The Canadian Journal of Surgery*, 23 (July 1980), 401-04.

In 1902 A. G. Nichols of McGill University first described an islet cell adenoma. Not until 1923 was the clinical syndrome of hyperinsulinism suspected. At Toronto General Hospital in 1929, Dr. R. R. Graham resected the pancreas of a 54 year old woman, removing an islet cell carcinoma. The woman survived another twenty years. Hyperinsulinism had also caused hypoglycemia.

Horwitz, Norman H. "Sir Geoffrey Jefferson on Invasive Pituitary Adenomas." *Journal of Neurosurgery*, 42 (February 1975), 244.

In 1940 Sir Geoffrey Jefferson made his presidential address to the Royal Society of Medicine in Great Britain, in which he spoke of his experience with invasive adenomas of the anterior pituitary. His work was important for two reasons: he described the clinical symptoms of individuals suffering from this tumor, making diagnosis easier, and he showed that the operative mortality in these patients increases tenfold when compared with patients suffering from localized pituitary tumors.

Klawans, Harold L. "The Acromegaly of Maximinus I: The Possible Influence of a Pituitary Tumor on the Life and Death of a Roman Emperor." In F. Clifford Rose and W. F. Bynum. *Historical Aspects of the Neurosciences*. New York: 1982. Pp. 317-26.

(See Chapter 3: Maximinus I).

Lips, C. J. M., et al. "Central Registration of Multiple Endocrine Neoplasia Type 2 Families in The Netherlands." *Henry Ford Hospital Medical Journal*, 32 (1984), 236-37.

Since 1981 the Dutch have been conducting, through the Danish Tumor Registry, a long-range study on inherited tendencies to develop Multiple Endocrine Neoplasias of the Type 2 variety. They predict that eventually they will identify 500 to 700 high-risk individuals and offer those people cyclical diagnostic examinations to catch the disease at an early stage.

Satoh, O. "Transsphenoidal Surgery for Pituitary Tumors: Historical Perspectives and Present Trends." *No Shinkei Geka,* 12 (January 1984), 7-26.

(See Chapter 23: Satoh).

Sindelar, William F., Timothy J. Kinsella, and Robert J. Mayer. "Cancer of the Pancreas. Historical Considerations." In Vincent P. DeVita, Jr., Samuel Hellman, and Steven A. Rosenberg. *Cancer. Principles & Practice of Oncology.* 1985. Pp. 691-92, 722-23.

(See Chapter 12: Sindelar, Kinsella, and Mayer).

Sipple, John H. "Multiple Endocrine Neoplasia Type 2 Syndromes: Historical Perspectives." *Henry Ford Hospital Medical Journal,* 32 (1984), 219-22.

In 1959, as a young medical student, John Sipple participated in an autopsy on a 33 year old male who had been hypertensive after surgery for arteriovenous malformations of the brain. He had died of cerebral hemorrhage. The autopsy revealed large, bilateral pheochromocytomas and a 2 centimeter, pale mass in each lobe of the thyroid gland, as well as a nodular enlargement of the only parathyroid gland he could find. A search of the 500 cases in the literature on pheochromocytoma revealed an incidence of thyroid carcinoma far in excess of statistical expectations. Sipple published an article on his findings in a 1961 issue of the *American Journal of Medicine.* Since then Multiple Endocrine Neoplasia Type 2 Syndrome has also been known as Sipple's syndrome.

Thompson, J. "Tumours of the Thyroid Gland. Introduction. Historical Notes." *Monographs of Neoplastic Diseases of Various Sites,* 6 (1970), 1-11.

Parry described the first case of hyperthyroidism in 1786, and in 1850 Curling offered the first published account of myxedema. In 1882 Reverdin performed a thyroidectomy and produced myxedema in the patient, and in 1890 Murray and Howitz successfully used thyroid extract in treating the disorder. Thyroidectomies had been performed for hundreds of years, but Theodor Kocher, a surgeon in Berne, Switzerland, pioneered the modern era and advocated subtotal thyroidectomies for carcinoma when possible since the procedure prevented the development of myxedema.

van Heerden, Jonathan A. "First Encounters With Pheochromocytoma." *American Journal of Surgery,* 144 (August 1982), 277-79.

The first successful resection of a pheochromocytoma was performed by Roux in Lausanne, Switzerland, in 1926, and the first such procedure in the United States was performed shortly thereafter by C. H. Mayo at the Mayo Clinic. The patient was Mother Joachim, a Roman Catholic nun who came to the clinic suffering from headaches, fatigue, severe hypertension, and nausea. Exploratory surgery revealed a lemon-sized tumor on the left adrenal, which Mayo felt resembled a brain tumor. He performed the resection and the tumor proved to be a malignant enlargement of the ganglion resting on a renal vessel. After the operation the patient recovered from the symptoms and survived for eighteen years.

Zamora, Jose L. "Cystic Neoplasms of the Pancreas. Evolution of a Concept." *American Journal of Surgery*, 149 (June 1985), 819-23.

Jean Cruveihlier first described a pancreatic cyst in 1816, and the first report of a pancreatic cystic tumor came in 1867. It was not until the end of the nineteenth century that physicians began to understand the nature of pancreatic disease, particularly the diverse origins of cystic lesions. In 1907 A. W. Mayo Robson and P. J. Cammidge divided pancreatic cysts into congential, hydatidic, neoplastic, hemorrhagic, retention cysts, and pseudocysts, and their classification system is still used today. It was not until the 1970s that the two forms of neoplastic disease of the pancreas were classified: benign, microcystic adenoma and malignant, mucinous cystadenoma-cystadenocarcinoma.

In the seventeenth and eighteenth centuries the major treatment for abdominal cysts was puncture and external drainage. The first surgical resection of a solid pancreatic tumor was performed in 1882, and in 1894 Theodor Billroth performed the first total pancreatectomy. The discovery of insulin in 1922 made total pancreatectomy a reasonable treatment.

IV DIAGNOSIS AND TREATMENT

22 Diagnostic

Angrisani, V. "L'introduzione della técnica microscopia nello studie delle neo-plasie meligne." *Pagine di Storia della Medicina*, 12 (September-October 1968), 66-74.

The Dutch scientist Zaccharias Janssen developed the first microscope in 1590, and Galileo developed another version in 1610. Early in the eighteenth century another Dutch physician began using the microscope regularly for tissue studies. Systematic biological studies using the microscope began with the work of the Italian scientist, Marcello Malpighi, late in the seventeenth century. Real optical improvements in the microscope, however, did not occur until the early 1800s when several British and German manufacturers perfected the instrument. The consequences of the technological improvements were enormous, because Johannes Müller and other German pathologists developed the cell theory of tissue structure shortly after the new microscopes appeared in the 1820s. The cellular theory of cancer was the beginning of modern oncology.

Baker, Harvey W. "Needle Aspiration Biopsy: An Introduction." *CA-A Cancer Journal for Clinicians*, 36 (March-April 1986), 69-70.

The needle biopsy was first developed by Hayes Martin of the Memorial Hospital for the Treatment of Cancer and Allied Diseases. Widely considered as the father of head and neck surgery in the treatment of cancer, Martin began advocating needle aspiration biopsies in the early 1930s. His research confirmed the ability to secure reliable tissue samples for cytological examination through needle aspiration biopsies of the cervical lymph nodes, but he also recommended the procedure for tumors of the breast, bone, lung, thyroid, mediastinum, and soft tissues. The pathologist who examines the tissue must know the anatomic site of the aspirations and the structures traversed by the needle. Martin recommended an 18 gauge needle, but contemporary practice favors the finer 21 or 22 gauge needle.

Becker, V. "Carl Ruge: 100 Jahre Stückchen-Diagnose." *Archiv fur Gynaekologie*, 227 (September 1979), 193-204.

(See Chapter 6: Hertig).

Bloomberg, Allan Ellia. "Thoracoscopy in Perspective." *Surgery, Gynecology & Obstetrics*, 147 (1978), 433-43.

The thorascope is a direct descendent of the cystoscope, an instrument invented by Bozzini in 1806 with which he attempted to look inside the urinary bladder using a candle as a light source. But he was hampered by the inability to project light into deep areas. In 1853 Desormeaux used a bright flame produced by a mixture of alcohol and turpentine to provide a better light source. In 1883 Newman incorporated the newly invented Edison light bulb into a cystoscope. The prototype of the modern cystoscope was born when the light bulb was added to the Nitze-Leiter endoscope. By the late 1930s the double cannula technique for intrapleural pneumonolysis had superseded the single cannula procedure. In the 1960s thoracic specialists were combining thorascopy and pleural biopsy to diagnose malignant diseases of the chest and distinguish between them and tuberculosis. Illumination of the chest was greatly advanced in the 1960s and 1970s with the new fiberoptic technology.

Bradbury, Steven. *The Evolution of the Microscope*. New York: 1967.

(See Chapter 22: Angrisani).

Bradbury, Steven, and G. L'E. Turner. *Historical Aspects of Microscopy*. Cambridge: 1967.

(See Chapter 22: Angrisani).

Carmichael, Erskine. "Dr. Papanicolau and the Pap Smear." *The Alabama Journal of Medical Science*, 21 (January 1984), 101-04.

(See Chapter 2: PAPANICOLAU, GEORGES: Carmichael, Erskine).

Candiani, G. B. "The Classification of Endometriosis: Historical Review and Present Status of the Art." *Acta European Fertility*, 17 (March-April 1986), 85-92.

(See Chapter 6: Candiani).

"Cuthbert Esquire Dukes (1890-1977)." *European Journal of Surgical Oncology*, 13 (February 1987), 77.

(See Chapter 6: "Cuthbert Esquire Dukes (1890-1977)").

Dehner, Louis P. "Classic Neuroblastoma: Histopathologic Grading as a Prognostic Indicator. The Shimada System and Its Progenitors." *The American Journal of Pediatric Hematology/Oncology*, 10 (1988), 143-54.

(See Chapter 10: Dehner).

De Moulin, Daniel. "Microscopie en Kankerdiagnostick in de Eerste Helft van de Negentiende Eeuw." *Tijdschrift voor de Geschiedenis der Geneeskunde, Nafuurwetenschappen, Wiskunde en Techniek*, 6 (1983), 99-107.

(See Chapter 22: Angrisani).

Dmochowski, Leon L. "Viruses and Tumors in the Light of Electron Microscope Studies: A Review." *Cancer Research*, 20 (August 1960), 977-1015.

The electron microscope was first developed in the 1930s by Knoll and Ruska at the University of Berlin in Germany, but it was the research program of Leon L. Dmochowski, beginning in the 1940s, which launched the modern era of research into tumors and tumor viruses. Because it can see beyond the wave lengths of visible light, the electron microscope provided unprecedented examination of cellular structures. Early in the twentieth century the use of cell-free filtrates provided confirmation of the viral etiology of some animal tumors, but not until the development of the electron microscope did the field of virology really have its beginning, and not until the 1950s did the belief in viruses as an important oncogenic factor in human cancers receive wide acceptance and trigger a new research effort on the causes of cancer.

Dooley, T. S. *Needle Biopsy*. Glasgow: 1974.

(See Chapter 22: Baker).

Egan, Robert L. "Evolution of the Team Approach in Breast Cancer." *Cancer; Diagnosis, Treatment, Research*, 36 (November 1975), 1815-22.

(See Chapter 22: Puretz).

Glasscock, Michael E. "History of the Diagnosis and Treatment of Acoustic Neuromas." *Archives of Otolaryngology*, 88 (December 1968), 578-85.

(See Chapter 14: Glasscock).

Härting, Paul. *Das Mikroscop*. Berlin: 1970.

(See Chapter 22: Angrisani).

Hertig, Arthur T. "Early Concepts of Dysplasia and Carcinoma *In Situ* (A Backward Glance at a Forward Process)." *Obstetrical and Gynecological Survey,* 34 (November 1979), 795-803.

(See Chapter 6: Hertig).

"The History of Mammography." *Cancer Bulletin,* 17 (July-August 1965), 84-85.

In 1913 Albert Salomon published his study of roentgenographic examination of 3,000 amputated breasts, hoping to identify identifiable characteristics of carcinomas. S. L. Warren published similar reports on 119 patients in 1930. In 1951 R. Leborgue of Uruguay described the multiple punctate calcifications which are almost pathognomonic of a malignant tumor. In 1960 R. L. Egan of M. D. Anderson Hospital and Tumor Institute in Houston began the modern era of mammography.

Hunter, John A. A. and Karl Holubar, eds. "In Praise of Alexander Breslow." *American Journal of Dermatopathology,* 6 (Summer 1984), Suppl. 1, 151-57.

(See Chapter 18: Hunter and Holubar).

Hutter, Robert V. P. "Lobular Carcinoma *in Situ.*" *CA-A Cancer Journal for Clinicians,* 32 (July-August 1982), 232-33.

(See Chapter 11: Hutter).

Jewett, Hugh J. "Historical Development of the Staging of Bladder Tumors: Personal Reminiscences." *Urological Survey,* 27 (April 1977), 37-40.

(See Chapter 20: Jewett).

Karpov, N. A. "Iz istorii diagnostiki raka gortani." *Zhurnal Ushnykh, Nosovykh, i Gorlovykh Boleznei,* 1 (January-February 1979), 81-82.

The major diagnostic innovations in the history of oncology have been the development of the microscope in the nineteenth century, which permitted the birth of cellular pathology; the discovery of x-rays in the 1890s, which led to the rise of radiology and radiotherapy; the post-World War II use of radioisotopes and nuclear medicine; the development of fiberoptics and accurate lymphangiography in the 1960s; and the invention of computer axial tomography in the 1970s.

Koprowska, I. "Concurrent Discoveries of the Value of Vaginal Smears for Diagnosis of Uterine Cancer." *Diagnostic Cytopathology,* 1 (July-September 1985), 245-48.

(See Chapter 6: Koprowska).

Kramer, W. "On the Classification of Tumours of the Peripheral Nervous System." *Psychiatria, Neurologia, Neurochirurgia,* 72 (1969), 65-75.

(See Chapter 10: Kramer).

"Medical Uses of Radioisotopes." *Cancer Bulletin,* 6 (March-April 1954), 29.

The first biological tracer study was done by Hevesy in 1924 using radioactive lead to study the absorption of that element by plants. Several years later S. Weiss and H. L. Blumgart in Boston used it to study the velocity of blood in humans. After World War II new radioisotopes became available: strontium for surface lesions; iodine for hypothyroidism and thyroid carcinoma; and phospherous for chronic leukemia.

Melicow, M. M. "Carcinoma *in Situ*: An Historical Perspective." *Urology Clinic of North America,* 3 (February 1976), 5-11.

(See Chapter 13: Douglass).

Mildner, T. "Versuche zur Krebs-Diagnostik und Therapie vor 200 Jahren." *Deutsch Medizinische Journal,* 17 (5 March 1966), 141-44.

(See Chapter 1: Fisher and Hermann).

Naylor, B. "The History of Exfoliate Cancer Cytology." *Medical Bulletin,* 26 (1960), 289-96.

(See Chapter 13: Douglass and Chapter 3: PAPANICOLAOU, GEORGES: Carmichael).

Nelson, Rodney B. "History." In *Endoscopy in Gastric Cancer.* New York: 1979. Pp. 1-5.

Until the development of fiberoptics in the 1950s, endoscopy was a crude science frought with the dangers of inaccurate diagnoses. In 1868 Kussmaul tried to observe the stomach of a carnival sword swallower, using a rigid metal tube, and in 1881 Mikulicz successfully observed the lining of a patient's stomach using a similar instrument. A variety of experiments took place until the 1920s, when Robert Schindler developed a workable, rigid instrument. Then in the 1930s Schindler developed a straight instrument with a short metal portion connected to a flexible tube containing lenses for transmitting light. Modern gastroscopy was born. Fiber optics—the ability to transmit light and images along coated glass or plastic fibers—became a diagnostic boon in 1958 when B. I. Hirshowitz developed a fiberoptic gastroscope. Soon after instrument manufacturers were developing scopes with visual images of remarkable clarity. Because of high rates of upper gastrointestinal carcinomas in Japan, the Japanese led the way in the development of fiber optic endoscopes in the 1960s. By the late 1960s American technology was able to mass produce high quality instruments which greatly assisted physicians in distinguishing between benign and malignant lesions of the stomach.

Pressman, David. "The Development and Use of Radiolabeled Antitumor Antibodies." *Cancer Research*, 40 (August 1980), 2960-64.

(See Chapter 24: Pressman).

Puretz, Donald H. "Mammography. History, Current Events, and Recommendations." *New York State Journal of Medicine*, 76 (November 1976), 1985-91.

(See Chapter 11: Puretz).

"Roentgen, Forssell and Madame Curie." *Cancer Bulletin*, 14 (May-June 1962), 47-48.

W. E. Baensch, a prominent faculty member of the Georgetown University Medical School, recalls his early years as an assistant to Wilhelm Conrad Roentgen at the University of Munich in 1913 and Madame Marie Sklodowska (Curie) at Paris in the 1920s.

Rosen, Peter Paul. "Specimen Radiography and the Diagnosis of Clinically Occult Mammary Carcinoma. A Brief Historical Review." *Pathology Annual*, 15 (1980), 225-37.

Recent technical advances have permitted the radiologist to detect carcinomas that were inapparent to the patient and the physician—clinically occult carcinoma. Albert Salomon of the University of Berlin was the first to use specimen radiography when he began studying breast lesions in 1913, and during the 1920s Dominguez did similar work in Uruguay. Cutler began transillumination of the breast in 1929, and Warren and Fray began radiologic studies of the breast in the 1930s. These early mammographic studies generated skepticism from surgeons and pathologists who doubted that radiologists would ever be able to distinguish between benign and malignant lesions. In the 1940s studies began which carefully correlated radiologic and histopathologic conclusions. Radiologic appearance of calcified lesions has been studied extensively. Today specimen radiography is essential to the management of nonpalpable breast lesions found by mammography because it provides two pieces of information. It is the only method for proving that the lesion discovered by mammography was removed, and it is a most efficient technique for pinpointing such an area for histologic examination by the pathologist.

Rosenblatt, Milton B. and James R. Lisa. "Diagnostic Progress in Lung Cancer: Historical Perspective." *Journal of the American Geriatric Society*, 16 (August 1968), 919-29.

The inherent characteristics of lung cancer—insidious onset, variability of physical signs, resemblance to other pulmonary diseases, and inaccessibility of the lesion to direct examination—have contributed to the previously very slow progress in clinical detection of the disease. For more than a century the autopsy remained the chief source of diagnostic confirmation. It was not until the 1930s that technical procedures were perfected and made generally available for the clinical diagnosis of lung cancer.

During the first half of the nineteenth century practically all the classical symptoms of lung cancer were fully established. The specific symptoms of the tumor such as cough, hemoptysis, dyspnea, and stridor were emphasized by Hughes, Bell, Bouillard, and Hayfelder. The neurologic and vascular syndromes produced by extrapulmonary metastases were described by MacLachlan, Hare, Burrows, Moneret, Fleury, and Lanceraux. Stokes and Graves identified unilateral dullness and absent breath sounds with bronchial obstruction in differentiating lung cancer from other pulmonary diseases like tuberculosis, pneumonia, and pleurisy.

The possibility of diagnosing lung cancer by examination of the sputum was nurtured for a century before coming to fruition in the 1940s with the perfection of Papanicolaou's cytologic technique. The early endeavors by Andral in 1821 and Walsh in 1843 involved microscopic study of expectorated lung tissue, a procedure hampered by the lack of effective staining techniques and the infrequent occurrence of tumor tissue in the expectorate. In 1887 Hampeln demonstrated that lung cancer could be diagnosed clinically by the examination of expectorated tissue. In 1895 Betschart identified lung cancer cells as large round cells with oversized nuclei and keratinized cytoplasm. In 1899 Hermann established criteria for differentiating between malignant squamous cells and benign squamous epithelium from the buccal cavity.

In 1901 Weinberger succeeded in producing x-ray pictures of the lung on photographic plates. By the 1920s and 1930s, as radiologic techniques improved, the diagnoses of lung cancer increased dramatically. The development of the bronchoscope by Killian in 1900 and Jackson in the 1930s had a similar impact on the clinical diagnosis of lung cancer. Progress in exploratory thoractomy for lung cancer followed the advances in surgery for non-malignant disease, and in 1933 Graham and Singer performed the first successful pneumonectomy for lung cancer. Other developments include lymph-node biopsy and aspiration biopsy, both of which permitted diagnosis without invasive surgery.

Ross, W. M. "Carcinoma of the Breast in the Section of Radiology." *Journal of the Royal Society of Medicine*, 73 (October 1980), 734-38.

(See Chapter 11: Ross).

Rywlin, Arkadi M. "Non-Hodgkin's Malignant Lymphomas. Brief Historical Review and Simple Unifying Classification." *The American Journal of Dermatopathology*, 2 (Spring 1980), 17-24.

(See Chapter 17: Rywlin).

Schindler, Robert. "La evolución de la gastroscopia." *Medicina Germano Hispano America*, 1 (1924), 690.

(See Chapter 22: Nelson).

von Haam, Emmerich. "The Historical Background of Oral Cytology." *Acta Cytologica*, 9 (1965), 270-72.

(See Chapter 6: von Haam).

Walk, L. "The History of Gastroscopy." *Clinical Medicine*, 1 (1966), 209.

(See Chapter 22: Nelson).

Witkowski, Jan A. "Experimental Pathology and the Origins of Tissue Culture: Leo Loeb's Contribution." *Medical History*, 27 (July 1983), 269-88.

(See Chapter 7: Witkowski).

Wolff, William I. "The Impact of Colonoscopy on the Problem of Colorectal Cancer." *Progress in Clinical Cancer*, 7 (1978), 51-69.

Endoscopic examination of the rectum and bowel goes all the way back to Hippocrates, who regularly used a rectal speculum to search for disease. The modern era of internal examination of the rectum and bowel began in 1853 with Desormeaux's invention of an examining tube. In 1903 Howard Kelly invented the rigid proctosigmoidoscope. Fiberoptics, a method of transmitting light and optical images along coated glass or plastic fibers, became important to medicine in 1958 when Hirshowitz invented a gastroscope. By construction of endoscopes in which each of hundreds of thousands of fibers in a colonoscope occupies the same relative position at each end of the bundle, it became possible to transmit back to an eyepiece an exact image of the illuminated surface. Work on such instruments went ahead in Japan in the early 1960s because of the high incidence of stomach cancer there and the need for better gastroscopes. By the late 1960s researchers in the United States, led by William Wolff, had developed a new colonoscope which could reach the entire colon, greatly enhancing the ability to achieve early diagnosis of colon carcinomas.

Wood, David A. "Clinical Classification of Cancer. Purposes and Methods: Historical Perspective." *Oncology: Proceedings of the Tenth International Cancer Congress*, IV (1970), 128-33.

Clinical staging systems are reliable only if certain basic rules are observed. First, the clinical classification for a given cancer location must be applicable to all cases, regardless of the treatment used. Second, all classifications must be based on clinical examination of the patient before treatment; otherwise there can be no comparison of the results of treatment. Third, a classification cannot be changed once it is made. Finally, clinical staging cannot be merged or combined with other sorts of staging, or the integrity of the clinical staging is violated. During the twentieth century oncologists from around the world have worked to develop an international system of clinical classification. A number of organizations and congresses were involved, including the Cancer Commission of the Health Organization of the League of Nations in the 1920s; the International Committee for Stage-Grouping in Cancer and for Presentation of the Results of Treatment of Cancer (ICPR), which began meeting in London in 1950; and the International Union Against Cancer in the late 1950s. What emerged was the "TNM System," in which "T" represented the degree of local extension of the tumor, "N" the condition of the regional lymph nodes, and "M" the presence or absence of distant metastases.

Yeh, Samuel D. J. "Nuclear Medicine and Cancer Research in the People's Republic of China." *American Journal of Chinese Medicine*, 7 (1979), 149-55.

(See Chapter 5: Yeh).

23 Surgery

Absolon, K. B., and M. J. Absolon, eds. "Resection of the Cancerous Pylorus Performed by Professor Billroth (With 5 Woodcuts and 3 Lithographs)." *Review of Surgery*, 25 (November-December 1968), 381-408.

(See Chapter 23: Brunschwig and Simandi).

Absolon, K. B., and John Keshishian. "First Laryngectomy for Cancer as Performed by Theodor Billroth on December 31, 1873: A Hundred Year Anniversary." *Review of Surgery*, 31 (March-April 1974), 65-70.

(See Chapter 23: Schechter and Morfit).

Austoker, J. L. "The 'Treatment of Choice': Breast Cancer Surgery 1860-1985." *Society for the Social History of Medicine Bulletin*, 37 (December 1985), 100-07.

(See Chapter 11: Handley).

Baker, Harvey W. "The General Surgeon and Cancer." *The American Journal of Surgery*, 139 (May 1980), 606-07.

The author complains about the growing influence of radiotherapists and chemotherapists and the declining role of surgery in cancer treatment. It all began with the 1942 experiments with nitrogen mustard therapy at Yale University by Alfred Gilman and Louis Goodman. Surgeons must not relinquish the leadership role in cancer treatment. More patients are cured by surgery than any other cancer therapy. Surgeons must know the limits of chemotherapy and radiotherapy, and must not retreat from basic surgical procedures, even though they should reevaluate the superradical operations which became increasingly popular in the 1940s and 1950s. He supports the idea of the team approach to cancer therapy, although he relegates radiotherapy and chemotherapy to adjuvant roles. Until alternate therapies demonstrate their capacity to destroy occult malignancies, most cancer treatment must start with surgery.

Biagini, R., and P. Ruggieri. "Resezione di bacino per tumore osseo. Primo caso presso l'Instituto Ortopedico Rizzoli nel 1914." *Chirurgia Organisazione*, 71 (January-March 1986), 69-73.

Until just recently, the treatment of choice for most bone tumors was a radical amputation of the affected area whenever possible, especially if it involved an extremity. One of the first surgical resections, without amputation, in Italy was performed on a teenaged boy in 1914. He was suffering from what was probably an osteogenic sarcoma. Not until the 1980s, however, with new surgical and radiotherapy techniques as well as more predictive histological grading of tumors, did alternatives to amputation become realistic in some osteogenic sarcoma cases.

Breasted, James H. *The Edwin Smith Surgical Papyrus*. 1930.

The Edwin Smith Papyrus is a surgical document written in Egypt in approximately 1,600 B. C. In addition to describing a variety of Egyptian medical treatments, it describes breast tumors and says that there is no treatment for lesions which are hard, painless, cool to the touch, and not secreting fluid, as opposed to inflammatory lesions. For inflammatory lesions, they recommend cauterization or excision. For what was obviously malignant tumors, they advocated no treatment at all.

Breen, R. E. and W. Garnjobst. "Surgical Procedures for Carcinoma of the Rectum: A Historical Review." *Diseases of the Colon and Rectum*, 26 (October 1983), 680-85.

(See Chapter 23: Polglase and Chapter 23: Hughes).

Brewer, Lyman A. "Historical Notes on Lung Cancer Before and After Graham's Successful Pneumonectomy in 1933." *The American Journal of Surgery*, 143 (June 1982), 650-59.

(See Chapter 15: Brewer).

Brock, Russell. "Thoracic Surgery and the Long-Term Results of Operation for Bronchial Carcinoma." *Annals of the Royal College of Surgeons*, (October 1964), 195-213.

It was not until the late 1920s that the first successful lobectomies for lung carcinoma were performed and not until 1933 that Evarts Graham performed the first successful pneumonectomy for bronchial cancer. Lobectomy had become a fairly routine procedure by the mid-1930s. By the years of World War II enough procedures had been performed to accumulate meaningful data about long-term survival. On younger patients with good respiratory capabilities, pneumonectomy is preferable to lobectomy because it offers a better chance of removing occult tumor cells. The classical operation is the best: removal of the diseased lung, the affected viscus and its fascial connections, the anterior and posterior fatty tissues and lymph nodes, the right or the left tracheobronchial group of nodes, and most of the tracheobronchial group. Also it is important not to disturb the hilar structures by routinely securing the vessels within the pericardium and excising an area of pericardium.

Brunschwig, Alexander and Edith Simandi. "First Successful Pylorectomy for Cancer." *Surgery, Gynecology & Obstetrics*, 92 (March 1951), 375-79.

Early in 1880 Theodor Billroth of the University of Vienna performed the first successful pylorectomy for carcinoma on a 43 year old female. She survived the surgery but died 4 months later of widespread metastases. The article contains a translation of Billroth's notes about the case as well as his follow-up on the patient.

Butterfield, W. C. "Tumor Treatment, 3000 B.C." *Surgery*, 60 (August 1966), 476-79.

The Edwin Smith Papyrus, written in Egypt in 1,600 B.C. using documents from 3,000 B.C., is the oldest known surgical treatise. It offered no hope for curing breast cancer, which was already recognized as a solid tumor not related to trauma, fever, or ulcers. Egyptian physicians had a crude sense of tumors that did not arise from inflammatory or traumatic origin. They recognized the utility of surgery on benign lesions but generally felt that the outlook was hopeless for individuals suffering from malignant tumors. Egyptian physicians were also careful to note that no surgery at all was better for the patient than surgery on a lesion which had already ulcerated and become clearly out of control.

Colcock, B. P. "Surgical Progress in the Treatment of Rectal Cancer." *Surgery, Gynecology & Obstetrics*, 121 (1965), 997-1003.

(See Chapter 23: Polglase and Chapter 23: Hughes).

Cole, Warren H. "Past, Present, and Future of Surgery and the Conquest of Cancer." *Nebraska Medical Journal*, 55 (December 1970), 715-20.

(See Chapter 23: Lawrence).

Collins, W. F. "Hypophysectomy: Historical and Personal Perspective." *Clinical Neurosurgery*, 21 (1974), 68-78.

(See Chapter 26: "Some Aspects of Hormonal Therapy").

Corman, Marvin L. "Classic Articles in Colonic and Rectal Surgery. Robert Fulton Weir, 1838-1927." *Diseases of the Colon and Rectum*, 25 (July-August 1982), 503-07.

(See Chapter 2: WEIR, ROBERT FULTON: Corman).

Cosbie, W. G. "Surgery for Ovarian Tumor." *Applied Therapeutics*, 9 (June 1967), 547.

(See Chapter 13: Cosbie).

"The Development of Head and Neck Surgery." *Cancer Bulletin*, 5 (May-June 1953), 68-69.

Celsus (100 A.D.), a Roman physician, first described surgical excision of lip and facial carcinomas. In Arabia, Avicenna (980-1037) routinely performed surgery for removal of tongue carcinomas. Until the eighteenth century, however, there were no new techniques in head and neck surgery. Aseptic modern surgery began in the nineteenth century. In 1842, Crawford Long used ether as an anesthetic for removing a "vascular tumor" of the neck. Pioneers in head and neck surgery included Auguste B. Berard (excision of the parotid gland); Nicholas Senn (resection of the mandible and maxilla); Henry T. Butlin (removal of the tongue and lymph nodes); and John Bland-Sutton (surgical resection for bronchiogenic carcinoma).

Duncum, Barbara M. *The Development of Inhalation Anaesthesia with Special Reference to the Years 1846-1900*. London: 1947.

(See Chapter 23: Gillespie).

Dymarskii, L. Iu. "K istorii razvitiia khirurgicheskogo lecheniia raka molochnoi zhelezy, machinaia s drevnogo Egipta i do nashikh dnei." *Khirurgiia*, 4 (April 1981), 111-16.

(See Chapter 23: Butterfield and Chapter 23: Breasted).

"Early Pulmonary Surgery." *Cancer Bulletin*, 11 (November-December 1959), 114-15.

Until the latter half of the nineteenth century, acute empyema was the only illness justifying thoracic surgery. Kronlein, a Swiss surgeon, resected a portion of a lung in 1884 for a patient whose lung had been invaded by a rib sarcoma. Kummel reported a lung resection in 1910 for a patient suffering from a carcinoma, but the patient died post-operatively. Surgical mortality rates were deemed too high until developments in the 1920s improved the patient's odds of surviving the operation. The first successful total pneumonectomy was done in 1931 by Rudolph Nissen on a 12 year old female with diffuse bronchiectasis of the left lung. In

1933 Evarts Graham did it in a one-stage procedure for carcinoma. Although various surgical penetrations of the thorax had occurred since the Greeks, it was not considered a realistic option until the twentieth century. The major problems which had to be overcome included successful ligation of the pulmonary artery, routine closure of the brachial stump, improved anesthetic techniques, especially endotracheal anesthesia, prevention of lung collapse, x-ray diagnosis of lesions, and blood transfusions. In 1939 Churchill and Belsey began to approach lung surgery in terms of segmental rather than lobe resection. Each lobe is divided into segments depending on the distribution of the bronchi and their pattern of branching. This innovation provided for the salvation of tissue in lung resections.

Ellis, H. "Eponyms in Oncology. William Ernest Miles (1869-1947)." *European Journal of Surgical Oncology*, 12 (March 1986), 85.

William Miles, a London surgeon, pioneered the wide excision surgical procedure for carcinoma of the rectum. The approach was through the abdomen and involved removal of the terminal pelvic colon, rectum, and anus to prevent recurrence and lymphatic metastasis. His resection technique, although radical, greatly reduced local recurrence rates for the disease and became the treatment of choice for rectal carcinoma in the early twentieth century.

"Eponym: Wertheim's Operation." *Cancer Bulletin*, 17 (March-April 1965), 45.

Ernst Wertheim (1864-1920), a Prague surgeon, performed the first of his series of radical hysterectomies for cervical cancer in 1898. He published his results of work on 500 patients in 1911, but because mortality rates from the surgery were above ten percent, the surgery was largely abandoned as the treatment of choice once intracavitary radium became available after 1915. The Wertheim procedure, with some modifications, was revived late in the 1930s by Joe Meigs when surgical techniques reduced the operating theater mortality rates.

"Evolution of Gastric Surgery." *Cancer Bulletin*, 11 (January-February 1959), 2-3.

In 1881 Theodor Billroth performed the first successful partial gastrectomy on a 43 year old female suffering from pyloric carcinoma. Although the surgery was a pioneering effort, the patient died 4 months later of metastatic disease in the liver. In the surgery Billroth extirpated the tumor and anastomosed the duodenum to the end of the lesser curvature of the stomach. In 1885 he removed so much of a patient's stomach that the resection involved an anastomosis of the stomach to the jejunum. Early in the 1900s surgeons changed the Billroth procedure to suture or clamp the stomach in order to narrow the opening and make the duodenum connection.

"Evolution of Surgical Intervention in Rectal Carcinoma." *Cancer Bulletin*, 13
(May-June 1961), 45-48.

The first successful surgical resection of a rectal carcinoma was performed by
Jacques Lisfranc in 1826. In 1883 Vincenz Czerny used the combined abdominal and perineal approach. Paul Kraske in 1885 developed a procedure which
preserved the perianal skin and the external sphincter. In 1908 William Ernest
Miles, recognizing that rectal carcinomas spread by direct extension, venous invasion, and lymphatic drainage, recommended the extensive abdominoperineal
resection and removal of the pelvic mesocolon. That surgical approach now bears
his name. The Miles procedure greatly reduced the rate of localized recurrence,
although it removed so much tissue that it often complicated the quality of life for
the surviving patient. Since then, surgeons have learned that the anal sphincter
can usually be saved in cases where the tumor is situated above the peritoneal
reflexion.

Fasching, W. "Der Beitrag der II. Chirurgischen Universitätsklinik Wien zur
Behandlung des Kolorektalen Karzinoms." *Wien Klinische Wochenschrift*,
91 (2 February 1979), 68-74.

Colorectal surgery for carcinoma at the University of Vienna has followed the
patterns developed by the leading British and German surgeons of the late nineteenth and twentieth centuries: Vincenz Czerny and the abdominal and perineal
surgical approach; Paul Kraske and the preservation of the sphincter; William E.
Miles and the radical abdominoperineal resection; and Cuthbert Dukes's demonstration in the 1930s that lymphatic drainage downward in rectal carcinoma was
unusual, limiting resections of the sphincter and improving the post-surgery quality of life for the patient.

Firmin, F. "Cancer de la joue et autoplastie in l'an 1838. Opération de génioplastie
pratiquée par M. Roux de Brignolles." *Annales de chirurgie plastique*, 27
(1982), 91-93.

(See Chapter 14: Firmin).

Fisher, Bernard. "The Revolution in Breast Cancer Surgery: Science or Anecdotalism." *World Journal of Surgery*, 9 (1985), 655-66.

(See Chapter 11: Fisher and Gebhardt).

Fisher, Bernard, and Mark C. Gebhardt. "The Evolution of Breast Cancer
Surgery: Past, Present, and Future." *Seminars in Oncology*, 5 (December
1978), 385-94.

(See Chapter 11: Fisher and Gebhardt).

Funk, T. G. "Uterine Fibromyome und Blutungen als Indikation für eine Bi-
laterale Oophorektomie im Spaten 19. Jahrhundert." *Medizinhistorisches
Journal*, 21 (1986), 159-71.

In the late nineteenth century physicians routinely performed bilateral oophorectomies as well as hysterectomies in women suffering from uterine fibromas and
vaginal bleeding. As gynecological understanding developed in the early twentieth century it became clear that removal of the uterus was sufficient in most cases
of benign and malignant uterine disease, eliminating the need for consistent use
of the bilateral oophorectomy.

German, William J., and Stevenson Flanigan. "Pituitary Adenomas: A Follow-
Up Study of the Cushing Series." *Clinical Neurosurgery*, 10 (1964), 72-81.

(See Chapter 10: German and Flanigan).

Gilbertsen, V. A. "Contributions of William Ernest Miles to Surgery of the Rectum for Cancer." *Diseases of the Colon and Rectum*, 7 (September-October
1964), 375-80.

William Ernest Miles (1869-1947), a London surgeon, was concerned about the
high rates of local recurrence and metastasis after surgery for colorectal cancer. He
carefully studied the lymphatic drainage patterns in carcinoma of the rectum. He
advocated and performed more radical surgery removing the anus, rectum, mesocolon, and a surrounding margin of healthy tissue using an abdomino-perineal
approach. It was a radical surgical approach but it did reduce the likelihood of
local recurrence and eventual metastasis. Miles's technique became the preferred
procedure in the early 1900s.

Gillespie, Noel A. "The Evolution of Endotracheal Anaesthesia." *Journal of the
History of Medicine*, 1 (October 1946), 583-94.

The development of endotracheal anesthesia was essential to lung surgery because it prevented pulmonary collapse once the thorax was opened and allowed
for aspirated removal of pus, blood, and mucus. The first written accounts of artificial ventilation of the lungs appeared in 1667. In 1869 Friedrich Trendelenberg
invented the inflatable cuff, a thin rubber bag connected to a trachiotomy tube.
In 1880 William Macewen of Glasgow first used true endotracheal anesthesia by
passing a tube into the trachea through the glottal opening. He wanted to remove a malignant tongue tumor and prevent the patient from ingressing blood
during surgery. By the 1890s a variety of tubes were in surgical use. Early in the
1900s Franz Kuhn in Germany regularly used intubation to maintain clear passages and aspirate excess fluids. In 1907 Bartelemy and Dufour in France invented
"endotracheal insufflation"—blowing air under positive pressure down a narrow
tube and allowing returning gases to escape between the wall of the trachea and

the tube. S. J. Meltzer and J. Auer perfected endotracheal insufflation to maintain chest pressure. Endotracheal insufflation, however, allowed for drainage of fluids during surgery into the lungs, and after World War I inhalation through a nasal tube replaced that procedure. All these developments paved the way for Evarts Graham's successful one-stage pneumonectomy for lung carcinoma in 1933.

Glasscock, Michael E. "History of the Diagnosis and Treatment of Acoustic Neuromas." *Archives of Otolaryngology*, 88 (December 1968), 578-85.

(See Chapter 14: Glasscock).

Goldwyn, Robert M. "Theodore Gaillard Thomas and the Inframammary Incision." *Plastic and Reconstructive Surgery*, 76 (September 1985), 475-77.

(See Chapter 23: Goldwyn).

Graham, Evarts A. "A Brief Account of the Development of Thoracic Surgery and Some of Its Consequences." *Surgery, Gynecology & Obstetrics*, 104 (February 1957), 241-50.

The major developments in the history of thoracic surgery are: 1) the invention in 1909 of insufflation intratracheal anesthesia which prevented lung collapse when the chest cavity was opened; 2) the sophistication of the one-stage lobectomy in the late 1920s and 1930s; 3) the development of improved bronchograms with the use of lipiodol in the 1920s; and 4) the first successful, total pneumonectomy in 1933.

Granshaw, L. "Clinical Research: The Case of St. Mark's Hospital, London, and Colo-Rectal Surgery." *Society for the Social History of Medicine Bulletin*, 37 (December 1985), 50-53.

(See Chapter 23: Polglase).

Greenwood, Ronald D. "Surgical Treatment for Facial Hemangiomas." *Alabama Medicine*, 54 (August 1984), 27.

(See Chapter 18: Greenwood).

Gruber, D., R. Hofmann, and E. Ehler. "Cancer Mammarum Infructose Extirpatus bei C. E. Eschenbach 1755." *Zentralblatt für Chirurgie*, 96 (30 October 1971), 1526-30.

Recognizing that the only hope for a cure of breast cancer was elimination of the lesion, the German physician C. E. Eschenbach surgically excised a large breast carcinoma from a young female patient in 1755. He also noticed hard masses of tissue in the axilla, indicating lymphatic involvement.

Hardy, K. J. "Bowel Surgery: Some 18th and 19th Century Experiences." *The Australian and New Zealand Journal of Surgery*, 58 (April 1988), 335-38.

In 1833 J. F. Reybard, a physician in Lyon, France, performed a one-stage sigmoid colectomy to remove a three-inch carcinoma from the patient. At the same time, he removed six inches of bowel together with a V-shaped margin of mesentery.

Hargrove, W. C., M. H. Gertner, and W. T. Fitts. "The Kraske Operation for Carcinoma of the Rectum." *Surgery, Gynecology & Obstetrics*, 148 (June 1979), 931-33.

The surgeon Paul Kraske is primarily remembered for his 1885 contribution to surgical excision for rectal carcinoma. At a time when the treatment of choice was wide surgical excision, based on the technique of William Ernest Miles, Kraske developed a technique for removing the tumor and a safe margin of healthy tissue while preserving the perianal skin and the external sphincter. The quality of life for the surviving patient was substantially improved by Kraske's innovation.

Harrison, R. Cameron and F. Miks. "Canadian Contributions Towards the Comprehension of Hyperinsulinism: The First Successful Excision of an Insulinoma." *The Canadian Journal of Surgery*, 23 (July 1980), 401-04.

In 1902 A. G. Nichols of McGill University first described an islet cell adenoma. Not until 1923 was the clinical syndrome of hyperinsulinism suspected. At Toronto General Hospital in 1929, Dr. R. R. Graham resected the pancreas of a 54 year old woman, removing an islet cell carcinoma. The woman survived another 20 years. Hyperinsulinism had also caused hypoglycemia.

Harvey, A. McGehee. "Early Contributions to the Surgery of Cancer: William S. Halsted, Hugh H. Young, and John G. Clark." *The Johns Hopkins Medical Journal*, 135 (December 1974), 399-417.

All three men were on the staff of the Johns Hopkins Hospital and the Johns Hopkins University Medical School. Halsted was responsible for the development of the radical mastectomy and the first surgeon to use rubber gloves in surgery; Hugh H. Young was the father of modern urology and responsible for developing the perineal prostatectomy; and John G. Goodrich developed the first successful removal of the uterus. All three men practiced in the late nineteenth and early twentieth centuries.

"Hempelvectomy." *Cancer Bulletin*, 10 (January-February 1958), 22-23.

Theodor Billroth first attempted a hempelvectomy (amputation at the hip) in 1891, but the patient did not survive the surgery. In 1895 and 1897 Girard performed the first successful hempelvectomies. In 1909 Ransohoff performed the first successful hempelvectomy in the United States. Because mortality rates exceeded 75 percent, however, the procedure was largely abandoned until the mid-1930s when G. Gordon-Taylor revived it for upper-thigh and pelvic bone tumors as well as for soft-tissue sarcomas too large for wide excision. Improved techniques for antisepsis and blood-transfusion greatly reduced surgical mortality rates.

Hill, G. J. "Historic Milestones in Cancer Surgery." *Seminars in Oncology*, 6 (1979), 409-27.

(See Chapter 23: Rosenberg).

"History of Bone Tumors." *Cancer Bulletin*, 16 (March-April 1964), 36.

(See Chapter 9: "History of Bone Tumors").

Hollinger, P. H. "The Historical Development of Laryngectomy." *Laryngoscope*, 85 (February 1975), 287-353.

(See Chapter 23: Schechter and Morfit).

Horwitz, Norman H. "Sir Geoffrey Jefferson on Invasive Pituitary Adenomas." *Journal of Neurosurgery*, 42 (February 1975), 244.

(See Chapter 10: Horwitz).

Hughes, E. S. R. "The Development of a Restorative Operation for Carcinoma of the Rectum." *The Australian and New Zealand Journal of Surgery*, 51 (April 1981), 117-19.

In the 1950s Theodore Bacon led the way in broadening the speciality of proctology from exclusive concern with the anal canal to the entire area of colonic and rectal diseases. He also led the way in convincing colorectal surgeons to accept carcinomas of the middle third of the rectum for sphincter-saving procedures rather than routine abdominoperineal resections with permanent colostomies in all cases. Between 1950 and 1980 in Australia, the trend was toward more and more sphincter-saving operations. Today almost all are sphincter-saving. This trend was made possible by four developments. First was the successful introduction of anterior resection and end-to-end anastomosis. The second factor was the development and adoption of the pull-through excision for middle-third rectal tumors. Third, the use of the E. E. A. autostapling device permitted more sphincter-saving procedures. Finally, experience has shown that small, superficial, circumscribed and non-invasive carcinomas can be treated by local excision or fulguration with every prospect of permanent cure without recourse to more radical procedures which compromise the quality of life for the patient after the operation.

Hunter, John A. A. and Karl Holubar, eds. "In Praise of Alexander Breslow." *American Journal of Dermatopathology*, 6 (Summer 1984), Suppl. 1, 151-57.

(See Chapter 18: Hunter and Holubar).

Imanaga, H. "Honoring Theodor Billroth by Attaining a Hundred Years Since His First Success in Gastric Cancer Resection." *Nippon Gans Chiryo Gakkai Shi*, 16 (June 20, 1981), 405-08.

(See Chapter 23: Brunschwig and Simandi).

Kambouris, Angelos A. "The Current Controversies in Surgical Management of Early Breast Cancer." *Henry Ford Hospital Medical Journal*, 32 (1984), 39-45.

(See Chapter 11: Kambouris).

Katsuki, H., and Y. Yamaguchi. "History of Surgical Treatment of Lung Cancer." *Japanese Journal of Thoracic Surgery*, 27 (August 1974), 533-42.

In the early nineteenth century lung cancer was recognized as a rare, untreatable, and universally fatal disease. Surgery was all but impossible because of the problem of lung collapse when pressure was equalized by cutting open the thoracic cavity. Early in the 1900s S. J. Meltzer and J. Auer demonstrated that respiration could be maintained by pushing air intratracheally under positive pressure. With the fear of pulmonary collapse and asphyxia eliminated, surgical procedures developed rapidly. In 1908 Ferdinand Sauerbach performed the first lobectomy. On April 5, 1933, Evarts A. Graham successfully performed the first one-stage pneumonectomy for lung cancer with individual ligation of the hilar structures.

Kirchner, John A. "A Historical and Histological View of Partial Laryngectomy." *Bulletin of the New York Academy of Medicine*, 62 (October 1986), 808-17.

In 1853 Gordon Buck, a New York surgeon, first operated on a laryngeal carcinoma. Complete resection was impossible, given the size of the tumor. H. B. Sands, another New York surgeon, performed the first successful resection of a laryngeal carcinoma in 1863. But for decades the laryngofissure was marked by high surgical mortality rates and frequent local as well as metastatic recurrences. Also, there were no specific tests for tuberculosis, syphilis, and cancer, the three chronic, ulcerative laryngeal diseases. Koch's first report on the tubercle bacillus came in 1882 and the Wasserman test for syphilis appeared in 1906. Although Rudolf Virchow's *Cellular Pathology* appeared in 1856, biopsy was a controversial diagnostic technique, especially after Virchow's negative examination in Frederick III's laryngeal carcinoma was widely reported in the lay and medical press. Not until the 1920s, with more careful patient selection, did surgical mortality rates improve. By the 1950s the bilateral anterior thyrotomy made safe the resection of tumors at the anterior commisure. Theodor Billroth had performed the first genuine hemilaryngectomy in 1878 and the first total laryngectomy in 1874. The first practical approach to resection of the supraglottic larynx and lateral pharyngeal wall was performed by Wilfred Trotter in 1913.

Lawrence, Walter. "The Scope of Surgical Oncology." *The Australian and New Zealand Journal of Surgery*, 52 (August 1982), 325-30.

Historically surgeons were usually the physicians called upon to deal with solid tumors since the therapeutic approach to cancer in the past was philosophically aligned with the concept that cancer is a localized process. The surgical approach, beginning in the nineteenth century, was to remove the cancer with an envelope of normal tissue, sometimes with dissection of the adjacent regional lymph nodes. In the 1930s and 1940s ancillary advances in medical care, such as blood transfusion, nutritional support, improved anesthesia, and antibiotics allowed safe expansion of the operative attack on cancer. Such operations as pneumonectomy, esophagogastrectomy, hepatic lobectomy, pelvic exenteration, and internal lymph node dissection became possible. But by the 1950s it was clear that surgical resection for cancer had been exploited to the utmost and that there were few untried extensions of the operative approach that were likely to reap major benefits. Surgeons must now work with radiotherapists, chemotherapists, and immunotherapists in a teamwork approach to treating neoplasms.

Lewison, Edward F. "Breast Cancer Surgery from Halsted to 1972." *Proceedings of the National Cancer Conference*, 7 (1973), 275-79.

(See Chapter 11: Lewison).

Lichenstein, L. "Progressi nella diágnosi e terapía del tumori scheletrici negli ultimi 30 anni." *Chirurgía Degli Organi di Movimento*, 59 (1971), 313-31.

(See Chapter 9: Lichenstein).

Mason, James B. "Cancer Control and the College." *Bulletin of the American Academy of Surgeons*, 41 (1956), 157-65.

Since its founding in 1915 the American Academy of Surgeons has conducted a public health campaign to educate the public about the warning signs of cancer and the need for early diagnosis. That campaign has helped improve survival rates in recent years because of early diagnosis of more tumors. (Also see Chapter 23: Raven).

MacMahon, Charles E., and John L. Cahill. "The Evolution of the Concept of the Use of Surgical Castration in the Palliation of Breast Cancer in Pre-Menopausal Females." *Annals of Surgery*, 184 (December 1976), 713-16.

(See Chapter 11: MacMahon and Cahill).

Mendelson, B. C. "The Evolution of Breast Reconstruction." *The Medical Journal of Australia*, 9 (January 9, 1982), 7-8.

(See Chapter 11: Mendelson).

Mendelson, Isaac. "Theodor Billroth and the Beginning of Gastric Surgery." *Journal of the Mount Sinai Hospital,* 24 (March-April 1957), 112-19.

(See Chapter 23: Schechter and Morfit).

Minton, John P. "The Laser in Surgery." *American Journal of Surgery,* 15 (June 1986), 725-29.

In 1963 John Minton began testing a surgical laser on metastatic tumors in experimental animals. At the time he was a surgical resident at Ohio State University. The laser provides a rapid, precise, and bloodless method of tissue cutting, vaporization, and destruction of tumor. It will prove to be especially useful for tumors in the oral cavity, nasopharynx, hypopharynx, and vocal cords. Eventually, it will have a wide application in surgical oncology.

Missotten, F. E. "Historical Review of Pharyngo-Oesophageal Reconstruction After Resection for Carcinoma of the Pharynx and Cervical Oesophagus." *Clinical Otolaryngology,* 8 (October 1983), 345-62.

(See Chapter 12: Gibbon).

Moore, Francis D. "Surgery." In John Z. Bowers and Elizabeth F. Purcell, eds. *Advances in American Medicine: Essays at the Bicentennial.* New York: 1976. Volume 2. Pp. 614-84.

Surgery was basically limited to surface lesions until the advent of anesthesia in the 1840s. John Warren of the Massachusetts General Hospital in Boston used sulphuric ether to anesthetize a patient before removing a tumor of the jaw. The use of anesthesia permitted heroic operations of deep-seated lesions and tumors, but the patients often died of massive post-surgical infections. Oliver Wendell Holmes in the 1850s began arguing that infection could be prevented by more sanitation care in surgery, as did Ignaz Semmelweis in Vienna. But the great development in nineteenth century surgery was the contribution of Joseph Lister, the English surgeon, to surgical procedure. Although his ideas spread slowly in the United States after 1876, the use of antiseptic surgery greatly reduced post-operative mortality rates from infection. The stage was set for the birth of modern surgical oncology. Modern surgical oncology began in the United States at the Johns Hopkins University Medical School where William Stewart Halsted pioneered the notion of *en bloc* resection of tumors, with healthy margins, to prevent local recurrences of malignancies. Halsted is remembered for pioneering the use of asepsis as well as the development of the radical mastectomy, which bears his name. Surgery was also greatly aided by Wilhelm Roentgen's development of the x-ray as a diagnostic tool. The combination of anesthesia, antisepsis, asepsis, *en bloc* resection, and radiology all contributed to the development of the modern discipline of surgical oncology.

Murley, Reginald. "Breast Cancer: Keynes and Conservatism." *The British Journal of Clinical Practice*, 40 (February 1986), 49-58.

Geoffrey Keynes of the St. Bartholomew's Hospital pioneered the idea of using radiotherapy instead of or in addition to radical surgery for the treatment of breast cancer in the 1930s. One of his associates, Robert McWhirter, by the late 1930s was advocating simple mastectomy and radiotherapy instead of the Halsted radical mastectomy because he felt long-term survival rates were the same while quality of life was substantially improved. Keynes's work inspired a new approach to breast cancer treatment by the 1950s, with the radical mastectomy declining somewhat in use and simple mastectomies or local excisions combined with radiotherapy increasing. The development of megavoltage external electron beam therapy in the 1950s and 1960s strengthened that approach. The routine use of oophorectomy, adrenalectomy, and hypophysectomy in pre-menopausal women also declined unless distant metastases were already clinically evident.

Murley, Reginald. "Breast Cancer: Keynes and Conservatism." *Transactions of the Medical Society*, 99-100 (1982-1984), 1-13.

(See Chapter 11: Murley).

Nayakama, K. "Progress in the Surgery of Oesophageal Carcinoma." *Nippon Kyobu Geka Gakkai Zasshi*, 23 (April 1975), 350-52.

(See Chapter 12: Gibbon).

Neel, H. B. "Historical Perspectives and Development of Cryosurgery for Cancer." Ph.D. Dissertation. University of Minnesota. 1976. Pp. 3-14.

The use of liquid nitrogen as a surgical tool was developed in the 1960s. Its leading advocate and finest technician was R. C. Marcove. Liquid nitrogen was applied to the tumor either as a spray or as a liquid inside a solid probe. By the 1970s it was being used for low-grade chondrosarcomas, low-grade intramedullary cartilage tumors, giant cell bone tumors, skin lesions, small ocular melanomas, and retinoblastomas. The advantages of cryosurgery are preservation of tissue and avoidance of resection.

Nissen, Rudolph. "Historical Development of Pulmonary Surgery." *American Journal of Surgery*, 89 (January 1955), 9-15.

(See Chapter 15: Brewer).

Pearce, J. M. S. "The First Attempts at Removal of Brain Tumors." In F. Clifford Rose and W. F. Bynum. *Historical Aspects of the Neurosciences*. New York: 1982. Pp. 239-42.

(See Chapter 10: Pearce).

Perel, L. "Historique de la reconstruction du sein après ablation pour cancer." In *Proceedings of the XXIII International Congress of the History of Medicine.* London: 1974. Pp. 1170-71.

(See Chapter 11: Mendelson).

Polglase, A. L. "Rectal Excision for Cancer 1880 to 1980." *Medical Journal of Australia,* 10 (January 1981), 3-4.

Segmental excision for cancer of the rectum with end-to-end anastomosis first became popular in the 1880s. The technique involved a sacral incision with resection of the coccyx and the last two sacral segments. It was popular until early in the 1900s. J. P. Lockhart-Mummery developed a two-stage perineal excision of the rectum, but it sacrificed the sphincter. William Ernest Miles abandoned the perineal approach because of recurrent tumors in the rectal mesentery. Miles performed radical wide excision of the rectum and inferior mesenteric artery. It too sacrificed the sphincters. In the 1930s C. Dukes and H. Westhues demonstrated that downward lymphatic spread of the disease was unusual so sphincter sacrifice was unnecessary. In 1948 C. F. Dixon of the Mayo Clinic treated rectosigmoidal carcinoma with an anterior resection and reestablishment of bowel continuity by sutures.

Polk, H. C. "Surgical Treatment for Carcinoma of the Colon and Rectum: Its Evolution in One University Hospital." *Archives of Surgery,* 91 (1965), 958-62.

(See Chapter 23: Polglase).

Pratt, Joseph H. "Ephraim McDowell. The First Five Cases of Ovariotomy, 1809 to 1818." *Mayo Clinic Proceedings,* 52 (February 1977), 125-28.

(See Chapter 13: Pratt).

Raven, Ronald W. "The Surgeon and Oncology." *Clinical Oncology,* 10 (December 1984), 311-18.

The landmarks in oncological surgery include Billroth (1881) and the subtotal gastrectomy; Halsted (1890) and the radical mastectomy; Schlatter (1897) and the total gastrectomy; Von Mickulicz (1898) and the oesophagogastrectomy; Wertheim (1900) and the radical hysterectomy; Miles (1908) and the abdominoperineal excision of the rectum; Torek (1913) and the oesophagectomy; Trotter (1913) and the partial pharyngectomy; and Graham and Singer (1933) and the pneumonectomy. The major conceptual breakthrough in surgery was William Stewart Halsted's notion of the *en bloc* resection for carcinomas and sarcomas. The basic sciences necessary for the understanding of oncology are pathology, endocrinology and metabolic medicine, clinical pharmacology, epidemiology, genetics, immunology, computer sciences and medical statistics, radiobiology, radiation physics, and anthropology. The major concerns of the twenty-first century in cancer care will be prevention; hormonal mechanisms for cancers of the breast, ovary, testicle, prostate, and corpus uteri; surgery for small, solid tumors, cancer complications, debulking operations, and tumors of the brain and spinal cord; radiotherapy for squamous cell carcinoma of the skin, larynx, and upper alimentary tract cancers; chemotherapy for leukemia, lymphomas, and chorioepitheliomas; metastatic cancers; and immunotherapy with monoclonal antibodies.

Raven, Ronald W. "Radical and Extended Radical Surgery for Cancer. Historical Background and Perspective." *Oncology: Proceedings of the Tenth International Cancer Congress*, IV (1970), 197-203.

Surgical excision for treatment of cancer was really the only effective treatment until the development of radiotherapy and chemotherapy in the twentieth century. In the nineteenth century, however, surgery was limited by the lack of understanding about the nature of infection, anesthesia, and blood transfusion. The development of anesthesia in the 1840s led to more extensive surgical procedures, while the use of antisepsis and asepsis in the 1880s and 1890s greatly reduced post-operative mortality rates. In the 1930s the development of effective blood transfusion techniques provided for hemorrhage control, while the rise of the antibiotics in the 1940s made further gains in reducing operative infection rates. All of these technical advances paved the way for the appearance of the superradical surgical tradition of the 1940s and 1950s—the hemicorporectomy, hempelvectomy, superradical mastectomy, complete pelvic exenteration, and the wide resection of head and neck tumors. By the end of the 1950s, as survival data began to accumulate, it became clear that the superradical procedures at best achieved only marginal improvements in cure rates but severe declines in the post-operative quality of life. By the 1960s and 1970s the superradical options were taken less and less frequently, with combined surgery and radiotherapy replacing them.

Ravitch, Mark M. *A Century of Surgery: History of the American Surgical Association*. Philadelphia: 1981.

(See Chapter 30: Ravitch).

Ravitch, Mark M. "Carcinoma of the Breast. The Place of the Halsted Radical Mastectomy." *The Johns Hopkins Medical Journal*, 129 (October 1974), 202-11.

In the 1890s, through surgical experience and clinical follow-up, William Halsted of the Johns Hopkins University Medical School developed the surgical procedure for breast cancer which now bears his name. By 1890 he knew that a lymph node dissection of the axilla was essential to patient survival, and by the mid-1890s he was removing the pectoralis major muscle as a means of reducing local recurrences of the disease. Occasionally he also performed more radical procedures involving removal of the pectoralis minor muscle and dissection of the supraclavicular glands. In the 1940s and 1950s the radical procedure became popular for a time, with the addition of an extensive mediastinal and pleural procedure. Medical debate in the 1970s revolved around several important questions: 1) a modified radical mastectomy with excision of the breast and axillary contents but without resection of the muscles; 2) irradiation alone; 3) simple mastectomy alone; or 4) simple mastectomy combined with irradiation or just a lumpectomy. Today, nearly ninety years after Halsted began developing his procedure, medical debate still centers on his approach to breast cancer.

Robinson, James O. "Treatment of Breast Cancer Through the Ages." *The American Journal of Surgery*, 15 (March 1985), 317-33.

(See Chapter 11: De Moulin).

Rosenberg, P. J. "Total Laryngectomy and Cancer of the Larynx. A Historical Review." *Archives of Otolaryngology*, 94 (October 1971), 313-16.

(See Chapter 23: Schechter and Morfit).

Rosenberg, Steven A. "Principles of Surgical Oncology. Historical Perspectives." In Vincent P. DeVita, Jr., Samuel Hellman, and Steven A. Rosenberg. *Cancer. Principles & Practice of Oncology.* 1985. Pp. 215-16.

The earliest description of surgical treatment of tumors is found in the Edwin Smith Papyrus from Egypt (1600 B.C.), but the modern era of elective surgery began in America in 1809 when Ephraim McDowell removed a large ovarian tumor from a female patient. He subsequently performed thirteen ovarian resections. The development of general anesthesia and the idea of antisepsis permitted surgeons to make quantam leaps forward in the middle of the nineteenth century. The major milestones in surgical oncology are:

1. The elective ovarian resection by Ephraim McDowell in 1809.

2. The use of ether anesthesia by John Collins Warren in 1846.

3. The introduction of antisepsis by Joseph Lister in 1867.

4. Performance of the first gastrectomy, laryngectomy, and esophagectomy by Theodor Billroth between 1850 and 1880.

5. William Halsted's practice of aseptic surgery in the 1880s.

6. The development of thyroid surgery by Theodor Kocher in the 1880s.

7. The development of the radical mastectomy by William Halsted in 1890 and his belief that the *en bloc* resection was the only way of removing malignant tissue and preventing local recurrence.

8. The performance of the first oophorectomy by G. T. Beatson in 1896.

9. The performance of the first radical prostatectomy by Hugh H. Young in 1904.

10. The performance of the first radical hysterectomy by Ernst Wertheim in 1906.

11. The performance of the first abdominoperineal rectal resection by W. Ernest Miles in 1908.

12. The development of the cordotomy for pain control by E. Martin in 1912.

13. The development of brain surgery by Harvey Cushing between 1910 and 1930.

14. The performance of the first successful resection of the thoracic esophagus by Franz Torek in 1913.

15. The first successsful resection for pulmonary metastases by G. Davis in 1927.

16. The performance of the first successful pneumonectomy by Evarts Graham in 1933.

17. The performance of the first successful pancreaticoduodenectomy by A. O. Whipple in 1935.

18. The performance of the adrenalectomy for prostate cancer by Charles B. Huggins in 1945.

Satoh, O. "Transsphenoidal Surgery for Pituitary Tumors: Historical Review and Present Trends." *No Shinkei Geka*, 12 (January 1984), 7-26.

The transsphenoidal approach for surgical removal of pituitary tumors was pioneered by Harvey Cushing in the 1920s and 1930s. Employing a nasal speculum, Cushing approached the pituitary through the sellar floor. The approach was very useful in that it did not disturb other cranial structures and leave neurological disfunctions. The transsphenoidal approach was largely abandoned in the 1950s and 1960s but then revived in the 1970s by Guiot and Hardy. In 1979 Zervas developed a technique for electrical coagulation of the tumor using a transsphenoidal approach.

Scanlon, E. F. "The Evolution of Surgical Oncology." *Cancer*, 37 (January 1976), 58-61.

(See Chapter 23: Raven).

Schechter, David Charles, and H. Mason Morfit. "The Evolution of Surgical Treatment of Tumors of the Larynx." *Surgery*, 57 (March 1965), 457-479.

The Egyptians first mentioned tumors of the larynx, and during the Middle Ages there were occasional references. In the nineteenth century the systematic study of laryngeal lesions began in the major European medical schools. As a result of autopsies, descriptions of laryngeal carcinomas became more and more common and detailed. The first surgery for laryngeal neoplasms was performed in 1750 by G. Koderik. In 1776 Vicq d'Azyr approached the larynx surgically by making an incision between the thyroid cartilage. Pierre J. Desault called this procedure a laryngotomy in 1798. This infrathyroid approach prevailed by the middle of the nineteenth century. The development of the mirrored laryngoscope in the second half of the nineteenth century led to new surgical treatment of throat cancers. In 1873 Theodor Billroth performed the first successful laryngectomy for cancer, removing the two upper tracheal rings, the cricoid, the thyroid, both arytenoid cartilages, and the lower third of the epiglottis. Partial laryngectomy, or hemilaryngectomy, was first performed in 1878 by David Foulis of Glasgow. Still, death rates were high from hemorrhagic shock, asphyxiation, or pneumonia from aspiration, sepsis, inanition, or despair. Real improvements in the procedure came with Themistokles Gluck's 1899 operation, in which he released the larynx and upper portion of the trachea from their bed, closed the hypopharyngeal defect, severed the trachea from the larynx, and then brought the tracheal stump to the outside of the neck and sutured it to the skin. This greatly reduced the drainage of blood into the lungs. In the modern period refined surgical techniques, radiotherapy, and improved classification of tumors have all improved survival rates.

Schober, K. L. "Das Chirurgische Erbe. Theodor Billroth und die Karzinomchirurgie des Intestinaltrakte." *Zentralblatt für Chirurgie*, 106 (1981), 693-99.

Theodor Billroth, the famed University of Vienna physician and father of modern surgery, performed the first successful resection of an intestinal carcinoma in 1881. The patient survived the operation but subsequently died of metastatic disease.

Schreiber, H. W. "Wo Steht die Carcinom—Chirurgie des Magens 100 Jahre Nach der ersten Erfolgreichen Magenresektion durch Theodor Billroth." *Langenbecks Archiv Chirurgie*, 358 (1982), 53-55.

(See Chapter 23: Brunschwig and Simandi).

Shelley, Harry S. "The Enlarged Prostate. A Brief History of its Treatment." *The Journal of the History of Medicine and Allied Sciences,* 24 (October 1969), 452-73.

Although Morgagni described prostatic enlargement in the mid-1750s, with involvement of the seminal vesicles, the first genuine description of a prostatic carcinoma was given by George Langstaff of London in 1817. In 1847 Benjamin Brodie described prostatic carcinoma and metastasis to the vertebra. Theodor Billroth performed the first perineal prostatectomy for carcinoma of the prostate in 1867, but the patient died of metastatic disease a year later. Hugh Young of Johns Hopkins developed his radical perineal prostatectomy in 1904. The operation involved removal of the entire prostate gland, the seminal vesicles, and a small cuff of bladder, with the bladder then sutured to the cut end of the urethra. That became the surgery of choice until the 1940s when Terrence Millin developed his retropubic approach. In 1956 Brice Vallett of the United States began employing the transsacral prostatectomy. Another important development in the treatment of prostate cancer was Charles Huggins's realization in the early 1940s that some prostatic carcinomas were androgen dependent. Castration or estrogen therapy could retard growth and relieve the pain of bony metastases.

Shimkin, Michael B. "Pneumonectomy and Lobectomy in Bronchogenic Carcinoma." *Journal of Thoracic and Cardiovascular Surgery,* 44 (1962), 503-19.

In 1912 H. M. Davies, a London surgeon, performed the first lobectomy for lung cancer, but the patient died from surgical complications, particularly the collection of excess fluids and pus in the chest cavity. A number of German, British, and American surgeons performed lobectomies in the 1910s and 1920s, but the surgical mortality rates exceeded fifty percent. Harold Brunn developed the successful, one-stage lobectomy and published his technique in 1929. The first successful pneumonectomy for lung carcinoma was performed by Evarts A. Graham of Washington University in St. Louis in 1933.

Sisson, G. A., J. C. Goldstein, and G. D. Becker. "Surgery of the Limited Lesions of the Larynx (Past and Present)." *Otolaryngology Clinics of North America,* 3 (October 1970), 529-41.

(See Chapter 23: Schechter and Morfit).

Stallworthy, J. A. "Surgery of Endometrial Cancer in the Bonney Tradition." *Annals of the Royal College of Surgeons of England,* 48 (May 1971), 293-305.

(See Chapter 13: Stallworthy).

Stehlin, John S., Jr., et al. "Treatment of Carcinoma of the Breast." *Surgery, Gynecology & Obstetrics*, 149 (December 1979), 911-22.

(See Chapter 11: Stehlin).

Stell, P. M. "The First Laryngectomy for Carcinoma." *Archives of Otolaryngology*, 98 (November 1973), 293.

(See Chapter 23: Schechter and Morfit).

Swanson, Neil A. "The Evolution of Mohs' Surgery: Introduction." *Journal of Dermatologic Surgery and Oncology*, 8 (August 1982), 650.

(See Chapter 18: Swanson).

Taylor, William B. "Mohs' Chemosurgery, Fixed Tissue Technique." *Journal of Dermatologic Surgery and Oncology*, 8 (August 1982), 650-51.

(See Chapter 18: Taylor).

Triebel, C. "Geschichte und Entwicklung der Nachgehenden Krankenfursorge in Berlin." *Offentliche Gesundheitswesen*, 48 (February 1986), 92-96.

The article deals with the development of post-operative surgical care for cancer patients, before and after the appearance of asepsis and antiseptic care. As a result of new concerns about infection, post-operative mortality rates were dramatically reduced, making surgery a much more reasonable approach in treating cancer patients and permitting the development of more and more radical procedures.

Tromovitch, Theodore A. "Mohs' Surgery, Fresh-Tissue Technique." *Journal of Dermatologic Surgery and Oncology*, 8 (August 1982), 651-53.

(See Chapter 18: Tromovitch).

Tsuchiya, R. "History of the Pancreactomy—With Special Reference to Pancreatic Cancer." *Nippon Geka Gakkai Zasshi*, 86 (April 1985), 375-80.

(See Chapter 12: Zamora).

Vasquez, Albaladejo G., and Ferrer R. Sospedra. "Evolución de las técnicas quirúrgicas en el cancer de mamá." *Revista Espania de Oncologia*, 28 (1981), 83-94.

(See Chapter 11: Lewison).

Weir, N. F. "Theodor Billroth: The First Laryngectomy for Cancer." *Journal of Laryngology and Otology*, 87 (December 1973), 1161-69.

(See Chapter 14: Schechter and Morfit).

Winkler, R., and H. P. Eichfuss. "Geschichte der Dickdarmchirurgie. Teil I. Klinik, Pathologie, Diagnostik—Dargestellt am Beispiel des Karzinoms. Historisches und Entwicklungstendenzem." *Medizinische Welt*, 28 (25 March 1977), 591-602.

(See Chapter 23: Rosenberg).

Winkler, R., and H. P. Eichfuss. "Geschichte der Dickdarmchirurgie. Teil II. Palliative Opérationen—Dargestellt am Beispiel des Karzinoms. Historisches und Entwicklungstendenzen." *Medizinische Welt*, 28 (4 November 1977), 1810-19.

(See Chapter 23: Rosenberg).

Wright, James R., Jr. "The Development of the Frozen Section Technique, the Evolution of the Surgical Biopsy, and the Origins of Surgical Pathology." *Bulletin of the History of Medicine*, 59 (Fall 1985), 295-326.

(See Chapter 6: Wright).

Zamora, Jose L. "Cystic Neoplasms of the Pancreas: Evolution of a Concept." *American Journal of Surgery*, 149 (June 1985), 819-23.

(See Chapter 12: Zamora).

24 Radiotherapy

Baker, Harvey W. "The General Surgeon and Cancer." *The American Journal of Surgery*, 139 (May 1980), 606-07.

(See Chapter 23: Baker).

Barkley, H. Thomas, Jr. "Accelerated Treatment." *Cancer*, 55 (May 1, 1985), 2112-17.

Before World War II most therapeutic courses in radiotherapy were given in periods of fourteen days or less. After the war routine treatments were given over thirty-five to fifty-six days, allowing for higher doses with modest fraction sizes, tolerable acute effects, better local control, and acceptable late normal tissue effects. Early attempts to accelerate treatment sought to achieve this by reducing the overall time and increasing the fraction size, but the result was unacceptable late tissue and frequently intolerable acute tissue effects. Current attempts toward acceleration have utilized multiple fractions per day, but in order to produce acceptable late tissue effects and tolerable acute effects, a considerable reduction in total dose or a lengthy split in treatment has been required. Today accelerated treatment should be given only to tumors with demonstrably rapid growth by means of multiple fractions per day over an extended period.

Brunner, Barbara E. "Radiation Treatment." *Journal of the History of Medicine and Allied Sciences*, 33 (October 1978), 551.

Ivo Saliger did a lithograph in Germany during the 1930s. It shows a gas-filled tube emitting x-rays over a reclining feminine figure with a dark, death shadow standing nearby. Using chiaroscuro, the artist shows a radiotherapist extending life. The lithograph effectively communicates the significance of the roentgen ray as a new weapon against disease by showing the skeleton of death retreating from the x-ray machine.

Churchill-Davidson, Ian. "Radiotherapy and the Problem of Oxygen Enhancement." *Oncology: Proceedings of the Tenth International Cancer Congress,* III (1970), 300-07.

Oxygen enhancement of radiotherapy was first recognized in 1904 by R. Hahn, who observed that if ice water was applied during treatment, skin reaction was reduced. Five years later G. Schwarz reported that applying mechanical pressure had the same effect. Neither of them, however, understood that the lack of oxygen was the causative agent. In 1924 Jolly showed that blocking the blood supply reduced irradiation damage in the thymus of guinea pigs and rats. K. A. Hultborn noticed in 1952 that after irradiating carcinoma of the rectum before surgery, the tumor parts most likely to first show damage were in regions with the best blood supply. Between 1932 and 1934 H. G. Crabtree and W. Cramer irradiated thin slices of mouse sarcomas *in vitro* under aerobic and anaerobic conditions; when they reinoculated the tumors back into fresh host animals, they found a decrease in the radiosensitivity of the tumor cells irradiated anaerobically. L. C. Gray showed in 1953 that the relationship between oxygen and radiosensitivity applied to a wide variety of living cells, both normal and malignant. His findings led to the first use of oxygen in cancer radiotherapy of man—the work of Hultborn and Forssberg in 1954 on squamous cell carcinomas of the skin. Ian Churchill-Davidson in 1955 began to use hyperbaric chambers to fill patients with oxygen just before radiotherapy treatments because fully oxygenated tissues are more vulnerable to radiation.

Emmanuel, I. G. "Symposium on Pituitary Tumours: Historical Aspects of Radiotherapy, Present Treatment and Results." *Clinical Radiology,* 17 (1966), 154-60.

Victor Horsley in 1889 made the first unsuccessful attempt at removal of a pituitary tumor, but between 1904 and 1906 he performed ten more operations, and only two of the patients died. In 1907 Schloffer made the first successful partial removal of a pituitary tumor through the transsphenoidal approach. The first successful use of radiotherapy on pituitary tumors came in 1909 when two French physicians, Gramegna and Beclere, used an early Crookes Tube with a tube voltage not exceeding 80 KV and a long glass cylinder used intra-orally. They used the beam on a 45 year old woman, treating her for one hour, twice a week, over a four-week period. She experienced temporary regression of her tumor. Beclere later that year used a five-field approach which looked forward to later beam directed radiotherapy. The patient, a 16 year old girl suffering from giantism, recovered and was still alive thirteen years later. In 1925 Dott, Bailey, and Cushing advocated post-operative radiotherapy for all pituitary patients as a means of reducing local recurrence. They applied a radium source to the roof of the mouth. Rawlings first reported the use of radon seeds in 1929. Although Cushing was an outstanding surgeon, he became a strong advocate of adjuvant radiotherapy. In 1939 Henderson, after reviewing Cushing's patient records, began to advocate radiotherapy as a necessary post-operative treatment to reduce local recurrence. By the 1940s the treatment of choice for chromophobe adenoma was an intracranial surgical resection followed by radiotherapy. During the 1940s the era of megavoltage radiotherapy began. Linear accelerators, electron beams, cyclotrons, and synchrocyclotrons all had a great impact on treatment of pituitary adenomas. By the 1960s some cancer centers were reporting a 90 percent recurrence-free rate in chromophobe adenomas treated with surgery and radiotherapy.

Ginzton, Edward L., and Craig S. Nunan. "History of Microwave Electron Linear Accelerators for Radiotherapy." *International Journal of Radiation Oncology, Biology, and Physics*, 11 (February 1985), 205-16.

Between 1935 and 1945 the basic theoretical understanding and practical application of microwave systems was established, and in the next fifteen years physics research laboratories manufactured 4 MeV linacs (linear accelerators) and installed them in hospitals. Varian Associates manufactured a fully rotational 6 MeV linac in 1962 and a fully rotational in-line standing wave 4 MeV X-ray linac in 1969. Between 1950 and 1985 the microwave electron linear accelerator has been gradually supplanting other forms of technology for external beam radiotherapy. Henry S. Kaplan of Stanford University played a critical role in the early development of clinical treatment. Kaplan introduced scientific discipline to supervoltage radiotherapy techniques, increasing the dosages through fractionated schedules and increasing the clinical radiation fields. As a result the electron linear accelerator has become the machine of choice in cancer radiotherapy.

Hafermann, M. "External Radiotherapy." *Urology*, 17 (April 1981), 15.

(See Chapter 20: Hafermann).

"The History of Mammography." *Cancer Bulletin*, 17 (September-October 1965), 84-85.

(See Chapter 11: "The History of Mammography").

Hodges, Paul C. *The Life and Times of Emil H. Grubbe.* Chicago: 1964.

Emil H. Grubbe was a 21 year old, part-time medical student in Chicago in 1896. To support himself he was employed manufacturing Crookes vacuum tubes. When he heard of Wilhelm Roentgen's discovery of x-rays using tubes similar to the Crookes vacuum tubes, Grubbe began experimenting with the invention. He noticed burns developing on his hands, and one of his professors concluded they were x-ray burns. On January 29, 1896, he treated one of the doctor's patients, a woman suffering from a recurrent breast carcinoma, with x-rays, and followed up with seventeen more treatments on the woman. It was the birth of modern radiotherapy. Grubbe spent the rest of his life working with radiotherapy, usually treating skin lesions, and he died in 1960.

Johns, H. E. "The Physicist in Cancer Treatment and Detection." *International Journal of Radiation Oncology, Biology, and Physics*, 7 (June 1981), 801-08.

In the twentieth century the physicist has become a more and more important figure in both cancer diagnosis and treatment. On the diagnostic side, physicists have played the central role in the technological development of radiology, especially the recent inventions of high-resolution, low-dose x-ray pictures and computer axial tomography. Physicists have also played an important part in the rise of nuclear medicine and the use of radioisotopes in combination with radiology to diagnose tumor tissue. Finally, in the area of treatment, physicists are central to the development of dosimetry measurements in fractionated radiotherapy.

Johnson, F. Leonard. "Marrow Transplantation in the Treatment of Acute Childhood Leukemia. Historical Development and Current Approaches." *The American Journal of Pediatric Hematology/Oncology*, 3 (Winter 1981), 389-95.

(See Chapter 16: Johnson).

Kremkau, Frederick W. "Cancer Therapy with Ultrasound: A Historical Review." *Journal of Clinical Ultrasound*, 7 (August 1979), 287-300.

Jacques and Pierre Curie discovered the phenomenon of piezoelectricity in 1880. In 1920 Langevin learned how to use piezoelectric materials as sources of ultrasound. Therapeutic heating by means of ultrasound was suggested in 1932, and the first publication about the use of ultrasound for cancer therapy appeared in 1933 by A. Szent-Gyorgyi. There have been four main periods in the history of ultrasound therapy. During the first period (1933-1947), German and Japanese researchers launched the field with animal and clinical studies which showed some tumor regression under the impact of ultrasound. The second period (1948-1957) was conducted primarily by German investigators and resulted in the introduction of high intensity short-time ultrasound, ultrasound in combination with x-ray therapy, the reporting of metastatic resorption and host response, and formulation of the Erlangen resolution. The third period was a time of pessimism (1958-1972), marked by studies of experimental animal tumors. The fourth period (1972-present) has been characterized by studies of ultrasound in combination with chemotherapy and radiotherapy, which have shown some positive effect on melanoma in mice.

Lederman, Manuel. "The Early History of Radiotherapy: 1895-1939." *International Journal of Radiation Oncology, Biology, and Physics*, 7 (1981), 639-48.

The discovery of x-rays was announced by Wilhelm Roentgen on November 30, 1895, although J. Plucker, a German, had produced them as early as 1859 by passing a high voltage current through a vacuum tube. Sir William Crooke, commenting that Plucker's flourescent light appeared at the end of the tube, named it a cathode ray. E. H. Grubbe, a German emigrant living in Chicago, first used the x-rays to treat cancer patients in 1896 after noticing that frequent exposure to x-rays had caused a dermatitis on his hands. In 1896 both static machines and induction coils were available and capable of generating an electric current high in voltage but low in milliamperage. These sources of current, combined with Crooke's tubes, provided the first radiotherapy machines. Production ranged between 50 and 100 kilovolts. By 1904 special tubes were available for intracavity treatments, and the introduction of the Snook interruptorless transformer in 1907 allowed for higher energy outputs under better conditions of control. Great advances in radiotherapy were made between 1910 and 1920. In 1913 the Coolidge hot cathode tube appeared, and in 1921 J. T. Case invented an experimental apparatus capable of delivering 200 kilovolts at 8 milliamperes. From this the construction of deep therapy transformers with a capacity of 200 kilovolts at 5 to 30 milliamperes led to the standard 200 kilovolt machines which became the backbone of radiotherapy until World War II.

Radium therapy also moved forward during these years, especially after Pierre Curie and Becquerel discovered the biological affects of radium exposure. The first radium appliances were little more than containers in which radium salts were placed. Radium-containing tubes were placed in intracavity spaces (anus, mouth, vagina, etc.) and radium-containing needles were used interstitially around accessible tumors. The founding figure in interstitial therapy was W. C. Stevenson of Dublin, Ireland, who in 1916 described the technique of loading a glass capillary containing radon gas into a serum needle. In 1908 the Dominici tube, a platinum apparatus, helped absorb damaging alpha and beta emissions and allowed only gamma radiation to reach the patient's tissues.

The development of telecurietherapy, or the delivery of an external radium beam, made some progress in the 1920s and 1930s, from the use of radium collars in Europe to the employment of the "radium bomb" for gynecological cancers in the United States. The direction of a radiation beam from an internal radiation source out through a lead lined exit portal was attempted by Kronig in 1912 and Lysholm in 1915. Finally, in 1933 R. M. Sievert developed a reliable external beam machine to treat head and neck cancers, and in 1936 L. G. Grimmett invented the Radium Beam Therapy Research unit. The limitations imposed by restricted supplies of radium meant that until the invention of artificially produced gamma rays, treatment was limited to head and neck, skin, and external genitalia tumors.

Lenz, Maurice. "The Early Workers in Clinical Radiotherapy of Cancer at the Radium Institute of the Curie Foundation, Paris, France." *Cancer*, 32 (September 1973), 519-23.

Emile Roux, director of the Pasteur Institute, founded the Radium Institute in 1921. Marie Curie was its first director and she was also in charge of the physics department. Claudius Regaud, assisted by Antoine Lacassagne, headed the biological division. Henri Coutard later joined them. They approached radiotherapy using three different techniques: 1) external therapy, in which the lesion and a clinically uninvolved border were covered by a wax mold and radon or radium tubes were attached to the mold; 2) intracavity therapy, in which .5 mm platinum tubes of radium or radon were inserted into natural body cavities—mouth, uterus, and anus; and 3) interstitial therapy, in which .5 mm hollow platinum neeldes containing radium were inserted around the tumor. Also in the 1920s, Regaud and Lacassagne pioneered the idea of single courses of treatment with maximum dosages of rads fractionated over several days, reducing damage to healthy tissue.

"Medical Uses of Radioisotopes." *Cancer Bulletin,* 6 (March-April 1954), 29.

(See Chapter 22: "Medical Uses of Radioisotopes").

Murley, Reginald. "Breast Cancer: Keynes and Conservatism." *Transactions of the Medical Society,* 99-100 (1982-1984), 1-13.

(See Chapter 11: Murley).

Pressman, David. "The Development and Use of Radiolabeled Antitumor Antibodies." *Cancer Research,* 40 (August 1980), 2960-64.

In the 1890s French researchers J. Hericourt and C. Richet prepared antisera against human osteogenic sarcoma in a donkey and two dogs and claimed that these sera were effective in reducing two different neoplasms, a fibrosarcoma of the chest wall and a stomach cancer. Since then all attempts to use heterologous antitumor antisera have not been successful. Pressman began his work at the Department of Immunological Research at Roswell Park Memorial Institute in the 1940s and demonstrated that antibodies can be radioiodinated without destroying antibody activity. Antibodies capable of localizing in tumors were demonstrated—well enough to permit their use diagnostically by scanning for radioactivity and therapeutically by localizing sufficient radioiodine.

Puretz, Donald H. "Mammography. History, Current Events, and Recommendations." *New York State Medical Journal,* 76 (November 1976), 1985-91).

(See Chapter 11: Puretz).

"Roentgen, Forssell and Madame Curie." *Cancer Bulletin,* 14 (May-June 1962), 47-48.

(See Chapter 22: "Roentgen, Forssell and Madame Curie").

Rosen, Peter Paul. "Specimen Radiography and the Diagnosis of Clinically Occult Mammary Carcinoma. A Brief Historical Review." *Pathology Annual,*
15 (1980), 225-37.

(See Chapter 22: Rosen).

Shapiro, S. L. "Radiotherapy for Laryngeal Cancer." *The Eye, Ear, Nose, and
Throat Monthly,* 48 (March 1969), 174-78.

In 1903 William Pusey, a dermatologist at the University of Chicago, became
the first physician to treat an inoperable laryngeal carcinoma with x-ray therapy.
Early devices could not generate a current of more than 50-75 kilovolts, however,
limiting the effectiveness of the treatment. The invention of the Coolidge tube
in 1913 made possible the delivery of up to 200 kilovolts, and filtering techniques
improved the percentage depth dose. Although treatment of laryngeal carcinomas
increased, the results were disappointing, and deaths often occurred because of
cartilage necrosis and even electrocution. The first cures for laryngeal carcinoma
through radiotherapy were achieved by Henri Coutard at the Radium Institute
in Paris, where he developed the idea of fractionated doses of radiation, spread
out over several weeks with daily treatments, and delivered to a strictly delineated field. In the 1930s English physicians used intracavity radium treatments
through a fenestration of the thyroid cartilage. The modern era of radiotherapy
for laryngeal carcinoma began in 1929 with the establishment of an international
standard for radiation dose, the "roentgen" or "r", which measured the amount
of ionization within a definable unit of space. After World War II a new yardstick
appeared—the "rad"—which stated the amount of radiation actually absorbed
by tissues. Also, the development of megavoltage generators after World War II
greatly improved treatment capabilities. Finally, pathological staging systems for
laryngeal carcinoma have helped radiotherapists in planning treatment.

Stockwell, Richard M. "Irradiation and Thyroid Cancer. History and Current
Recommendations." *Connecticut Medicine,* 43 (February 1979), 63-67.

(See Chapter 14: Stockwell).

Streitmann, B. "Strahlentherapie der Tumoren im Kindesalter. Bericht über den
1. Roentgenbestrahlungsfall in Wien (Leopold Freund, 1896)." *Fortschrifte
auf dem Gebiete den Roentgenstrahlen und der Nuklearmedizin,* Supplement
163, 1973.

One year after Wilhelm Roentgen's discovery of x-rays in 1895, physicians
were already experimenting with x-ray therapy on cancerous lesions. In Vienna,
Leopold Freund in 1896 was already trying x-rays on skin and breast lesions and
noting reduction in tumor sizes.

Tateno, Y. "Historical Outline of Radiotherapy of Cancer." *Kango Gijutsu*, 21 (August 1975), 110-17.

(See Chapter 24: Trout).

Trout, E. Dale. "The History of High Energy Radiation Sources for Cancer Therapy." *Cancer Bulletin*, 8 (January-February 1956), 8-12.

Teletherapy is "distance" therapy where the source of radiation is placed up to 100 centimeters from the body. High energy radiation allows for a cancerocidal dose to deep-seated tumors with minimal damage to other tissues. The discovery of radium was first announced in December 1898, and by the early 1920s, the first radium teletherapy units were operating at what is now the Roswell Park Memorial Institute in Buffalo. The first x-ray treatments were given soon after Roentgen's discoveries in 1895. The Coolidge x-ray tube and mechanical rectifier in 1913 made possible the production of x-rays up to 140,000 volts. In 1922 deep therapy became available with Coolidge's 200,000 volt x-ray tube. In 1930 C. C. Lauritsen installed two 750,000 volt x-ray tubes at California Technological University. In 1934 Henry Schmitz installed an 800,000 volt unit at Mercy Hospital in Chicago. New developments rapidly followed, including the Charlton and Westendorp 2,000,000 volt unit in 1943. After World War II, the use of linear accelerators provided for developments in the 100,000,000 volt range.

Tschakert, H. "Funfjahresheilungsergebnisse bei der Strahlentherapie von 4347 Collum-Uteri-Karzinom im Zeitraum von 1928 bis 1977. Historischer Überblick über einen Berichyszeitraum eines Halben Jahrunderts." *Strahlentherapie Onkologie*, 162 (November 1986), 680-85.

Early in the 1900s the Wertheim surgical procedure for uterine and cervical carcinoma was largely abandoned because of new developments in radiotherapy. During the 1920s radium implants were used, with both intracavity and interstitial approaches, and by the 1930s the development of the 200 kilovolts external beam therapy was widely used. The use of fractionated doses of radiation exposure was also fine-tuned. Megavoltage external beam therapy came of age in the 1950s and 1960s when developments in high-energy physics permitted construction of new machines.

Vaeth, Jerome M. "Historical Aspects of Tylectomy and Radiation Therapy in the Treatment of Cancer of the Breast." *Frontiers in Radiation Therapy and Oncology*, 17 (1983), 1-10.

The relatively recent idea that women can be saved from disfiguring radical mastectomies rests on one assumption: ionizing radiations can sterilize adenocarcinoma of the breast and regional lymphatics. In January 1896 Wilhelm Roentgen announced his discovery of x-rays, and two months later Emil H. Grubbe, a medical student in Chicago, irradiated a women suffering from breast carcinoma. Just two years before, William Halsted had made the radical mastectomy the treatment of choice in breast carcinoma. J. L. Rauschoff in 1914 first treated breast carcinoma with radium applications. Credit for the development and practice of tylectomy and radiation therapy in a systematic fashion goes to Geoffrey Keynes of St. Bartholomew's Hospital in 1924. He began the routine practice of tylectomy followed by radium application to the entire breast and nodal drainage in operable carcinoma. Keynes believed in tumor removal followed by interstitial radium to the breast and regional lymph nodes. In the 1930s the work of Maurice Lenz first described the relationship between tumor size, radiation dose, and tumor sterilization. The first substantial radiation therapy challenge to the radical mastectomy came in 1949 when R. McWhirter published his results in the use of the simple mastectomy with postoperative medium-voltage x-ray therapy as a routine procedure in breast cancer treatment. Survival rates closely approximated those of the radical mastectomy.

Yeh, Samuel D. J. "Nuclear Medicine and Cancer Research in the People's Republic of China." *American Journal of Chinese Medicine*, 7 (1979), 149-55.

(See Chapter 5: Yeh).

25 Chemotherapy

Axelrod, Arnold R. "Cancer Chemotherapy—An Historical View." *Bulletin of the American Association of Industrial Nurses*, 16 (January 1968), 17-20.

Chemotherapy has been in existence for a century in the treatment of cancer. Potassium arsenite and Fowler's solution were used in the mid-nineteenth century, but it was not until World War II that chemotherapy entered the modern era. Screening processes using pharmacological agents on animals have been widespread. If therapeutic results are indicated, clinical trials then begin. Practical chemotherapy got underway during World War II when research attempts to develop antidotes for poisonous mustard gas resulted in the production of nitrogen mustard, a methyl-bisamine compound. It was found to have a therapeutic effect on Hodgkin's disease. Over the years modifications of nitrogen mustard resulted in chlorambusil, which proved effective in treating chronic lymphocytic leukemia; sarcolysin, effective for multiple myeloma; and busulfan for chronic granulocytic leukemia. In 1946 folic acid was discovered, and development of antifolic acid drugs—pterolyglumatic acid and methotrexate—followed. They proved therapeutic in leukemia and choriocarcinoma respectively. Since cancer cells seemed to require purines, more nucleic acids, chemists developed antipurine drugs—5-fluorouracil for advanced carcinoma of the colon. From the periwinkle plant came vincristine and vinblastine for Hodgkin's disease and acute leukemia.

Baker, Harvey W. "The General Surgeon and Cancer." *The American Journal of Surgery*, 139 (May 1980), 606-07.

(See Chapter 23: Baker).

Becker, H., and G. Schwarz. "Die Mistel (Viscum Album L.) als Krebstherapeutikum; ein Ueberblick über die Geschichte und Neuere Forschung." *Deutsche Apotheker Zeitung*, 112 (21 September 1972), 1462-65.

(See Chapter 25: Kardinal).

Brockman, R. W. "Drug Resistance: Clinical and Experimental. Historical Perspectives." *Oncology: Proceedings of the Tenth International Cancer Congress*, II (1970), 254-64.

From early in the twentieth century researchers knew that the appearance of bacteria and protozoa resistant to a particular drug therapy was inevitable. In cancer chemotherapy, that same conclusion became clear with the initial chemotherapy work of Huggins, Farber, Heilman, and Kendall. Resistance has been demonstrated to nearly all known anti-cancer agents. Early in the 1950s researchers demonstrated that resistance was a product of genetic mutation and selection in the cancer cell. If the number of tumor cells exceeds the statistical rate of cell mutation, the chemotherapy will fail because the tumor will mutate and become resistant. This finding led to the development of multiple chemotherapeutic approaches to the same tumor.

Brunner, K. W. "Grundsatze der Chemotherapeutischen Behandlung der Krebskrankhein." *Schweizerische Medizinische Wochenschrift*, 95 (1965), 789-99.

(See Chapter 25: Kardinal).

Burchenal, Joseph H. "The Historical Development of Chemotherapy." *Seminars in Oncology*, 4 (June 1977), 135-46.

(See Chapter 25: Kardinal).

Burzynski, S. R. "Antineoplastons: History of the Research." *Drugs Under Experimental and Clinical Research*, 12 (Suppl. 1, 1986), 1-9.

Antineoplastons are naturally-occurring peptides and amino acid derivatives which control neoplastic growth. Antineoplaston theories basically applied cybernetic notions of autonomous systems to the studies of peptides in human blood. The original research began in 1967 when researchers noticed significant differences in the peptide content in the blood serum of cancer patients compared to a control group. Similar peptide fractions were isolated from urine. For thousands of years around the world urine has been used for medicinal purposes, and the first modern study of growth-inhibiting substances in urine was conducted in 1937 by G. L. Rohdenburg. Research on antineoplastons led to the isolation of different peptide fractions from urine, which became named Antineoplaston A1, A2, A3, A4, and A5, all of which possessed high anticancer activity and low toxicity. The first active component was chemically identified as 3-phenylacetylamino-2, 6-piperidinedione and was named Antineoplaston A10. Two synthetic derivatives were named Antineoplaston AS2-1 and AS2-5. All of the antineoplastons were submitted for Phase 1 clinical studies on advanced cancer patients and proved to have few side effects and genuine anti-tumor properties.

Carter, Stephen K., and Milan Slavik. "Chemotherapy of Cancer." *Annual Review of Pharmacology*, 14 (1974), 157-83.

Since World War II there has been an extraordinary success in developing effective chemotherapy agents for a number of malignant tumors. Prolonged survival and cures have been achieved for choriocarcinoma through the use of methotrexate and dactinomycin; acute childhood lymphocytic leukemia through the use of daunorubicin, prednisone, vincristine, 6-mercaptopurine, methotrexate, BCNU, and adriamycin; Hodgkin's disease with HN2, vincristine, prednisone, procarbazine, and bleomycin; testicular tumors through use of dactinomycin, methotrexate, and chlorambusil; Wilms' tumor through adjuvant dactinomycin therapy, surgery, and radiotherapy; and neuroblastoma through adjuvant cyclophosphamide chemotherapy, surgery, and radiotherapy. Palliation and extension of life have been achieved in prostate carcinoma with estrogen therapy and orchiectomy and in breast cancer with androgen and estrogen therapy and chemotherapy with 5-fluorouracil, vincristine, prednisone, and methotrexate. The alkylating agents have shown some effect in treating ovarian carcinoma and multiple myeloma.

DeVita, Vincent T., Jr. "Principles of Chemotherapy. Historical Perspectives." In Vincent T. DeVita, Jr., Samuel Hellman, and Steven A. Rosenberg. *Cancer. Principles & Practice of Oncology*. 1985. Pp. 257-58.

Paul Ehrlich coined the term chemotherapy to describe the use of known chemicals to treat parasitic diseases. Between 1903 and 1915 he worked on developing chemotherapeutic agents by testing drugs on diseased animals. He synthesized a long series of organic arsenic compounds and discovered the drug salvarsan, which was effective against trypanosome infections and rabbit syphilis. The drug was the first man-made chemical found to be effective against human parasitic disease. It was an important milestone for future chemotherapeutic research because Ehrlich had proven that infectious diseases, particularly syphilis, could be cured in rodents and humans and that the rodent model predicted for human effectiveness. The first significant advance after Ehrlich's work came in 1926 with the discovery of penicillin and its clinical use between 1939 and 1943.

Cancer treatment research began in earnest at the turn of the century with three major developments. First, William Stewart Halsted in 1894 proposed *en bloc* surgical resections of tumors. Second, about the same time, Wilhelm Roentgen discovered x-rays and physicians were soon using them to treat localized lesions. Third, Paul Ehrlich in 1898 isolated the first alkylating agent. His use of rodent models for infectious diseases led George Clowes of the Roswell Park Memorial Institute in Buffalo to develop in-bred rodent lines that could carry transplanted tumors. These models served as the testing ground for potential chemotherapeutic agents. During World War II work with nitrogen mustard gas led to the effective testing of these agents on lymphoma victims. The modern era of chemotherapy was born when Sidney Farber discovered the effect of folic acid on lymphoblastic leukemia during the 1950s.

Einhorn, Jerzy. "Nitrogen Mustard: The Origin of Chemotherapy for Cancer." *International Journal of Radiation Oncology, Biology, and Physics*, 11 (July 1985), 1375-78.

In 1942 Alfred Gilman and Louis S. Goodman of Yale received government grants to develop antidotes for mustard gas chemical warfare. They examined the systemic effects of mustard gas on human beings and noted that rapidly growing lymphatic tissues were especially vulnerable to the mustard gases. They soon discovered that intravenous injections of nitrogen mustard produced remissions of murine lymphoma in mice. Clinical trials began late in 1942. Chemotherapy was born.

Elion, Gertrude B. "Mechanism of Action of Chemotherapeutic Agents. Historical Perspectives." *Oncology: Proceedings of the Tenth International Cancer Congress*, II (1970), 219-23.

Cancer chemotherapy was underway before the biochemistry of the neoplastic cell was understood on even a minimal level. In the early 1940s nucleic acid chemistry was a little backwater in which a few academic scientists labored quietly. The antimetabolite theory was proposed by P. Fields and D. D. Woods in 1940 to explain the antibacterial action of sulfonamides. Their theory made possible a biochemical approach to chemotherapy which might provide agents with known mechanisms of action. 6-Mercaptopurine was synthesized and found to have antipurine activity in micro-organisms in 1951, and by 1953 it had been shown to be active against acute lymphocytic leukemia in children. The antifolic acids also had their beginnings before the biosynthetic pathways for nucleic acids had been demonstrated. Sidney Farber discovered in 1948 that aminopterin, the 4-amino analog of folic acid, had antileukemic activity in children. The real understanding of the mechanism of action of antifolic acids as inhibitors of dihydrofolate reductase had to wait until the 1950s, which demonstrated that the biologically active forms of folic acid were tetrahydrofolic acid derivatives and that enzymatic reduction of folic acid *in vivo* was a prerequisite to the activity of the vitamin in the biosynthesis of purines and thymine.

Endicott, Kenneth M. "The Chemotherapy Program." *Journal of the National Cancer Institute*, 19 (1957), 275-93.

By the early 1950s it was clear to most oncologists that the nitrogen mustards and the antifolic acid drugs had great potential in cancer treatment, and that there might be other naturally occurring or synthetic drugs yet to be discovered which had tumorcidal capabilities. In 1954 Congress dramatically increased the budget of the National Cancer Institute and targeted a large proportion of the funds to the chemotherapy program. Kenneth Endicott, a pathologist with the United States Public Health Service, was selected to head up the chemotherapy program at the National Cancer Institute. In 1957 he established the Cancer Chemotherapy National Service Center to coordinate the work of the NCI, the major pharmaceutical companies, and universities in drug development and testing programs.

Freireich, Emil. "Intramural Therapeutic Research at the National Cancer Institute, Department of Medicine: 1955-1965." *Cancer Treatment Reports*, 68 (January 1984), 21-30.

The article reviews the work of the National Cancer Institute in the curative treatment of acute lymphocytic leukemia through methotrexate and mercaptopurine, as well as the new therapeutic techniques for lymphomas, chronic mylegenous leukemia, and choriocarcinoma.

Freireich, Emil. "Nitrogen Mustard Therapy." *Journal of the American Medical Association*, 251 (May 4, 1984), 2262-63.

The first clinical test of chemotherapy took place in 1942 on 67 patients by Drs. Alfred Gilman, Louis Goodman, William Dameshek, and Maxwell Wintrobe. The patients were suffering from a variety of tumors, and the study indicated that the nitrogen mustards had a therapeutic effect on lymphomas and Hodgkin's disease. Two of the authors—Wintrobe and Dameshek—eventually became nationally known experts in clinical hematology. Today chemotherapy is the treatment of choice in advanced lymphomas, acute leukemia, choriocarcinoma, and embryonal testicular cancer. Currently there are thirty chemical moieties commercially available which have significant therapeutic effects in patients with widespread clinical cancer.

Gilman, Alfred. "The Initial Trial of Nitrogen Mustard." *American Journal of Surgery*, 105 (1962), 574-78.

The first clinical trial of nitrogen mustard was performed by Gustav E. Lindskog, a surgeon at Yale, in December 1942. The patient suffered from a previously irradiated, rapidly progressive malignant lymphoma. Lindskog achieved a transient but complete remission and a second, short remission after renewed treatment before the patient died.

Goldin, Abraham. "Experimental Models and Clinical Trials: Screening Methodology. Historical Review and Perspectives." *Oncology: Proceedings of the
Tenth International Cancer Congress*, II (1970), 1-9.

Before World War II small-scale drug development programs were underway
by Boyland in Great Britain, where he used spontaneous breast tumors in mice,
by Furth in the United States, where he used experimental leukemia, and by
Lettre in Germany, where he employed bacterial polysaccharides on sarcomas.
World War II research showing the antitumor capabilities of nitrogen mustard
gave chemotherapy screening a real boost, and it gained momentum in the early
1950s when Sidney Farber showed that the antifolic acid antagonist, aminopterin,
was effective in treating acute lymphocytic leukemia. Major screening programs
were launched at the Memorial Sloan-Kettering Institute by Rhoads, Stock, and
Burchenal; at the National Cancer Institute with the extension of Shear's program to screen synthetic compounds and plant products; at the Chester Beatty
Research Institute in London by Haddow; at the Cancer Institute in Moscow by
Larionov; at the University of Tokyo by Yoshida; at the Children's Cancer Research Foundation in Boston by Farber; and at the Southern Research Institute
by Skipper. The establishment of the Cancer Chemotherapy National Service
Center at the National Cancer Institute then provided national coordination to
all these research efforts.

Goldin, Abraham. "Studies with High-Dose Methotrexate—Historical Background." *Cancer Treatment Report*, 62 (February 1978), 307-12.

(See Chapter 25: Snyder).

Greene, Frederick L. "A Review of the Historical Development and Results of the
Chemotherapy of Wilms' Tumor." *Southern Medical Journal*, 63 (December
1970), 1405-08.

(See Chapter 20: Greene).

Gross, R., and O. Claus. "Chemotherapie von Tumorleiden: Vergangenheit und
Gegenwart." *Medizinische Welt*, 33 (November 5, 1982), 1531-38.

(See Chapter 25: Kardinal).

Heller, John R. "Cancer Chemotherapy, History and Present Status." *Bulletin
of the New York Academy of Medicine*, 38 (May 1962), 348-63.

Medical treatment of cancer did not really begin until 1865 when Lissauer
first treated chronic myelocytic leukemia with arsenic in Fowler's solution. Many
ancients used ointments on external lesions, but the Arab physician Avicenna (b.
980) first advised the use of arsenic in treating carcinoma. After Lissauer various
quack treatments appeared as well. Early in the 1900s the use of heavy metals,
particularly selenium, to treat cancer became popular, and between 1896 and

1920 new research into hormone therapy emerged. Modern chemotherapy had its birth during World War II. Experimentation with mustard gas led to Cornelius Rhoads's identification of nitrogen mustard as a therapeutic agent in treating cancer. In 1947 Sidney Farber noted the effect of folic acid on children with acute leukemia. Today modern chemotherapy includes four categories of agents useful in treating cancer: 1) the antimetabolites, including such folic acid antagonists as methotrexate; 2) the alkylating agents, nitrogen mustard and its derivatives; 3) the antibiotics, namely the actinomycins; and 4) the adrenal steroids such as cortisone and hydrocortisone.

"History of the Cancer Chemotherapy Program." *Cancer Chemotherapy Report,* 50 (1966), 349-96).

(See Chapter 25: Kardinal).

Hitchings, George H. "Design of Cancer Chemotherapeutic Agents: Historical Review and Perspectives." *Oncology: Proceedings of the Tenth International Cancer Congress,* II (1970), 46-51.

(See Chaptr 25: Kardinal).

Ichikawa, A. "Discovery of the Effect of Bleomycin on Squamous Cell Carcinoma and the Development of Its Research." *Journal of the Japanese Medical Association,* 62 (15 July 1969), 153-58.

In 1955 the Japanese scientist Hidao Umezawa developed phleomycin and in 1966 the compound drug bleomycin. Bleomycin accumulated in the skin and was shown by Ichikawa to be effective in shrinking squamous cell carcinomas.

Jackson, Robert. "Medicine and History. How Caustics Were Used to Treat Skin Cancer." *The Journal of Dermatologic Surgery and Oncology,* 5 (December 1979), 949-50.

Caustic agents were used to treat skin cancer as far back as the eighteenth century, but three caustics were most commonly used in the early twentieth century. Zinc chloride made into a paste of flour and cocaine was applied to malignant skin lesions to mummify the tissue, after which it would be surgically removed. Potassium hydroxide was applied for two to three minutes on small lesions before it was neutralized with vinegar applications. Arsenic trioxide was applied to neoplasms for five to eight days before the malignant tissue was removed. Four other caustics—nitric acid, pyrogallic acid, alum, and acid nitrate of mercury—were also commonly used. By 1930, however, all of them were being employed with decreasing frequency in favor of x-ray therapy.

Jacobs, Edwin M., Franco M. Muggia, and Marcel Rozencweig. "Chemotherapy of Testicular Cancer: From Palliation to Curative Adjuvant Therapy."
Seminars in Oncology, 6 (March 1979), 3-13.

(See Chapter 20: Jacobs, Muggia, and Rosencweig).

Kardinal, Carl G. "Cancer Chemotherapy. Historical Aspects and Future Considerations." *Postgraduate Medicine*, 77 (May 1, 1985), 165-74.

Effective cancer chemotherapy was really unknown until after World War II.
Internal use of arsenicals was introduced by the Arab physician Avicenna around
1000 A.D. Throughout the centuries an infinite number of remedies have been
tried for cancer treatment. Modern chemotherapy was born in the 1940s with
the development of the alkylating agents. As part of studies of chemical warfare
and the effects of nitrogen mustard, Drs. Louis Goodman and Alfred Gilman at
Yale noticed therapeutic effectiveness of nitrogen mustard on mice afflicted with
lymphosarcoma. In the early 1940s Charles Huggins noticed the hormonal respon-
siveness of some prostate and breast cancers. In 1947 Sidney Farber discovered
that folic acid accelerated the leukemic process, so he administered metabolic antagonists to folic acid, especially aminopterin, to a child suffering from leukemia
and achieved a temporary remission of the disease.

During the 1950s multiple new cytotoxic drugs were synthesized, including
5-fluorouracil, 6-thioguanine, 6-mercaptopurine, actinomycin D, methotrexate,
and such alkylating agents as cyclophosphamide, melphalan, busulfan, and triethylenethiophosphoramide. There were two landmark developments in the 1950s.
One was the development of the clinical arm of the National Cancer Institute and
the other was the discovery that advanced metastatic gestational choriocarcinoma
in women could be cured by methotrexate. That work was done by Dr. Min Chiu
Li and Dr. Roy Hertz.

By the end of the 1960s all of the chemotherapeutic agents in common use
today had been synthesized, including the vinca alkyloids vincristine and vinblastine; the nitrosoureas BCNU, CCNU, and streptozotocin; the anthracyclines
daunorubicin and doxorubicin; procarbazine; cytosine arabinoside; bleomycin; cisplatin; and L-asparaginase. The two major developments of the 1960s involved
new understanding of the kinetics of cancer cells and the pharmacokinetics of
chemotherapeutic agents, and that chemotherapeutic agents could be used in
combination without undue toxicity. By the end of the 1960s chemotherapy
had become effective in curing acute lymphocytic leukemia, Hodgkin's disease,
Burkitt's lymphoma, and some embryonal testicular carcinomas.

During the 1970s curative chemotherapy protocols were developed for advanced testicular cancer, diffuse histiocytic lymphomas, Wilms' tumor, and some
embryonal rhabdomyosarcomas.

Larionov, L. F. "Razvitie khimioterapii raka v SSSR." *Voprosy Onkologii*, 13
(1967), 3-34.

(See Chapter 25: Perevodchikovo).

Li, Min Chiu. "The Historical Background of Successful Chemotherapy for Advanced Gestational Trophoblastic Tumors." *American Journal of Obstetrics and Gynecology*, 135 (September 15, 1979), 266-72.

Gestational trophoblastic tumors of the placenta in pregnant women are among the fastest growing tumors. During the 1950s Dr. Min Chiu Li and Roy Hertz found the antifolate drug methotrexate highly effective in treating even advanced, metastatic cases of the disease. Since then, advanced gestational trophoblastic disease has become one of the most curable tumors. Also see Chapter 25: Snyder.

Liebenov, T. and G. Ikonomov. "Comparaisons portant sur le traitement des tumeurs dans la medecine populaire Europeene et Bulgare (XIe-XVIe s.)." In *International Congress of the History of Medicine*. 1981. Volume 3. Pp. 224-26.

During the Middle Ages in Europe in general and Bulgaria in particular, cancer was known for its danger, and most scientists associated its origins with "black bile." Treatment for localized, superficial lesions was wide surgical excision combined with cauterization. Caustic pastes were also used, and most of the time they contained, among other things, arsenic. For more systemic disease, physicians recommended bleeding, herbal potions, and prayer. Popular treatments of cancer almost always involved topical applications of folk medicine.

MacGregor, Alasdair B. "The Search for a Chemical Cure for Cancer." *Medical History*, 10 (1966), 374-85.

As early as 1500 B.C. the Egyptians advised the use of arsenical ointments for treating ulcerated lesions, and over the years an enormous variety of anecdotal chemical treatments were attempted to cure neoplasms. The list of internal and external remedies included hemlock, belladonna, digitalis, antacids, tonics, arsenic, mercury, cod liver oil, flesh of the grey lizard, lead, iodine, gastric juice, carbonic acid, petroleum, tar products, potash, silver nitrate, and turpentine by 1800. The first steps toward modern chemotherapy came in 1898 when Ehrlich described the necrotic effects of an alkalyting agent, ethylinimine, on animal epithelial tissue. In 1916 Strobel advocated the use of potassium hydroxide and zinc chloride, instead of mastectomy, in treating breast cancer. The era of modern chemotherapy began during World War II with the development of the nitrogen mustards. Researchers discovered its cytotoxic effect on rapidly growing cells. Also, researchers in the 1940s discovered the effectiveness of the antimetabolite drugs on some tumors, particularly acute leukemia.

Perevodchikovo, N. I. "Brief Historical Statement: Chemotherapy of Malignant Tumors in the U.S.S.R." *National Cancer Institute Monographs*, 45 (March 1977), 181-82.

Chemotherapy research began in the Soviet Union in 1950 and was led by L. F. Larionov at the Leningrad Institute of Oncology. In 1952 the formation of the Institute of Experimental and Clinical Oncology further promoted chemotherapy research, as did the establishment of the All-Union Antitumor Chemotherapeutic Center in 1966.

Perevodchikovo, N. I., and A. M. Garin. "Osnovnye etapy razvitiia klinicheskoi khimioterapii opukholeĭ v SSSR." *Voprosy Onkologii*, 28 (1982), 31-38.

(See Chapter 25: Perevodchikovo).

Potter, V. R. "Years with Charles Heidelberger." *Carcinogenic Comparative Survey*, 10 (1985), 1-13.

Charles Heidelberger was a biochemist at the University of California at Berkeley, the University of Wisconsin, and the University of Southern California. His most important contribution to cancer research and treatment was the development of 5-fluorouracil, an antipyrimadine chemotherapeutic agent effective in treating some breast and gastrointestinal carcinomas.

Riddle, John M. "Ancient and Medieval Chemotherapy for Cancer." *Isis*, 76 (September 1985), 319-30.

The modern era of chemotherapy began with the nitrogen experiments of World War II, but for centuries physicians and lay healers have tried to use a variety of chemicals to treat cancer. Most of the drugs had no therapeutic effect, but recent tests of the antitumor capabilities of a number of ancient remedies have shown them to be active against tumors. The Greeks, for example, used some of the plant alkaloids, and Dioscorides recommended the bulb of narcissus for skin tumors. Narcissus contains colchicine which is used as a modern drug in chemotherapy. Unfortunately, when the United States Cancer Chemotherapy National Service Center began its plant screening program in the 1950s, it did not systematically research ancient and medieval writings and test the plants they recommended for use. Since many of them had at least some level of antitumor powers, much valuable time and money could have been saved.

Schepartz, Saul A. "Historical Overview of the National Cancer Institute's Fermentation Program." *Recent Results in Cancer Research*, 63 (1978), 30-32.

(See Chapter 30: Schepartz).

Schepartz, Saul A. "History of the National Cancer Institute and the Plant Screening Program." *Cancer Treatment Reports*, 60 (August 1976), 975-78.

A new excitement about chemotherapy led to the establishment of the Cancer Chemotherapy National Service Center in 1955. It was part of the National Cancer Institute. By 1958 it had already become a huge, industrial clearinghouse looking at drug development; it was closely allied with the major pharmaceutical companies and academic medicine. The systematic plant screening program began in 1961, and by 1974 the CCNSC had tested more than 80,000 plants for their anti-neoplastic characteristics.

Shabel, F. M. "Historical Development and Future Promise of the Nitrosources." *Cancer Chemotherapy Reports*, Suppl. (May 1973), 43-46.

(See Chapter 25: Kardinal).

Shimkin, Michael B., and George E. Moore. "Adjuvant Use of Chemotherapy in the Surgical Treatment of Cancer." *Journal of the American Medical Association*, 167 (1958), 1710-14.

Adjuvant chemotherapy is a term describing the use of chemotherapy in association with other treatment modalities—surgical resection and radiotherapy. During the 1940s and early 1950s it became clear that the nitrogen mustards and the folic acid antagonists had therapeutic effects on some of the leukemias and lymphomas, but the viability of chemotherapy on solid tumors remained yet to be proved. But in the 1950s the antimetabolites like methotrexate appeared to have an effect on some of the solid tumors, such as the choriocarcinomas. By the late 1950s surgeons were cautiously willing to consider the use of chemotherapy following a surgical resection if the histology and stage of the tumor indicated the likelihood of metastasis and if there was experimental evidence that a particular chemical agent was capable of inducing a regression of the tumor or the destruction of clinically occult cells. By the late 1950s and early 1960s chemotherapy had joined surgery and radiotherapy as a major treatment modality, and the notion of the team approach to cancer treatment received a dramatic boost.

Snyder, R. D. "Some Aspects of the Development of Methotrexate Therapy." *Clinical and Experimental Pharmacology and Physiology*, 5 (1979), 1-4.

The first use of antifolate therapy was in the 1940s when dietary measures were employed to render leukemia patients folate deficient. Shortly thereafter, aminopterin was synthesized and shown to be effective in producing remissions in acute leukemia. It was soon replaced by the introduction of methotrexate. In the 1960s studies showed that patients with trophoblastic disease had active responses to methotrexate therapy. Over the years experimentation with doses had led to more and more powerful regimens designed to destroy tumor cells without permanently damaging normal tissues. Methotrexate has also been shown to be active in patients suffering from squamous cell tumors of the head and neck and osteogenic sarcomas. In the 1960s vincristine and later adriamycin was added to the regimen but has complicated the long-term evaluation of methotrexate effectiveness. A number of factors have been identified as important in the delivery of methotrexate therapy. They include the volume of the dose, the route of administration, the schedule and rate of administration, the rescue technique which may or may not selectively rescue normal cells, and the use of agents which increase drug uptake.

Sugiura, Kanematsu. "Reminicences and Experience in Experimental Chemotherapy of Cancer." *Medical Clinics of North America*, 55 (May 1971), 667-82.

With a scholarship from railroad magnate E. E. Harriman, Kanematsu Sugiura came to the United States and earned a degree in chemistry from the Polytechnic Institute of Brooklyn in 1915 and a master's degree from Columbia University in 1917. He specialized in biochemistry and went to work on the chemotherapy of cancer for the Harriman Research Laboratory. During the 1910s and 1920s most of the experimental research on animal tumors was done using inorganic compounds such as copper sulfate, calcium chloride, arsenic trioxide, etc. They were far too toxic, although some of them had modest antitumor capabilities. In those early experiments chemotherapists also worked on the connections between diet and neoplasms. Experimental chemotherapy received its real boost during and just after World War II when the antitumor properties of nitrogen mustard and the antifolic acids was discovered. During the last twenty years more than one thousand chemicals as well as crude extracts of biological materials have been tested against a spectrum of 43 mouse, rat, hamster, and chicken tumors. Of the alkylating agents tested, cyclophosphamide was the most effective on tumors, followed by 1,3-bis(2-chloroethyl)-1-nitrosourea, triethylene thiophosphoramide, and sarcolysin. Of the pyrimidine analogs, 5-fluorouracil was the most potent. Methotrexate was the most effective of the antimetabolites. 6-Mercaptopurine was the best of the purine analogs. The best steroid therapy involved hydrocortisone. Of the antibiotics, mitomycin C had the greatest anti-tumor properties, along with fumagillin.

Suraiya, J. N. "Chemotherapy of Cancer—25 Years of Progress." *Indian Journal of Cancer*, 9 (December 1972), 296-301.

(See Chapter 25: Kardinal).

Swann, John Patrick. "Paul Ehrlich and the Introduction of Salvarsan." *Medical Heritage*, 1 (March/April 1985), 137-38.

Paul Ehrlich (1854-1915) had a profound interest in the chemical basis of biological phenomena and is considered the father of chemotherapy. In 1907 he announced his receptor theory, arguing that a drug molecule possesses certain atomic groups responsible for binding it to a chemically allied site in the microorganism invading the body, and for poisoning the organism once it is bound. The aim of Ehrlichian chemotherapy was to design a chemical with 1) a binding group corresponding to a chemoreceptor in the parasite; 2) a chemical group that will destroy the parasite; and 3) much greater receptivity for the chemoreceptors of the pathogen than for the receptors in the host's normal cells. These same principles all became the foundation for cancer chemotherapy after World War II.

Vaeth, Jerome M. "Role of the Pharmacist in Cancer Care Throughout History." *Frontiers in Radiation Therapy and Oncology*, 25 (1981), 1-4.

Ancients developed a variety of herbal potions and caustic pastes to treat cancer, but it was not until nineteenth century developments of chloroform, opium, cocaine, and ether that pharmacology really became useful in cancer treatment.

Wright, Jane C. "Cancer Chemotherapy: Past, Present, and Future." *Journal of the National Medical Association*, 76 (August 1984), 773-84.

Over the centuries there have been thousands of anecdotal chemical treatments for cancer, but the first systematic, clinical trial of a drug for treating cancer was Lissauer's use of potassium arsenite, or Fowler's solution, on a leukemia patient. The first major development in hormonal therapy came in 1896 when George Thomas Beatson advocated oophorectomy for breast carcinoma. The first clinical reports of androgenic therapy proving beneficial for metastatic breast carcinoma were by Loeser (1939) and Ulrich (1939). In 1941 Charles Huggins developed the use of androgen deprivation through orchiectomy for prostatic carcinoma. In 1944 Haddow first reported regressions in metastatic breast carcinomas following the use of estrogens.

The modern era of chemotherapy began during World War II with the discovery of the nitrogen mustards. Cornelius Rhoads soon reported the ability of the nitrogen mustards to inhibit animal lymphomas. In 1946 Gilman and Philips reported improvements in patients with lymphosarcoma treated with tris-nitrogen mustard. Research in the 1950s produced a variety of new alkylating agents, including triethylenethiophosphoramide, triethylenemelamine, chlorambusil, cyclophosphamide, sarcolysin, melphalan, busulfan, and carmustine. The alkylating agents produced remissons in lymphomas, Hodgkin's disease, chronic leukemias, ovarian cancer, breast cancer, oat-cell carcinoma of the lung, lymphoepithelioma of the nasopharynx, Kaposi's sarcoma, multiple myeloma, and neuroblastoma.

The antimetabolites—folic acid antagonists, purine antagonists, and pyrimidine antagonists—are another major group of chemotherapeutic drugs. In 1948

Sidney Farber demonstrated the effectiveness of folic acid antagonists on acute leukemia. By 1960 methotrexate was clearly effective on patients with mycosis fungoides, choriocarcinoma, chorioadenoma, squamous cell carcinomas, and breast carcinoma. Of the purine antagonists, the most important was 6-mercaptopurine, which is antileukemic in children. The most effective pyrimidine antagonist is fluorouracil for gastrointestinal adenocarcinomas and cytosine arabinoside for acute mylogenous leukemia.

Antitumor antibiotics constitute another major group of chemotherapeutic agents. Actinomycin is effective in treating Hodgkin's disease, rhabdomyosarcomas, adenocarcinomas, and squamous cell carcinomas; mithramycin for embryonal testicular cancer and glioblastoma; adriamycin for a wide variety of tumors; bleomycin for squamous cell carcinomas and lymphomas; streptozotocin for islet-cell cancer of the prostate; and daunomycin for leukemia.

The plant alkaloid drugs—vincristine, vinblastine, vindesine, etoposide, and teniposide have proven effective in treating lymphomas, leukemia, Hodgkin's disease, and breast, ovarian, testicular, and choriocarcinomas. The enzyme drug asparaginase is effective against leukemia. Cisplatine, an inorganic metal salt, has proven therapeutic against squamous cell carcinomas, uterine and bladder tumors, osteogenic sarcomas, and neuroblastomas.

Zubrod, C. Gordon. "Approaches to Cancer Chemotherapy. Historical Perspectives." *Oncology: Proceedings of the Tenth International Cancer Congress,* III (1970), 337-43.

(See Chapter 25: Zubrod).

Zubrod, C. Gordon. "Historic Milestones in Curative Chemotherapy." *Seminars in Oncology,* 6 (December 1979), 490-505.

The major milestones in the history of curative chemotherapy are: 1) the discovery of such highly active drugs as the alkylating agents (nitrogen mustard, the folate antagonists (aminopterin and methotrexate), the corticosteroids, mercaptopurine, actinomycin, and L-Asparaginase between 1940 and 1955; 2) the establishment of effective drug development programs and the discovery of such new active agents as vinblastine, vincristine, procarbazine, cytosine arabinoside, daunorubicin, bleomycin, cisplatinum diamminedichloride, and fluorouracil between 1955 and 1965; 3) the cure of metastatic choriocarcinoma by methotrexate in 1956; 4) the cure of Burkitt's lymphoma in 1965; 5) the use of the L1210 model and cellular kinetics leading to combination chemotherapy for cure of acute lymphocytic leukemia of children, lymphomas, testicular cancer, and childhood neoplasms between 1962 and 1975; and 6) the development of adjuvant chemotherapy, first started in 1957, which demonstrated effectiveness on Wilms' tumor, large growth fraction cancers, and breast cancer.

Zubrod, C. Gordon. "Origins and Development of Chemotherapy Research at the National Cancer Institute." *Cancer Treatment Reports*, 68 (January 1984), 9-19.

Research in the chemotherapy of cancer at the National Cancer Institute had its beginnings in 1935 while the Institute was still in its early beginnings at Harvard. The US Public Health Service had created the Office of Field Investigations in Cancer under Joseph Schereschewsky in 1927, and it remained in Cambridge until 1939, when it was moved to Bethesda, Maryland, as part of the newly formed NCI in 1939. Between 1945 and 1948 the NCI screened more than 3,000 agents for their antitumor qualities. The Clinical Center was opened in 1953 and began treating patients. In 1955 the NCI established the Cancer Chemotherapy National Service Center. Late in the 1950s NCI researchers played a pioneer role in the cure of choriocarcinoma with methotrexate. The NCI also played a key role in the development of chemical treatments for acute lymphocytic leukemia and Hodgkin's disease.

Zubrod, C. Gordon. "The Cure of Cancer by Chemotherapy—Reflections on How It Happened." *Medical and Pediatric Oncology*, 8 (1980), 107-14.

Since 1956 ten cancers have proven to be curable by drugs: choriocarcinoma, Burkitt's lymphoma, acute lymphocytic leukemia, Hodgkin's disease, histiocytic lymphoma, Wilms' tumor, rhabdomyosarcoma, embryonal testicular cancer, Ewing's sarcoma, and ovarian cancer in children. Since the World War II discovery at Yale of the effectiveness of nitrogen mustard therapy, thirteen other drugs have been shown to retard tumor growth: cyclophosphamide, actinomycin D, methotrexate, mercaptopurine, prednisone, procarbazine, vincristine, asparaginase, adriamycin, fluorouracil, cisplatin, bleomycin, and cytarabine.

Zubrod, C. Gordon, Saul A. Schepartz, and Stephen K. Carter. "Historical Background of the National Cancer Institute's Drug Thrust." *National Cancer Institute Monograph*, 45 (March 1977), 7-11.

Since its creation in 1937 the National Cancer Institute has been the primary agency through which the United States government has sought to marshall biomedical research toward the goal of controlling human cancer. Modern chemotherapy research began with the nitrogen mustard research of World War II, and after the war, Memorial Sloan-Kettering, under Cornelius Rhoads, became the leading chemotherapy center in the world. In 1955 the National Cancer Institute founded the Cancer Chemotherapy National Service Center to manage NCI chemotherapy research, coordinate national chemotherapy efforts, and engage in contract research.

Zubrod, C. G., S. Schepartz, J. Leiter, J. M. Endicott, L. M. Carrese, and C. G. Baker. "The Chemotherapy Program of the National Cancer Institute: History, Analysis, and Plans." *Cancer Chemotherapy Reports*, 50 (1966), 349-540.

(See Chapter 25: Zubrod).

26 Hormonal Therapy

"Adrenalectomy." *Cancer Bulletin*, 5 (September-October 1953), 116-17.

(See Chapter 20: "Adrenalectomy").

Besson, A., R. Chabloz, and F. Saegesser. "Pheochromocytomes sporadiques, familiaux ou associes a une neurocristopathie. 27 Observations dont 26 chirurgicales (1926 a 1985)." *Schweizerische Rundshau für Medizin Praxis*, 74 (November 12, 1985), 1267-82.

(See Chapter 21: Brennan and Macdonald).

Brennan, Murray F., and John S. Macdonald. "Cancer of the Endocrine System." In Vincent DeVita, Jr., Samuel Hellman, and Steven A. Rosenberg. *Cancer. Principles & Practice of Oncology*. 1985. Pp. 1179-1241.

(See Chapter 21: Brennan and Macdonald).

Collins, W. F. "Historical and Personal Perspective." *Clinical Neurosurgery*, 21 (1974), 68-78.

(See Chapter 26: "Some Aspects of Hormonal Therapy").

d'Auteuil, Pierre and J. Lemay. "La thérapeutique endocrinienne du cancer du sein: Un historique." *Union médicale du Canada*, 114 (February 1985), 139-45.

(See Chapter 11: d'Auteuil and LeMay).

Furth, Jacob. "Hormones and Cancer: Clinical and Experimental. Historical Perspective." *Oncology: Proceedings of the Tenth International Cancer Congress*, I (1970), 288-99.

In 1896 George Beatson introduced the notion of hormonal control of human breast cancer when he recommended ovariectomy. Subsequent research on breast cancer in mice at the Jackson Memorial Laboratory by Loeb, Lacassagne, Little, and Bittner focused on the question of ovarian hormones, a specific milk virus, and genes. Rous, Berenblum, and others developed the concept of latent cancer cells, and Wooley discovered that the adrenal gland compensates for lack of ovarian hormones. Charles Huggins introduced adrenalectomy as a treatment for human breast cancer. Recognition of the physiology of the pituitary led Luft and Ray to introduce hypophysectomy for breast cancer control. Such radical surgical procedures did not begin to end until the 1950s when synthetic hormones were developed.

German, William J., and Stevenson Flanigan. "Pituitary Adenomas: A Follow-Up Study of the Cushing Series." *Clinical Neurosurgery*, 10 (1964), 72-81.

(See Chapter 10: German and Flanigan).

Gilbertsen, V. A. "Beatson's Contribution to Cancer Research." *Surgo*, 32 (1964), 17-19.

(See Chapter 11: Goldenberg).

Goldenberg, Ira S. "Hormones and Breast Cancer: Historical Perspectives." *Surgery*, 53 (February 1963), 285-88.

In 1889 A. Schinzinger of Germany first noted that the prognosis was poor in young breast cancer patients and a little better in post-menopausal women. He advocated removal of the ovaries to "bring about breast atrophy," which he felt would also shrink tumors. At the same time Scottish surgeon George Beatson came to the same conclusion. Soon castration was widely used for women with inoperable lesions. In 1905 Foveau de Courmelles of France began radiation castration. After World War II Charles Huggins of Chicago used adrenalectomy and hypophysectomy for advanced breast cancer. About 20 to 30 percent of women with breast cancer will improve with such treatment.

Jensen, Elwood V. "Hormone Dependency of Human Breast Cancers." *Cancer*, 46 (December 15, 1980), 2759-61.

(See Chapter 11: Jensen).

Lips, C. J. M., et al. "Central Registration of Multiple Endocrine Neoplasia Type 2 Families in The Netherlands." *Henry Ford Hospital Medical Journal*, 32 (1984), 236-37.

(See Chapter 21: Lips).

MacMahon, Charles E., and John L. Cahill. "The Evolution of the Concept of the Use of Surgical Castration in the Palliation of Breast Cancer in Pre-Menopausal Females." *Annals of Surgery*, 184 (December 1976), 713-16.

Astley Cooper in 1836 described the metastatic lesions of breast cancer and their likelihood of spreading to the lung, vertebra, and ovary, along with "an increase in size of the primary lesion premenstrually with some diminution in the size after cessation of the menses." A. Schinzinger of Friedborg, Germany, noted in 1889 that the survival rates for breast carcinoma were worse among younger victims and speculated that castration might prematurely age the patient and cause a shrinkage of all breast tissue, malignant as well as normal. The birth of hormonal therapy for breast cancer, however, began with the work of George Thomas Beatson of Glasgow, Scotland. Early in his career Beatson learned that lactating cattle, if their ovaries were removed, would continue giving milk all of their lives. He also noted histologic changes in the lactating breast after pregnancy, especially the proliferation of epithelial cells, and he thought they resembled carcinoma cells. In 1895 he performed a bilateral oophorectomy on a young woman with advanced, inoperable, ulcerating breast carcinoma. She initially underwent a complete regression of the tumor, although it recurred nearly four years later and killed her. Oophorectomy became very common between 1900 and 1910, declining then when ovarian radiation became more popular. Not until 1953, when Charles Huggins explained the benefits of oophorectomy and adrenalectomy, did surgical castration become common again for treatment of advanced, pre-menopausal breast carcinoma.

Simmer, H. H. "Kastration Beim Mammakarzinom: Eine Retrospektive." *Muenchener Medizinische Wochenschrift*, 120 (24 November 1978), 1555.

(See Chapter 11: Simmer).

Simmer, H. H. "Oophorectomy for Breast Cancer Patients: Its Proposal, First Performance, and First Explanation as an Endocrine Ablation." *Clio Médica*, 4 (1969), 227-47.

George Thomas Beatson, a Scottish physician, had noticed behavioral and tissue changes in farm animals undergoing castration, and he had read the work of English physician E. Nunn that breast tumors sometimes regressed temporarily in women undergoing a rapid menopause. In 1896 Beatson performed a bilateral oophorectomy on a pre-menopausal woman with an inoperable breast carcinoma. Her tumor went into a rapid, but temporary, remission. By the early 1900s the bilateral oophorectomy was a common procedure for inoperable breast cancers in pre-menopausal women.

Sipple, John H. "Multiple Endocrine Neoplasia Type 2 Syndromes: Historical Perspectives." *Henry Ford Hospital Medical Journal*, 32 (1984), 219-22.

(See Chapter 21: Sipple).

"Some Aspects of Hormonal Therapy." *Cancer Bulletin*, 18 (July-August 1966), 70-72, 79.

The existence of a functional relationship between the prostate and the testes was first recorded in 1837 by the French surgeons D'Etoilles and Civiale. They unintentionally performed a bilateral orchiectomy during an operation for hernia and observed the shrinking of the prostate. The use of castration for malignant disease of the prostate began in 1941 when Charles Huggins developed the concept of androgen deprivation therapy. Approximately 65 percent of patients will benefit from the procedure. Huggins then learned that for some patients the elimination of the adrenal sex steroids through bilateral adrenalectomy is helpful in reducing prostatic tumors.

The relationship between the ovaries and breast cancer was first observed in 1882 by the English physician R. Nunn when he noted a patient's breast tumor shrank considerably after the sudden onset of menopause. In 1889 Schinzinger, a German surgeon, postulated a relationship between breast cancer and hormonal activity. In 1896 George Beatson reported the success of castration on some women suffering from breast carcinoma. By the 1940s oophorectomy was considered an important treatment for pre-menopausal women suffering from breast cancer.

Recently some interest has been shown in the control of advanced endometrial cancer by the use of progestins. Younger women are more likely to respond to the therapy.

van Heerden, Jonathan A. "First Encounters with Pheochromocytoma." *American Journal of Surgery*, 144 (August 1982), 277-79.

(See Chapter 10: van Heerden).

27 Immunotherapy

Bartlett, Gerald L. "Milestones in Tumor Immunology." *Seminars in Oncology*, 6 (December 1979), 515-25.

In the twentieth century there have been several major milestones in the evolution of immunology and neoplastic disease. They are as follows:

1. The concept that tumors possessed antigens not found in normal cells.

2. Immunodeficient or immunosuppressed patients had a greater risk of developing malignancies than immunocompetent patients.

3. The concept of tumor antigens was most clearly established by the ability to induce tumors in syngeneic animals. New techniques of *in vitro* analysis of immunity to histocompatibility antigens allowed for greater efficiency, sensitivity, replication, and quantitative abilities as well as to clinical applications.

4. A variety of new extraction methods have allowed for the isolation of various tumor specific transplantation antigens.

5. The diversity of antigens on chemically or physically induced tumors, and the absence of effective tumor specific transplantation antigens on naturally occurring tumors, are obstacles to practical immunoprophylaxis of non-viral cancer. The prospects for immunologic prevention of viral tumors is more optimistic because of the virus-related specificity of tumor transplantation antigens.

6. Another level at which tumor immunology can fight malignant disease is in the early diagnosis of cancer, either by detecting antigenic tumor products, using standardized antisera as the diagnostic reagents, or by detecting evidence of host immunity (antibodies or sensitized cells) to tumor antigens, using standardized antigens as the diagnostic probes.

Currie, G. A. *Cancer and the Immune Response.* 1974.

(See Chapter 27: Currie).

Currie, G. A. "Eighty Years of Immunotherapy." *The British Journal of Cancer,*
26 (June 1972), 141-53.

Evidence for the existence of tumor-associated antigens in animal systems and
of host reactions to them is now vast and convincing. In the last two decades of
the nineteenth century the recognition of immunity to bacterial infections led to
the postulate that tumors possessed distinct antigens capable of eliciting host
reactions. All animal experiments performed at this time involved the use of
transplantable tumors in randomly-bred or recently captured wild animals. The
absence of inbred strains of experimental animals invalidated all these experiments
as the resistance of an animal to a transplantable tumor contained an element of
allograft rejection. This problem was not recognized at the time, so beginning
in 1880 a series of cancer treatments with vaccines spread throughout Europe,
beginning in Germany. Most of the treatments involved injecting tumor cells or
tumor cell extracts into patients with metastatic disease. Although temporary
remissions were sometimes described, the treatments were generally abandoned
as ineffective.

Specific passive immunotherapy treatments also began in the late nineteenth
century. In these trials experimental animals such as sheep, horses, goats, and
rabbits were immunized with fragments of the patient's tumor and the resulting
antiserum was either fractionated and then used or administered as a whole serum.
The first documented form of this therapy came in France in 1895 with the work
of Hericourt and Richet. They employed antiserum raised in dogs and monkeys.
Since then there have been a variety of similar experimental treatments.

There have also been attempts to increase immunological reactivity in a non-
specific manner. In 1938 the Soviet researcher Fedyushin suggested developing
antisera from the human reticuloendothelial system and injecting it in low doses to
tumor patients. Mathe in 1969 began treating acute lymphoblastic leukemia with
BCG applied to large skin abrasions. Another bacteria, Corynebacterium, was
used by Halpern in 1972 in patients receiving combined cytotoxic chemotherapy.

Specific adoptive immunotherapy is a relatively recent phenomenon. Nadler
and Moore in 1969 cross-immunized patients with the same type of tumor and
then exchanged their blood supplies. Other researchers administered thoracic
duct lymphocytes from patients immunized with tumor. The administration of
large numbers of non-sensitized lymphoid cells as a form of therapy began in the
1960s, and the most important of these was the treatment of leukemia by total
ablation of the bone marrow and reconstitution with allogenic marrow.

In and of themselves, immunotherapeutic approaches to cancer have achieved
only temporary regressions, but combined with surgery, radiotherapy, and chemotherapy, immunotherapy will certainly play an important role in cancer treatment
in the future.

Klein, Eva. "Tumor Antigens: Clinical and Experimental." *Oncology: Proceedings of the Tenth International Cancer Congress*, I (1970), 226-35.

The development of tumor immunology has proceeded in three phases. During the first phase of the late nineteenth and early twentieth centuries, the so-called transplantable tumors were used which grew also in allogenic recipients. Their progressive growth was frequently taken as proof for host-tumor compatibility, and the high levels of resistance that could be attained by various forms of immunization generated the belief that tumor cells carry specific and strong antigens and that an immunologic solution to cancer was near. That conviction was destroyed in the 1930s and 1940s when experiments with inbred mouse strains demonstrated that tumor antigenicity could not be demonstrated. The Mendelian segregation of histocompatibility genes governed the transplantability of neoplastic as well as of normal tissues. The transplantable tumors grew across genetic barriers not because they lacked the relevant histocompatibility antigens, but because they avoided the host response, and preimmunization against the relevant histocompatibilty antigens caused their rejection. This finding led to the opinion that all tumor rejection responses were probably transplantation artifacts and to gloomy conclusions about the role of immunology in cancer research and therapy. A new era started in the 1950s after the experiments of Gross and Foley. They ligated isografted, methylcholanthrene-induced sarcomas in C3H mice, inducing tumor necrosis.

Panem, Sandra. *The Interferon Crusade*. Washington, D.C.: 1984.

During the 1960s and 1970s most of the genetic research on cloning was carried out by a small group of genetic academicians; interferon research was financed largely by grants from the National Institutes of Health. In 1975 Dr. Mathilde Krim of the Memorial Sloan-Kettering Institute organized a professional meeting to discuss promising Swedish research on the effectivness of human interferon against osteogenic sarcomas. The meeting triggered great public interest in interferon, expansion of NIH funding for interferon research, and dramatic increases in industrial research aimed at artificially producing interferon, since extracting it from human blood supplies was prohibitively expensive. In 1979 several groups announced the successful production of human interferon through recombinant DNA research. The increased supplies of the drug allowed for much more research. Subsequent clinical research, however, has eliminated the drug as a cancer panacea, although its usefulness when combined with more standard surgical, radiotherapeutic, and chemotherapeutic modalities is important.

Prehn, Richmond T. "Tumor-Specific Antigens. Historical Review and Perspective." *Oncology: Proceedings of the Tenth International Cancer Congress*, I (1970), 188-91.

In 1900 expectations about the prospects for tumor immunology were very high following the tremendous success of vaccination against some infectious diseases. It was clear that immunization could prevent the growth of transplantable animal tumors and, consequently, the immunologic prevention of cancer seemed imminent. By the 1920s, however, doubts appeared when it was demonstrated that immunization with embryonic or even normal adult tissues could inhibit cancer growth. Confidence in immunology began to decline, especially when researchers realized, with the development of inbred animal strains, that they had been confusing immunologic reactions with homograft rejection.

In 1957, however, faith in immunology began to increase again with the demonstration of true tumor-specific antigenicity in 3-methylcholanthrene induced mouse sarcomas. Today it is seriously suggested by many immunologists that cellular immunity has as its *raison d'être* the suppression of neoplasia. Cancer may be largely a vertebrate diseas_h this prob

lem. Neoplasia probably occurs frequently in all vertebrates, but it is usually promptly suppressed by an immunologic surveillance mechanism. When that mechanism fails, clinically manifest tumors appear.

Southam, Chester M. "History and Prospects of Immunotherapy of Cancer: An Introduction." *Annals of the New York Academy of Science*, 277 (1976), 1-6.

Although reports on immunotherapy and cancer appear in the literature sporadically beginning in 1910, the real birth of the field does not occur until the 1970s. Most researchers assumed that immune reactions were excited by and directed against foreign materials, not against one's own body cells. Since cancer was a derangement of the patient's own cells, it seemed for years that immunotherapy was not going to be a fruitful endeavor. The great barrier to the concept of tumor immunology in the first half of the twentieth century was the tacit assumption that a cell could not carry an antigen which differed from the normal cells of the body in such a way that it would be recognized as foreign and excite an immune response from the body. But transplantation studies in the 1970s by Gross, Foley, Prehn, Main, and Klein proved conclusively that tumors growing in the original host, or in hosts that were genetically identical to the original host, excited immune responses that would prevent the growth of tumor cells and exert no effect on normal tissues. These syngenetic tumor transplantation studies thus demonstrated simultaneously the existence of tumor-specific antigens and specific antitumor immunity.

Southam, Chester M. "Relationships of Immunology to Cancer: A Review." *Cancer Research*, 20 (1960), 271-91.

(See Chapter 27: Southam).

Thomas, Lewis. "Immunology." In John Z. Bowers and Elizabeth F. Purcell, *Advances in American Medicine: Essays at the Bicentennial.* New York: 1976. Volume 2. Pp. 459-83.

Paul Ehrlich was the first to describe a chemical basis for the selective, specific binding of antigens and antibodies through what he called the side-chain theory of a molecular fit between the two. The experimental research on tumor transplantability of M. A. Novinsky inspired hopes for specific mechanisms of tumor immunology and immunotherapy. Ehrlich speculated that specific antibodies should protect against cancer. Research has shown that there are high rates of cancer in children with immunodeficiency syndromes; that patients carrying kidney homografts from donors with cancer of other organs often develop cancer at the graft site during immunosuppressive treatment, and those tumors disappear when immunosuppressant drug therapy stops; that some cancer patients show immunological impairment by slow reactions in skin tests; and that some tumors spontaneously regress and disappear. Future research will try to find ways of helping the patient's own immunological system recognize tumor cells as foreign.

Trentin, John J. "Approaches to Immunotherapy: Clinical and Experimental. Historical Perspectives." *Oncology: Proceedings of the Tenth International Cancer Congress*, II (1970), 295-302.

Late in the nineteenth century and early in the twentieth century hopes for immunotherapy got off to a false start when immunity was demonstrated in transplantable tumors in non-inbred (non-histoisogenic) animals. Actually, the immunity appeared because of the genetic and normal tissue disparity between the transplanted tumor and the recipient. To clearly prove cancer-specific antigenecity, it is necessary to work within a histoisogenic tumor transplant donor-recipient system or to demonstrate immunity of an individual animal or patient against its own tumor in the absence of immunity against its normal tissues. Such conclusive evidence did not begin to accumulate until recent years. In 1953 E. J. Foley showed immunizaton against early transplant generations of a methylcholanthrene-induced tumor. R. T. Prehn's and J. M. Main's experiments in 1957 ruled out residual heterozygosis by skin transplantability. C. J. Klein showed in 1960 the specific nature of the antigenecity of methyl-cholanthrene-induced tumors with *in vitro* neutralization of sarcoma cells by lymph node cells of immune, but not of non-immune isologous mice. In the 1960s researchers learned that the following human tumors generated tumor specific antigens: Burkitt's lymphoma, nasopharyngeal carcinoma, melanoma, neuroblastoma, lung adenocarcinoma, colon adenocarcinoma, Wilms' tumor, osteosarcoma, and several soft-tissue sarcomas.

28 Unorthodox Treatments

Baylen, Joseph O. "The Mattei Cancer Cure: A Victorian Nostrum." *Proceedings of the American Philosophical Society*, 113 (April 1969), 149-76.

Casare Mattei was born on January 11, 1809, in Bologna, Italy, to a wealthy, landed family. In the 1850s he became a follower of Samuel Hahnemann, founder of the nineteenth century homeopathic medicine movement. He developed a series of herbal remedies—what he called "Electro-Homeopathic" medicines. Lady Walburga Paget, wife of Sir August Paget, the British ambassador to Vienna, believed that her husband had been cured of cancer by Mattei ointments. She popularized the Mattei claims throughout Great Britain in the 1890s, forcing skeptical British physicians to arrange clinical trials of the treatment. All patients with genuine malignant lesions died of metastatic disease. Mattei died in 1896 and the treatment disappeared early in the 1900s.

Cole, David. "Doctrinal Deviance in New Zealand Medical Practice: Some Historical Comments." *New Zealand Medical Journal*, 98 (1985), 541-45.

In 1867 New Zealand required registration of all orthodox medical practitioners to provide quality assurance to the consuming public. In recent years there have been three unorthodox medical practitioners which have been investigated and restricted by public health officials. In the 1970s the Medical Council of New Zealand moved against Vlastimil Byrch, who had invented medical credentials, including his medical degree. Back in the 1920s Dr. Dundas Mackenzie lost his license to practice medicine for using he so-called "Abrams Box," an "electronic dynamizer," to cure cancer. Finally, Dr. Eva Hill brought the "cancer cure" of Harry M. Hoxey of the United States to New Zealand in the 1950s.

Darby, W. J. "Etiology of Nutritional Fads." *Cancer*, 43 (May 1979), 2121-24.

(See Chapter 28: Kardinal and Chapter 28: Fishbein).

Farrow, Ruth T. "Odyssey of an American Cancer Specialist of a Hundred Years Ago." *Bulletin of the History of Medicine*, 23 (1949), 236-52.

(See Chapter 2: FELL, JESSE WELDON: Farrow).

Fishbein, Morris. "History of Cancer Quackery." *Perspectives in Biology and Medicine*, 8 (1965), 139-66.

In the United States during the twentieth century there have been a number of people offering false cures for cancer. The most influential of them have been:

1. L. D. Rogers founded the National Medical University of Chicago as well as the American Cancer Research Society at the turn of the century. Rogers treated patients with injections of their own blood after he had "incubated and energized" it. He then claimed that the injected blood had special immunological properties capable of attacking tumor tissue.

2. Arthur d'Collard of Richmond, Virginia, practiced what he called "poropathy," something similar to chiropractic medicine in which internal tumors were "cured" through spinal manipulations.

3. Albert Abrams of San Francisco was at one time a respected physician and pathologist. But in 1910 he developed what he called "spondylotherapy" for cancer. It resembled a chiropractic treatment. Later he developed his electronic "dynamizer" to help physicians diagnose and cure cancer. It had absolutely no therapeutic value, but Abrams managed to sell the devices to unorthodox medical practitioners throughout the English-speaking world.

4. In the 1920s Lester Tilton of Chicago introduced his "Blood Poison Treatment" for cancer, an escharotic containing zinc. Tilton was convicted of violating the Medical Practice Act of Illinois and imprisoned.

5. William Koch, a graduate of the University of Michigan, announced in 1919 that he had discovered a cure for cancer through "recrystallized synthetic antitoxin." Throughout the 1920s and 1930s the Koch treatment was extremely popular among cancer patients and their families, even though it had no therapeutic value. Eventually Koch left his business in Detroit and set up practice in Sao Paulo, Brazil.

6. In the 1930s Norman Baker, a radio broadcaster from Muscatane, Iowa, set up the Baker Hospital to treat cancer patients with two drugs: an arsenic powder and a concoction of various herbs and grasses. Baker eventually set up treatment centers in a variety of places, including Mexico, before being arrested and convicted of fraud in Arkansas.

7. Thomas Glover, a physician in Toronto, Canada, announced a new treatment for cancer in 1920. The Glover serum was created by taking blood and tumor tissue from cancer victims, injecting them into a horse, waiting a week, taking blood specimens from the horse, and then injecting this "antiserum" into the same cancer patients. Glover later worked for the Hygienic Laboratory, which eventually became the National Institutes of Health, testing his serum, but co-workers could never substantiate his claims.

8. Max Gerson, a physician who died in 1959, established a sanitarium in New York City which claimed to cure cancer through nutritional therapy— a diet consisting of liver, vitamins, fresh vegetables, fruit juices, and periodic enemas.

For the other examples of cancer quackery Fishbein discusses, see Chapter 28: Kardinal.

Haneveld, G. T. "Compression as a Treatment of Cancer: A Historical Survey." *Archivum Chirurgicum Neerlandicum*, 3 (1979), 1-8.

For a time in the seventeenth and eighteenth centuries some reputable physicians advocated compression as a treatment for cancer, especially for cancer of the breast. Some of them viewed the tumor as a single pathological entity which could be damaged and then "die" from a vigorous, manual compression regimen; others believed such a treatment could press poisonous fluids from the tumor, bringing upon its death. The idea of compression as a treatment died out in the nineteenth century when cellular pathology advanced tumor biology and when the concept of metastasis emerged. Compression was then seen as a treatment more likely to accelerate metastasis than retard tumor growth.

Issels, Thomas G. *The Biography of a Doctor*. London: 1975.

(See Chapter 28: Thomas).

Janssen, W. F. "Cancer Quackery. Past and Present." *FDA Consumer*, 11 (July-August 1977), 27-32.

(See Chapter 28: Kardinal).

Janssen, W. F. "Cancer Quackery—The Past in the Present." *Seminars in Oncology*, 6 (1979), 526-36.

Over the years, although the promoted cancer cures have changed, the pattern remains the same. Promoters used testimonials rather than clinical trials to prove the efficacy of the cure; they claim government persecution of them and conspiratorial "cover-ups" of the benefits of the treatment; and they prey on patients for whom conventional medicine offers little hope. They also tend to use the most enflamed metaphors in their descriptions of orthodox cancer treatment. Most of the time their advertisements used "mutilation" as a synonym for surgery, "burning" for radiotherapy, and "poison" for chemotherapy.

Janssen, W. F. "The Cancer 'Cures': A Challenge to Rational Therapeutics." *Annals of Chemistry*, 50 (February 1978), 197A-202A.

(See Chapter 28: Kardinal).

Kardinal, Carl G. "Laetrile in Historical Perspective." *Missouri Medicine*, 77 (September 1980), 564-69.

Cancer patients are vulnerable to charlatans because only 40 percent of them are cured by standard therapy, and that therapy is often painful and disfiguring. In the last forty years unproven cancer treatments have assumed pseudoscientific dimensions, complete with their own jargon and testimonials. The major quack regimens in recent years have been:

1. The Koch Antitoxins. In the late 1930s and early 1940s William Koch, a Detroit physician, postulated that cancer came from the body's reaction to its own toxins. He began prescribing "glyoxide" (very pure, distilled water) to patients. Koch moved to Brazil in 1948.

2. Harry Hoxey's Herbal Tonic. In the 1950s Harry Hoxey argued that cancer developed because the body's fluids were chemically imbalanced. He prescribed "pink medicine" (pepsin and potassium iodide) and "black medicine" (a mixture of various flowers and tree barks) to more than 10,000 patients. Hoxey advertised widely over the radio until the FDA forced him to relocate to Tijuana, Mexico.

3. Krebiozen. In the 1960s Arthur C. Ivey of the University of Illinois began promoting Krebiozen as a cancer cure. The drug was supposedly an extract from the blood of a breed of Argentinian horses. The FDA banned the drug in 1969.

4. Laetrile. In the 1970s the most prominent of the unproven cancer therapies was laetrile, an extract from apricot pits. In 1980 the FDA began a study of the effectiveness of laetrile therapy on terminally ill cancer patients, but in 1984 the trials showed that laetrile had no therapeutic effects. Their results were confirmed in similar studies conducted by the National Cancer Institute.

Lerner, Irving J. "The Whys of Cancer Quackery." *Cancer*, 53 (February 1, 1984), 815-19.

Cancer quackery, especially the laetrile controversy of the 1960s and 1970s, depends on three factors. First, medical failure contributes to quack therapies. As late as 1983 most patients died of cancer, and until the rise of oncology as a discipline, physicians usually tried to dismiss their cancer patients because they could do so little for them. Rejected patients sought other healers. Even oncology

contributed because of the severity of many surgical, chemotherapy, and radiotherapy procedures. Second, there has been a public failure, a fear of cancer out
of proportion to its incidence. Public skepticism was also fueled by the antiestab-
lishment attitudes of the 1960s and 1970s because of Watergate and Vietnam.
The medical establishment came under some suspicion, especially compared to
the 1950s when people had faith in institutions. The third factor was the success
of the promoters of cancer cures. The John Birch Society helped make laetrile a
national issue when the FDA outlawed it, and laetrile advocates claimed cancer
was a vitamin deficiency which laetrile replaced.

Miller, Nancy J. and Josie Howard-Ruben. "Unproven Methods of Cancer Man-
     agement. Part I. Background and Historical Perspectives." *Oncology Nurs-
     ing Forum*, 10 (Fall 1983), 46-52.

Historically the tell-tale signs of cancer quackery are: 1) peculiar credentials
for a practitioner; 2) frequent use of conspiracy theories; 3) isolation from the
medical community; 4) constant use of testimonials rather than the results of scientific, clinical trials; 5) claims that the composition of the therapies is classified;
and 6) use of mechanical devices to effect a cure. In the last century the major
"quack cures" for cancer have been the Koch treatment, the Hoxey treatment,
and Krebiozen. Bizarre metaphysical and spiritual treatments have also appeared
recently.

Morris, Nathan. *The Cancer Blackout: Exposing the Official Blacklisting of
     Beneficial Cancer Research, Treatment, and Prevention.* New York: 1977.

The author argues that a conspiracy within the powerful medical establishment in the United States prevents "natural" and "non-invasive" cancer treatments from ever gaining acceptance. The American Medical Association, the
Food and Drug Administration, the National Cancer Institute, the research foundations, universities, pharmaceutical companies, Congress, and the press all con-
spire together to outlaw homeopathic remedies so they can establish a profitable
monopoly over the business of cancer in the United States, preventing the development of new, natural therapies which will reduce their profit levels.

Peterson, J. C., and G. E. Markle. "Politics and Science in the Laetrile Contro-
     versy." *The Social Study of Science*, 9 (1979), 139-66.

(See Chapter 28: Young).

Stoddard, George D. *Krebiozen, The Great Cancer Mystery.* Boston: 1955.

Early in the 1950s Professor Arthur C. Ivey, a noted biochemist at the University of Illinois, began promoting the drug "Krebiozen" as a cancer cure. Because
of his scientific credentials, Ivey's claims gained credence in the late 1950s and

1960s. The drug was an extract from the blood of Argentinian horses. The FDA did clinical trials on the drug in the 1960s, found it to be ineffective, and outlawed it in 1969.

Stokes, S. H. "Cancer Quackery: A Continuing Problem." *Journal of the Tennessee Medical Association*, 79 (July 1986), 415-21.

(See Chapter 28: Janssen and Chapter 28: Kardinal).

Thomas, Gordon. *Dr. Issels and his Revolutionary Cancer Treatment.* New York: 1973.

Thomas G. Issels was born in Monchen-Gladbach, Germany, on November 21, 1907. He attended six German medical schools before earning a degree from the Julio-Maximilian University at Wurzburg. Issels became preoccupied with cancer and frustrated at how little medicine could do for most patients. Eventually he began to practice unorthodox medicine, insisting on tonsillectomies and teeth extractions for cancer patients, hoping to remove sources of infection from the body system and give a boost to the immunological system. Issels began treating terminal cancer patients and his fame spread throughout Europe. Oncologists were extremely skeptical of his claims, and in 1970 the American Cancer Society added Issels to their list of unproven cancer claims.

Young, James Harvey. "Laetrile in Historical Perspective." In Gerald E. Markle and James C. Petersen. *Politics, Science, and Cancer: The Laetrile Phenomenon.* New York: 1980. Pp. 11-60.

Laetrile's history in the United States as a cancer treatment can be divided into three fundamental periods. During the first period in the 1950s laetrile was created by Ernest Krebs, Sr., a California pharmacist and physician with a history of unorthodox medical treatments. In 1951 Krebs announced that he had isolated a marvelous drug, which his son dubbed "laetrile," from the kernels of shelled apricot seeds. Krebs claimed that when the laetrile reached the site of a tumor, it was hydrolized by an enzyme, beta-glucosidase, releasing cancer-killing hydrogen cyanide. The enzyme accumulated in cancer cells more readily than in normal cells. Also, normal cells were protected by another enzyme, rhodanese, which detoxified any cyanide that might have reached them. So early in the 1950s Krebs was claiming to have discovered a new drug which targeted malignant cells while bypassing healthy tissue.

By the early 1960s the Food and Drug Administration as well as various state health agencies were attacking laetrile, claiming that clinical trials had failed to prove its effectiveness. At that point Andrew Robert McNaughton, a Canadian entrepreneur, took over the laetrile movement by establishing treatment centers in Canada and campaigning widely in the United States on behalf of the treatment. Articles in the Hearst newspapers, lobby groups like the International Association of Cancer Victims and Friends, and a variety of books appeared touting laetrile's effectiveness.

By the early 1970s the John Birch Society, an ultra-conservative, anti-Communist group, took up the laetrile battle, arguing that the Food and Drug Administration's campaign against the drug was a perfect example of bureaucratic tyranny, and that there should be complete freedom of choice in treatment selection by cancer patients. By that time laetrile had taken refuge in Mexico, where clinics appeared all along the borders of Texas, New Mexico, Arizona, and California. A new Committee for Freedom of Choice in Cancer Therapy claimed that "orthodox physicians were futilely cutting, burning, and poisoning their victims, and rejecting hopeful treatments like Laetrile for fear of doing themselves out of their jobs." The pro-laetrile movement had acquired considerable political power, despite the lack of clinical data to prove the claims of its advocates.

Young, James Harvey. *The Medical Messiahs. A Social History of Health Quackery in Twentieth Century America.* Princeton: 1977.

(See Chapter 28: Fishbein and Chapter 28: Kardinal).

V CLINICAL TREATMENT

29 Clinical Services

Abdurasulov, D. M. "Razvitie onkologicheskoi sluzbhy v Uzbekskoi SSR." *Voprosy Onkologii*, 15 (1969), 3-9.

The article provides a brief survey of the development of clinical oncology in the Uzbekistan Soviet Socialist Republic, with the focus on the events occurring in the years since the Bolshevik Revolution, especially the expansion of clinical services to larger numbers of people.

Bramberga, V. M. "Razvitie onkologii v Latviiskoi SSR." *Voprosy Onkologii*, 14 (1968), 6-13.

(See Chapter 29: Bramberga).

Bramberga, V. M. "Stanovlenie, sovremennoe sostoianie i perspektivy razvitiia onkologii v Latviiskoi SSR." *Voprosy Onkologii*, 28 (1982), 8-13.

The article provides a survey history of the development of clinical oncology in the Latvian Soviet Socialist Republic, particularly in the years since the Bolshevik Revolution.

Bratus, V. D., and I. T. Shevchenko. "Onkologicheskaia sluzhba v Ukrainskoi SSR za gody sovetskoi vlasti." *Voprosy Onkologii*, 16 (April 1970), 37-42.

The article surveys the development of clinical oncology in the Ukrainian Soviet Socialist Republic in the years since the Bolshevik Revolution and argues that medical services to the masses are infinitely superior than they were when the czars ruled Russia.

"Le cancer dans le monde. Quelques donees sur l'histoire du cancer dans l'état
du Texas." *Lutte cancer*, 42 (January-February 1965), 36-39.

The major development in the history of oncology in the state of Texas was
the founding of the M. D. Anderson Hospital and Tumor Institute in Houston and
its evolution into one of the premier cancer centers in the world, especially in its
commitment to radiotherapy.

Clarke, B. L. "Foundation of Cancer Treatment in Queensland." *Medical Journal
of Australia*, 2 (20 December 1969), 1271-74.

Ernest Sanford Jackson (1860-1938) was a physician trained at the University
of Melbourne. Concerned about the high incidence of skin cancers in Australia,
he organized a group of physicians and lay people into the Queensland Cancer
Trust in 1926. Their initial purpose was to raise money to purchase a radium
source to upgrade cancer treatment. Eventually the Queensland Cancer Trust
funded special clinical cancer services at most of the major hospitals in Queensland, Australia.

Colebach, John H. "Development of Pediatric Oncology in Australia." *The American Journal of Pediatric Hematology/Oncology*, 7 (Summer 1985), 175-81.

Until the 1930s pediatric oncology in Australia was the domain of pathologists,
led by Rupert A. Willis (1898-1980) at the University of Melbourne and Reginald
Webster (1889-1976) at the Royal Children's Hospital in Melbourne. Late in the
1930s radiotherapists began to have some success with low stage neuroblastomas,
gliomas, and Wilms' tumors. After World War II the work of the American physician Sidney Farber with the antifolic acids gave birth to modern chemotherapy
for acute lymphocytic leukemia in children. By the 1950s pediatric oncology had
emerged in Australia. In 1967 John Colebach was appointed director of the Hematology Research Clinic at the Royal Children's Hospital.

Costachel, O. "Cancer Treatment Facilities in Romania." *Oncology: Proceedings
of the Tenth International Cancer Congress*, III (1970), 427-33.

Surgical treatment was all that was available in Romania until 1912 when the
first radiotherapy equipment was set up in Bucharest. In the 1920s Aurel Babes
led the way in the development of cytological diagnosis of vaginal smears for cervical cancer, and in 1927 the Institute for the Study and Prophylaxis of Cancer
was established in Cluj under the direction of I. Moldovan. Since then the Institute at Cluj has evolved into a major cancer center. The Oncological Institute at
Bucharest, which has become the premier cancer research and treatment facility
in the country, was founded by the Ministry of Health in 1949.

Dedkov, I. P. "Razvitiie onkologii v Ukrainskoi SSR." *Klinik Khirurgiia*, 5 (May 1978), 1-5.

(See Chapter 29: Shevchenko).

Dorzhgotov, B. K. "Razvitie onkologicheskoi sluzbhy v Mongol'skoi Narodnoi Respublike." *Voprosy Onkologii*, 23 (1977), 27-29.

The article provides a brief survey of the development of clinical oncology in the Mongolian Soviet Socialist Republic. Because of the remoteness of the territory significant gains in cancer treatment did not emerge there until the 1960s. By the end of the decade patients had access to major surgical facilities, megavoltage radiotherapy equipment, and a variety of chemotherapy protocols.

Fanardzhian, V. A., A. P. Shishkin, and K. L. Bazikian. "Onkologicheskaia sluzhba v Armianskof SSR i etapy e razvitiia." *Voprosy Onkologii*, 16 (April 1970), 46-49.

The article provides a brief survey of the history of clinical and research oncology in the Armenian Soviet Socialist Republic since the time of the Bolshevik Revolution.

Gomez, P., and A. Rosado. "Unidad de investigacion clinica, Hospital de Oncología, Central Mexico Nacional, IMSS." *Archivos de investigacion de médica*, 12 (1981), 361-75.

For more than 30 years one of the major clinical cancer facilities has been the Oncology Hospital in Mexico City. Its major research effort has involved clinical trials on patients being treated with surgery, radiotherapy, and chemotherapy.

Hammes, S. E. "An Historical Examination of Nursing in Cancer with Implications for Development of the Cancer Nurse Specialist." Ed.D. Dissertation. University of Kansas. 1982.

(See Chapter 29: Hilkemeyer).

Hilkemeyer, Renilda. "A Historical Perspective in Cancer Nursing." *Oncology Nursing Forum*, 9 (Spring 1982), 47-56.

In the last 35 years oncology nursing has emerged as a subdiscipline in nursing. The term "oncological nursing" was first used in 1950 by the Department of Nursing Education at New York University. The first academic course devoted exclusively to cancer nursing was at Columbia University in 1946. By 1982 there were 16 universities offering master's degrees in cancer nursing. The American Cancer Society held the first National Cancer Nursing Conference in 1973. The first International Conference on Cancer Nursing was held in London in 1981. The 1970s and 1980s also found nurses more actively engaged in clinical research programs.

Kairakbaev, M. K. "Etapy razvitiia i stanovlenia onkologicheskoi sluzbhy v Kazakhskoi SSR za gody sovetskoi vlasti." *Voprosy Onkologii*, 18 (1972), 19-23.

(See Chapter 29: Suleimenov).

Kavtaradze, L. S., and K. F. Vepkhvadze. "Razvitie onkologicheskof pomoshchi
nasleniiu Gruzinskof SSR za gody sovetskof vlasti." *Voprosy Onkologii*, 16
(April 1970), 3-8.

The article provides a brief of the history of clinical oncology and cancer prevention education in the Georgian Soviet Socialist Republic since the time of the
Bolshevik Revolution.

Kuiatkhanov, B. A. "O stanovlenii onkologicheskoi sluzhby v Turkmenskoi SSR."
Voprosy Onkologii, 28 (1982), 25-28.

The article briefly describes the development of clinical oncological services
in the Turkmenistan Soviet Socialist Republic during the last half-century, em-
phasizing the benefits which the working classes now enjoy compared to medical
services under the czar.

Nugmanov, S. N. "Razvitie onkologii v Kazakhskoi SSR." *Voprosy Onkologii*, 14
(1968), 3-14.

The article provides a brief survey of the development of clinical oncology in
the Kazakhstani Soviet Socialist Republic in the fifty years since the Bokshevik
Revolution.

Paymaster, J. C., and P. Gangadharan. "The Development of Cancer Treatment
Facilities in India." *Oncology: Proceedings of the Tenth International Cancer
Congress*, III (1970), 412-420.

Because the infectious diseases still account for the majority of deaths in India,
oncological services have not received priority as a public health matter. By 1970
there were only five special cancer institutes performing research and treatment
of cancer, along with six regional cancer centers to deal with patients. The major
facility in India is the Tata Memorial Centre in Bombay.

Rutkowski, J. "Dzieje walki z rakiem na terenie Lodzi." *Archiwum Historii Me-
dycyny*, 32 (1969), 465-67.

The article provides a brief history of the anti-cancer activities of the territory
of Lodzi, Poland, particularly the efforts to help people recognize the importance
of early diagnosis of the disease as well as the development of surgical and radio-
therapuetic services.

Savchenko, N. E., and B. D. Shitikov. "Ob uspekhakh i tendentsiiakh razvitiia onkologicheskoi sluzhby v Belorusskoi SSR." *Voprosy Onkologii,* 28 (1982), 13-20.

(See Chapter 29: Savchenko and Aleksandrov).

Savchenko, N. E., and N. N. Aleksandrov. "Onkologicheskaia pomoshch' v belorusii do i posle velikoi oktiabr'skoi sotsialisticheskoi revoliutsii." *Voprosy Onkologii,* 15 (1969), 3-7.

The article briefly surveys the history of clinical oncology in Byelorussia before and after the Bolshevik Revolution, arguing that since the overthrow of the czar, the masses have enjoyed far greater access to competent medical treatment for cancer.

Shevchenko, I. T. "K istorii protivorakovoi bor'by na Ukraine." *Klinik Khirurgiia,* 5 (May 1982), 67-70.

(See Chapter 29: Shevchenko).

Shevchenko, I. T. "Razvitie onkologii na Ukraine za gody sovetskoi vlasti." *Klinik Khirurgiia,* 11 (November 1967), 1-8.

The article briefly surveys the history of clinical oncology in the Ukraine, with the emphasis on the years since the Bolshevik Revolution.

Shevchenko, I. T. "Stanovlenie i razvitie onkologii v Ukrainskoi SSR." *Voprosy Onkologii,* 13 (1967), 3-11.

(See Chapter 29: Shevchenko).

Sorochin, I. D. "Razvitie onkologicheskof pomoshchi naseleniiu Moldavskof SSR za gody sovetskoi vlasti." *Voprosy Onkologii,* 18 (1972), 15-19.

The article outlines the development of clinical oncology in the Moldavian Soviet Socialist Republic in the previous half-century and how large numbers of patients were able to avail themselves of surgery, radiotherapy, and chemotherapy treatments.

Suleimenov, A. A., S. B. Balmukhanov, and B. E. Abdrakhimov. "Onkologicheskaia sluzbha Kazakhstana za 60 let SSSR." *Voprosy Onkologii,* 28 (1982), 3-7.

The article describes the development of clinical oncological services in the Kazakstan Soviet Socialist Republic since the 1920s.

Telichenas, A. I., L. A. Gritsiute, and R. I. Skarulis. "Istoriia razvitiia onkologicheskoi sluzbhy v Litovskoi SSR." *Voprosy Onkologii*, 28 (1982), 8-11.

The article describes the development of clinical oncology services in the Latvian Soviet Socialist Republic, with the emphasis on the years since the Bolshevik
Revolution.

Vekilov, F. M. "Razvitie onkologii za gody sovetskoi vlasti v Azerbaidzhanskoi
SSR." *Voprosy Onkologii*, 16 (1970), 3-8.

The article outlines the development of clinical oncology in the Azerbajani
Soviet Socialist Republic between 1930 and 1980, particularly the delivery of surgical and radiotherapy services to cancer patients.

30 Cancer Institutions

Agranat, V. Z., and V. V. Starinskii. "Radioizotopnaia diagnostika v Moskovskom nauchno-
issledovatel'skom Onkologicheskom Institute im. P. A. Gertsen (K 75-letiiu
instituta)." *Meditsinskaia Radiologiia*, 23 (October 1978), 81-82.

The article provides a brief, outline history of the research and clinical uses
of nuclear medicine, particularly diagnostic radioisotopes, at the P. A. Gertsen
Oncological Research Institute in Moscow during the last 75 years.

Austoker, J. "The Politics of Cancer Research: Walter Morley Fletcher and the
Origins of the British Empire Cancer Campaign." *Society for the Social
History of Medicine Bulletin*, 37 (December 1985), 63-67.

(See Chapter 30: Duke).

Avdeev, G. A., V. Z. Agranat, and M. A. Volkova. "Die Entwicklung der
Strahlenbehandlung von Geschwülsten und der Nuklearmedizin im Moskauer
Wissenschftlichen Forschungsinstitut für Onkologie P. A. Herzen. Zum 75
Jahrestag des Instituts." *Radiobiologia, Radiotherapia*, 19 (October 1978),
535-39.

(See Chapter 30: Kapatsinskii).

Avdeev, G. I., A. I. Volegov, and G. I. Rozenbaum. "K istorii osnovaniia
Moskovskogo Nauchno-Issledovatel'skogo Onkologicheskogo Institute im. P.
A. Gertsen." *Voprosy Onkologii*, 24 (1978), 5-9.

(See Chapter 30: Kapatsinskii).

Baker, Carol B. "Cancer Research Program Strategy and Planning—The Use of Contracts for Program Implementation." *Journal of the National Cancer Institute*, 59 (August 1977), 651-59.

The article describes the process by which the National Cancer Institute made the transition from simply a cancer research facility itself to that of a cancer research center and the largest dispenser of research funds for cancer studies in the world.

Baud, Jean. "Historique de la ligue." *Lutte cancer*, 45 (1968), Suppl.: 15-19.

(See Chapter 30: *Ligue francais contra le cancer*).

Bernoulli, R. "Un Gran méconnu: Gustave Roussy." *Gesnerus*, 37 (1980), 34-46.

The Institut Gustave-Roussy is the major cancer center, for research as well as clinical treatment in France. It was founded in 1921 by Gustave Roussy (1874-1948), a professor of pathology and anatomy in the medical school at the University of Paris. Roussy first called it Le Fondation de l'Institut de Cancer. Early in the 1930s the Institut received its clinical and laboratory sections. It became known as the Institut Gustave Roussy in 1950. By that time it had been incorporated into the series of French cancer centers offering treatment facilities throughout the country.

Beumer, J. "Jules Bordet, 1870-1961." *Journal of General Microbiology*, 29 (1962), 1-13.

The Institut Jules Bordet is the premier cancer in Belgium. It was founded in 1925 by Jules Bordet, the renowned Belgian bacteriologist, and he directed the Institut until 1940. It has evolved into a major clinical and research facility.

Blokhin, N. N., N. N. Trapeznikov, and A. V. Chaklin. "Vsesoiuznomu onkologicheskomu naushnomu tsentru AMN SSSR 30 let." *Voprosy Onkologii*, 27 (1981), 81-87.

In 1951 the All-Union Oncological Scientific Center was established to serve the needs of cancer patients and their families in the Armenian Soviet Socialist Republic. It provides basic research, clinical research, and treatment to Soviet citizens there and has evolved into a comprehensive facility.

Brehant, Jean. "Les debuts de la lutte contre le cancer en France (1895-1930)." *Lutte cancer*, 45 (1968), Suppl., 11-14.

(See Chapter 30: *Ligue francais contre le cancer*).

Bricker, Eugene M. "Turmoibus Praeter Naturam." *Annals of Surgery,* 202 (September 1985), 265-77.

(See Chapter 30: Rusch).

Brunning, D. A. and C. E. Dukes. "The Origin and Early History of the Institute of Cancer Research of the Royal Cancer Hospital." *Proceedings of the Royal Society of Medicine,* 58 (1965), 33-36.

In 1851 William Marsden founded the Free Cancer Hospital, which evolved into the Royal Marsden Hospital. Cancer research began there in 1856. Its Cancer Hospital Research Institute was founded in 1909 and enlarged to become the Chester Beatty Research Institute in 1939. Alexander Haddow was appointed director of the Chester Beatty Institute in 1946, where he focused research in the areas of carcinogenesis and chemotherapy. Under Haddow's direction the Chester Beatty Institute became one of the most influential research oncology centers in the world.

"The Christie Hospital and Holt Radium Institute, Manchester." *Cancer Bulletin,* 13 (January-February 1961), 11.

The Christie Hospital and Holt Radium Institute serves the treatment needs of four million people in Wales and Western England. They concentrate primarily on radiotherapy. The Christie Hospital opened in 1892 to care for cancer patients, and radium treatments began in 1903. In 1921 Sir Edward and Lady Elizabeth Holt contributed a building for the Manchester District Radium Institute, the first real radiotherapy center in England. It was primarily a teaching institution.

Chrzanowski, A. "Polskie towarzystwo onkologiczne. Rys historyczny." *Polski Tygodnik Lekarski,* 21 (August 22, 1966), 1297-1300.

The article provides a brief history of the Polish Oncological Society and its efforts in the areas of public health education and support for clinical research and treatment.

Chrzanowski, A. "Karta z historii onkologii polskiej. Fundacja im. Jakuba hr. Potockiego." *Nowotwory,* 27 (July-September 1977), 255-59.

The article provides a brief history of the Jakuba Potockiego Foundation and its anti-cancer program.

Considine, Bob. *That Many Might Live: Memorial Center's 75-Year Fight Against Cancer*. New York: 1959.

In 1902 the family of Collis P. Huntington, the railroad magnate, bestowed a gift of $100,000 for the establishment of the Collis P. Huntington Fund for Cancer Research at the General Memorial Hospital in New York City. James Ewing, the noted cancer pathologist from Cornell University, became its first director. In 1918 James Douglas of the Phelps-Dodge Corporation donated $600,000, but he insisted that the hospital drop the name "General" from its title and treat only cancer patients. Early research focused on radiotherapy. In 1937 a grant from the Rockefeller Institute permitted the construction of a new hospital at East 67th and 68th Streets in New York City. James Ewing died in 1943 and Cornelius Rhoads became the new director. The institution evolved into the Memorial Sloan-Kettering Cancer Center, one of the premier research and clinical oncology institutions in the world.

Creech, H. J. "Historical Review of the American Association of Cancer Research, Inc., 1941-1978." *Cancer Research*, 39 (June 1979), 1863-90.

The American Association for Cancer Research was established in 1907, with James Ewing serving as its moving force and first president. Between 1907 and 1940, the association published two journals—*The Journal of Cancer Research* and *The American Journal of Cancer*. Beginning in 1941 the association changed the name of its journal to *Cancer Research*, which continues to be a major international journal in oncology. Over the years the association has seen its research focus change from surgical oncology and *en bloc* resection in the early twentieth century to radiotherapy in the 1920s and 1930s, chemotherapy in the 1940s, 1950s, and 1960s, and immunotherapy in the 1970s and 1980s. It also been active in research at the level of molecular biology.

Daillez, L. *Combat contre le cancer*. Paris: 1974. Pp. 252.

Throughout modern medical history French physicians and researchers have played an important role in the struggle to conquer neoplastic disease. In the Middle Ages, Henri de Mondeville (1260-1320) advocated surgery only with clean management of the wound, and Guy de Chauliac (1300-1370) called for wide surgical excision of tumors, application of caustic pastes, and bleeding. Ambroise Paré (1510-1590) also called for wide excision of operable tumors. Claude Gendron (1663-1750) rejected the notion that cancer was a humoral disease and instead approached it as a localized disease which, if excised early and completely, was curable. French surgeons Henri Le Dran (1685-1770) and Jean Louis Petit (1674-1750) advocated mastectomies for breast cancer along with removal of the regional lymph nodes when they were involved.

In the nineteenth century French physicians were prominent in surgery and pathology. Xavier Bichat (1771-1802) and Rene Laennec (1781-1826) both argued that tumors were not systemic in nature but arose from connective tissue.

Joseph Claude Recamier (1774-1852) understood the process of secondary cancers and coined the term "metastasis." Prominent nineteenth century French surgeons included Jacques Lisfranc, Jean F. Reybard, and Edouard Quenu.

In the twentieth century the fight against cancer in Paris has involved the radiological work of Marie and Pierre Curie, the public health crusades of the Ligue Française Contre Le Cancer, the viral theories of Amédée Borrel and Charles C. Oberling, and the endocrinal theories of Antoine Lacassagne.

Denoix, P., ed. *Soixante années de l'Institut Gustave Roussy.* 1982.

(See Chapter 30: Bernoulli).

Dohanany, L. "Anfange der Krebsbekampfung in der Tschecholowakei." In *The International Congress of the History of Medicine,* (1974), 250-54.

(See Chapter 30: Thurzo).

"Dr. Harold P. Rusch and the Wisconsin Clinical Cancer Center." *Wisconsin Medical Journal,* 78 (June 1978), 96-97.

(See Chapter 30: Rusch).

Dukes, C. E. "The Origin and Early History of the Imperial Cancer Research Fund." *Annals of the Royal College of Surgeons of England,* 36 (1965), 1165-69.

In 1902 the Royal College of Physicians of London and the Royal College of Surgeons of England joined hands in establishing the Imperial Cancer Research Fund, an institution devoted to statistical and experimental cancer research. Between 1902 and 1914 the fund was chaired by Dr. E. F. Bashford. He was succeeded by J. A. Murray in 1914, who served until 1935.

Dunn, Thelma, B. "Intramural Research Pioneers, Personalities, and Programs: The Early Years." *Journal of the National Cancer Institute,* 59 (August 1917), 605-16.

The article reviews the first 16 years of the National Cancer Institute in terms of its commitment to basic research. It focuses on the work of Dr. Carl Voegtlin as director of the NCI; Dr. Howard B. Anderson as head of biology (general biology, cytology, genetics, tissue culture, and virology); Dr. Jesse Greenstein in biochemistry; Dr. Murray Shear in chemotherapy; Dr. Egor Lorenz in biophysics; Dr. Harold Stewart in pathology; Dr. Julius White in physiology; and Dr. Roy Hertz in endocrinology.

"The Ellis Fischel State Cancer Hospital." *Cancer Bulletin*, 12 (July-August 1960), 73.

The Ellis Fischel State Cancer Hospital was established in 1940 in Columbia, Missouri, as a cancer treatment center for indigent patients. It evolved into a major cancer center.

Fath, Harold. *A Dream Come True: The Story of St. Jude's Children's Hospital.* 1983.

In the late 1930s a struggling comedian, Amos Jacobs, was distraught and dejected about life. In a prayer to St. Jude, the patron saint of lost causes, he promised to build a memorial for suffering people if he could just have success in his own life. The comedian changed his name to Danny Thomas and had great success. Twenty years after his prayer he donated $250,000 for the construction of St. Jude's Children's Hospital in Memphis, Tennessee. The hospital received its first patient in 1962 and specialized in the treatment of childhood leukemia. Later it evolved into a comprehensive cancer center for children. Throughout the 1980s Danny Thomas retained his connection with and commitment to St. Jude's, sponsoring an on-going fund-raising program to augment research grants from the National Cancer Institute.

"50-lecie zakładu Radiodiagnostyki Instytutu Onkologii im. Marii Sklodowskiej-Curie w Warszawie." *Polski Przeglad Radiologii*, 47 (July-August 1983), 261-62.

The article celebrates the 50th anniversary of the Radiation Department of the Marii Sklodowskiej-Curie Oncological Institute in Warsaw.

The First Twenty-Five Years of the University of Texas M. D. Anderson Hospital and Tumor Institute. Houston: 1964.

In 1941 the state of Texas provided $500,000 for a new cancer hospital within the University of Texas. The M. D. Anderson Foundation provided a matching grant of $500,000 if the hospital was built in Houston. The M. D. Anderson Hospital for Cancer Research of the University of Texas began clinical operations in 1942. Ernest Bertner was appointed the first director, and he was succeeded by R. Lee Clark in 1964.

"Forty Years of the Oncological Institute of Brno." *Neoplasma*, 22 (1975), 565-70.

From its establishment in 1935 the Oncological Institute of Brno, Romania, has evolved into a major cancer research and treatment center.

Frei, Emil. "Intramural Therapeutic Research at the National Cancer Institute, Department of Medicine: 1955-1965." *Cancer Treatment Reports*, 68 (January 1984), 21-30.

(See Chapter 22: Frei).

Gerster, John C. A. "A Tribute to the Founders of the American Society for the Control of Cancer." *Quarterly Review of the American Society for the Control of Cancer*, 8 (1943), 35-36.

(See Chapter 30: Triolo and Shimkin).

Hancock, R. L. "The High River Institute: A Theoretical Approach to Carcinogenesis." *Medical Hypotheses*, 5 (1979), 193-98.

The High River Institute of Alberta, Canada, was established in 1974 by local businessmen to provide a facility for the theoretical investigation of carcinogenesis. The institute functions today largely as a local organization engaged in public health awareness.

Hayward, Oliver S. "The History of Oncology. II. The Society for Investigating Cancer, London." *Surgery*, 58 (September 1965), 586-99.

(See Chapter: Schoenberg).

Heller, J. R. "The National Cancer Institute: A Twenty-Year Retrospect." *Journal of the National Cancer Institute*, 19 (1957), 147-90.

(See Chapter 30: Shimkin).

Holstein, John. *The First Fifty Years of the Jackson Laboratory.* 1979.

The Jackson Memorial Laboratory was founded in 1929 by Dr. Clarence Little at Bar Harbor, Maine. Little had been president of the University of Michigan, but he left in 1929 to build a genetics laboratory for cancer research on Mt. Desert Island at Bar Harbor. He retired in 1956, by which time the Jackson Laboratory had become a major cancer research facility.

Iarmonenko, S. P. "Klinicheskaia radiobiologiia—nauchnaia osnova luchevoi terapiia opukholei." *Meditsinskaia Radiologiia*, 27 (March 1982), 6-9.

(See Chapter 30: Agranat and Starinskii).

"Indian Cancer Research Centre." *Cancer Bulletin*, 12 (May-June 1960), 53.

The Indian Cancer Research Centre began in 1922 in Bombay as the Radium Service. In May 1941 the Tata Memorial Hospital was opened for cancer patients, and the Indian Cancer Research Centre was formally opened in 1952.

"Institut du Cancer, Louvain." *Cancer Bulletin*, 12 (September-October 1960),
    87.

The Institut du Cancer at Louvain, Belgium, was established in 1925 by phi-
lanthropist Ulmar Verdure and evolved into one of Belgium's principal cancer
centers.

"Instituto Nacional de Cancer." *Cancer Bulletin*, 14 (January-February 1962),
    20.

The Instituto Nacional de Cancer was opened in Rio de Janeiro in 1957 with
Antonio Pinto Vieira as director. The Instituto is a major teaching hospital and
research center.

Izsak, S. "L'institut pour l'etude et la prophylaxie du cancer de Cluj (1929),
    premier institut oncologique de roumanie." In *International Congress of the
    History of Medicine*. 1974. Pp. 1563-66.

Since its establishment in 1929 the Oncological Institute at Cluj has evolved
into a major treatment and research center concerning the causes and prevention
of neoplastic disease.

Jasinksi, W. "Działalnośe Instytutu Onkologii im. Marii Sklodowskiej-Curie w
    latach 1961-1972." *Nauka Polska*, 21 (1973), 78-90.

The article provides a brief history of the research and treatment activities of
the Sklodowskiej-Curie Institute in Poland.

Jeney, A. and K. Lapis. "A. Haddow es a Royal Cancer Hospital Chester Beatty
    intezetenek szerepe az 1950-1960—az evek daganat kutatasaban." *Orvosi
    Hetilap*, 126 (May 19, 1985), 1237-38.

(See Chapter 30: Brunning and Dukes).

Jones, Gertrude. *North Carolina History of the American Cancer Society*. Raleigh:
    1966.

From its founding in 1913 as the American Society for the Control of Cancer, the American Cancer Society has been the primary institution in the United
States in advertising public health concerns about cancer and lobbying for increased government funding for clinical, experimental, and research oncology. The
North Carolina branch of the American Cancer Society has functioned since 1938
as part of that larger, nationwide campaign to achieve, ultimately at least, the
elimination of neoplastic disease as a public health threat.

Kapatsinskii, E. V., and E. V. Kozlova. "Rol'moskovskogo Nauchno—issledovatel'skogo onkologicheskogo Instituta im. P. A. Gertsen v razvitii organizatsionnykh osnov onkologii." *Sovietskoi Zdravookhr*, 11 (1981), 50-52.

The P. A. Gertsen Oncological Research Institute in Moscow has played the leading role in providing the organizational direction for Soviet clinical oncology, dividing therapeutics into surgery, radiotherapy, chemotherapy, and immunotherapy sections and clinical stations into gynecology, head and neck, urology, neurology, heart and lung, circulatory, and bone.

Koszarowski, T. "Udział Instytutu Onkologii im. Marii Sklodowskiej-Curie w rozwóju społecznej walki z chorobami nowymi w polsce w latach 1945-1982." *Nowotwory*, 33 (January-March 1983), 7-12.

The article is a brief history of the Marii Sklodowskiej-Curie Oncological Institute in Poland between 1945 and 1982.

Ligue Nationale Française Contre le Cancer. *Cancer, 50 ans de lutte, espoir.* 1968.

In 1918, at the end of World War I, physicians and concerned French citizens established the French National League Against Cancer, a public education group advocating increased research, public health, and clinical treatment programs for cancer. During the past half-century, the League has become one of France's most important anti-cancer and cancer control lobbying organizations.

Little, Clarence C. "The American Society for the Control of Cancer—Past and Future." *Quarterly Review of the American Society for the Control of Cancer*, 8 (1943), 46-52.

(See Chapter 30: Triolo and Shimkin).

McPherson, Howard. *Second North Carolina History of the American Cancer Society*. High Point, N. C.: 1976.

(See Chapter 30: Jones).

"Middlesex Hospital." *Cancer Bulletin*, 11 (May-June 1959), 53.

The first cancer ward in any European hospital was established at Middlesex Hospital in London in 1792. Middlesex Hospital has been opened in 1745. John Howard, a surgeon, was the moving force behind establishment of the ward. There he could provide a service to cancer patients and have more opportunity to study the disease.

Mirand, E. A. *History of the Roswell Park Memorial Institute.* 1981.

(See Chapter 30: Murphy).

Murphy, Gerald P. "Roswell Park Memorial Institute: Genesis of a Cancer Center." *Oncology*, 37 (1980), 426-28.

The Roswell Park Memorial Institute in Buffalo, New York, was established in 1898 by an act of the New York legislature. It was the brainchild of Dr. Roswell Park. Park and its subsequent directors (Harvey Gaylord, 1904-1923; Burton T. Simpson, 1923-1943; William H. Wehr, 1943-1945; Louis Kress, 1945-1952; George Moore, 1952-1967; James T. Grace, 1967-1970; and Gerald P. Murphy, 1970-present) built Roswell Park into one of the premier cancer treatment centers in the world.

Nakahara, Waro. "A Pilgrim's Progress in Cancer Research, 1918 to 1974: An Autobiographical Essay." *Cancer Research*, 34 (1974), 1767-74.

The Japanese Foundation for Cancer Research was established in 1908. The foundation was the major source of research funds in Japan before World War II. American bombers destroyed the foundation building and hospital in Tokyo in 1945. The hospital reopened in 1946 and the research unit in 1953. The Japanese Foundation for Cancer Research became the nucleus of the Japanese National Cancer Center Research Institute and Hospital in 1962. Waro Nakahara served as director from 1953 to 1974.

Negru, I. "Profesorul Iuliu Moldovan creatorul primului instit oncologic in Romania." *Viata Medicina*, 30 (December 1982), 281-86.

(See Chapter 30: "Forty Years of the Oncological Institute of Brno").

Neiman, I. M. "K 50-letiiu sozya i vsesoiuznogo s'ezda onkologov (iz vospominanii uchastnika)." *Voprosy Onkologii*, 27 (1981), 88-89.

The article provides an outline history of the All-Union Oncological Society of the Soviet Union.

"The Netherlands Cancer Institute." *Cancer Bulletin*, 11 (September-October 1959), 85.

The Netherlands Cancer Institute was established in Amsterdam in 1913. Since that time it has evolved into one of the world's most outstanding clinical cancer facilities.

New York City Cancer Committee. *History of the American Society for the Control of Cancer, 1913-1943.* New York: 1913.

(See Chapter 30: Triolo and Shimkin).

"Onkoloski Institut." *Cancer Bulletin,* 11 (November-December 1959), 115.

The Oncological Institute of Ljubljana, in Slovenia, Yugoslavia, was established in 1938.

"The Paterson Laboratories, Manchester, England." *Oncology,* 38 (1981), 59-61.

Dr. Ralston Paterson, a radiation biochemist, and his wife Edith, a radiotherapist, founded the Paterson Laboratory in 1932 in the Manchester suburb of Withington. It was at first a research unit associated with the Christie Hospital and Holt Radium Institute. They retired in 1962. Professor Laszlo Lajthen became the new director.

Petrovskii, B. V., and B. E. Peterson. "Onkologicheskii Institut im. P. A. Gertsen i ego rol' v razvitii otechestvennoi khirurgii i onkologii." *Khirurgiia,* 11 (November 1978), 3-8.

(See Chapter 30: Kapatsinskii).

Peterson, B. E. "75 let moskovskomu mauchno-issledovatel'skomu onkologicheskomu institutu im. P. A. Gertsen i sovetskaia onkologicheskaia doktrina." *Sovetska Meditsin,* 8 (August 1978), 8-12.

(See Chapter 30: Kapatsinskii).

Poelman, J. R. *Het Carcinoid: Bijdrage tot de Klinick van de Carcinoide Tumoren.* Amsterdam: 1973. Pp. 3-12.

(See Chapter 30: "The Netherlands Cancer Institute").

Pozmogov, A. I., V. T. Demin, and L. F. Arendarevskii. "'Kievskomu nauchno—Issledovatel'skomu rentgenoradiologicheskomu i onkologicheskomu insitutut 60 let." *Vestnik Rentgenologii i Radiologii,* 3 (May-June 1980), 78-80.

Since its founding in 1920 the Scientific Radiology and Oncology Institute in Kiev has been a leading center in the Soviet Union for clinical research and treatment in radiotherapy.

"The Princess Margaret Hospital." *Cancer Bulletin*, 14 (September-October 1962), 93.

The Princess Margaret Hospital, part of the Ontario Cancer Institute in Toronto, Canada, was founded in 1958. Only cancer patients with tumors amenable to radiotherapy are admitted to the hospital.

"The Radiumhemmet." *Cancer Bulletin*, 11 (July-August 1959), 72.

The Radiumhemmet was founded in Stockholm in 1910 at the urging of John Berg, Sweden's leading surgeon and founder of the Swedish Anti-Cancer Society. It was a radiotherapy center with 16 beds and a roentgen laboratory. In 1937 the Caroline Hospital became the new home of the Radiumhemmet.

Rauscher, F. J. *The First Five Years of the National Cancer Program.* Bethesda: 1976.

(See Chapter 30: Kalberer and Newell).

Rauscher, Frank J. "The National Cancer Program and the National Cancer Act of 1971." *National Cancer Institute Monographs*, 40 (February 1974), 3-6.

(See Chapter 30: Rettig).

Ravitch, Mark M. *A Century of Surgery: History of the American Surgical Association.* Philadelphia: 1981.

Founded in 1880, the American Surgical Association has played an important role in promoting more effective treatment for cancer—through the *en bloc* resection and adjuvant radiotherapy and chemotherapy—and public health campaigns on the importance of early diagnosis.

Rettig, Richard A. *Cancer Crusade: The Story of the National Cancer Act of 1971.* Princeton: 1977.

A number of medical, political, social, and scientific trends merged in the late 1970s to create an extraordinary public interest in, and fear of, cancer. As the mortality rate from infectious diseases steadily dropped in the twentieth century, the incidence of cancer steadily rose, primarily because people were living longer and becoming subject to carcinogens and genetic damage for longer periods of time. More and more Americans were coming down with cancer or knew someone suffering from the disease. At the same time public faith in science, stimulated by the successes of the space program, reached unprecedented levels. The notion that "if we can put a man on the moon we can find a cure for cancer" became more and more compelling. Finally, there was a political motive for a new emphasis on cancer research. President Richard Nixon was jealous of Senator Ted

Kennedy's high profile on public health issues. Concerned that Kennedy might seek the presidency in 1972, Nixon wanted to upstage him on a major health issue, so in 1970 the president became a major advocate of the legislation which became the National Cancer Act of 1971.

Ross, Walter. *Crusade. The Official History of the American Cancer Society.* 1987.

In 1913 a group of physicians and health volunteers established the American Society for the Control of Cancer as a public education group to increase awareness about cancer. Its first president was George Clark. In 1943 its name was changed to the American Cancer Society. By then it was on its way to becoming one of the largest and most powerful health volunteer and interest groups in the United States.

"Roswell Park Memorial Institute." *Cancer Bulletin*, 13 (November-December 1961), 106.

(See Chapter 30: Murphy).

"The Royal Marsden Hospital." *Cancer Bulletin*, 14 (May-June 1962), 53.

The Free Cancer Hospital was founded in London in 1851 and headed by William Marsden. The present hospital was constructed in 1862. It became known as The Royal Marsden Hospital in 1954. Its associate unit, The Institute of Cancer Research, was established in 1909.

Ruchkovskii, B. S., and L. N. Guslitser. "K 60 letiiu kievskogo obshchestva bor'by so zlokachestvfennymi novoobrazovaniiami." *Vrachebnoe Delo*, 5 (May 1968), 124-25.

Founded in 1908, the Kiev Cancer Society has focused on providing public information and support for clinical research in oncology.

Rusch, Harold P. "The Beginnings of Cancer Research Centers in the United States." *Journal of the National Cancer Institute*, 74 (February 1985), 391-403.

The first center in the United States devoted specifically to cancer research was founded by Dr. Roswell Park in 1898 in Buffalo. It evolved into the Roswell Park Memorial Institute. The article discusses the history of James Ewing and the Memorial Sloan-Kettering Cancer Institute in New York City, the John Collins Warren Laboratories and Huntington Memorial Hospital of Harvard University, the Cancer Research Institute of the New England Deaconess Hospital, the Pondville

Hospital in Massachusetts, Sidney Farber and the Dana-Farber Cancer Institute in Boston, the Crocker Research Laboratory of Columbia University, the Fox-Chase Cancer Center in Pennsylvania, the Barnard Free Skin and Cancer Hospital in St. Louis, the Jackson Laboratory in Maine, the National Cancer Institute in Bethesda, Maryland, the Ellis Fischel State Cancer Hospital in Missouri, the McArdle Memorial Laboratory for Cancer Research at the University of Wisconsin, the M. D. Anderson Hospital and Tumor Institute in Houston, the Michigan Cancer Center, the Kettering-Meyer Laboratory of the Southern Research Institute in Birmingham, Alabama, the Fels Research Institute of Temple University, the Ben May Laboratory of the University of Chicago, and the St. Jude's Children's Research Hospital in Memphis, Tennessee.

Rusch, Harold P. "The First Forty Years of the McArdle Laboratories." *Wisconsin Medical Alumni Quarterly*, 13 (Fall 1973), 2-6.

In 1934 Michael W. McArdle, a wealthy businessman from Chicago, donated the funds for the construction of the McArdle Memorial Laboratory for Cancer Research. It was constructed at the site of the medical school of the University of Wisconsin at Madison. Harold P. Rusch became its first director. With a grant from the National Institutes of Health in 1961, the new McArdle Institute for Cancer Research was constructed. Today the facility has become the University of Wisconsin Cancer Center.

"St. Rose's Free House." *Cancer Bulletin*, 11 (January-February 1959), 31.

St. Rose's Free House for Incurable Cancer was established in New York City in May 1899. It was founded by Rose Lathrop and Alice Huber. It was the first hospital for indigent cancer patients in the United States.

Savitskii, A. I., and A. V. Chaklin. "Istoriia razvitiia vsesoiuznogo obshchestva onkologov." *Voprosy Onkologii*, 13 (1967), 3-13.

(See Chapter 30: Neiman).

Schepartz, Saul A. "Historical Overview of the National Cancer Institute's Fermentation Program." *Recent Results in Cancer Research*, 63 (1978), 30-32.

It was not until after World War II that several scientific discoveries occurred which greatly increased the interest in chemotherapy. First was the well-known accidental discovery of the effects of mustard gas on blood elements that led to nitrogen mustard and opened the entire field of the aklylating agents. Second were the folic acid studies that led to the development of aminopterin and the antimetabolites. Finally, there was the rapid expansion of antibiotic research and the discovery that some antibiotics had tumorcidal effects. The actinomycins were especially potent. Because the only real testing program was going on at the Sloan-Kettering Institute, and its resources were not sufficient to keep up with demand, the National Cancer Institute established the Cancer Chemotherapy National Service Center in 1955. The CCNSC was designed to establish experimental tumors for screening agents submitted by chemists, prepare additional quantities of certain chemical compounds for further testing, development of new synthetic drugs, research into chemical dose formulations, the evaluation of endocrine agents, the implementation of toxicological and pharmacological studies, generate studies on the biochemical mechanisms of active drugs, and development of clinical resources for the testing of old and new agents.

Schepartz, Saul A. "History of the National Cancer Institute and the Plant Screening Program." *Cancer Treatment Reports*, 60 (August 1976), 975-78.

(See Chapter 25: Schepartz).

Schmidt, Benno C. "Five Years Into the National Cancer Program: A Retrospective Perspective—the National Cancer Act of 1971." *Journal of the National Cancer Institute*, 59 (August 1977), 687-92.

Between 1971 and 1976 the budget of the National Cancer Act increased from $180 million to $815 million. Just over 50 percent of the budget was spent on basic research. Fundamental research is the key to the future. The United States has also increased the number of comprehensive cancer centers from three to nineteen.

Schoenberg, Bruce S. "A Program for the Conquest of Cancer: 1802." *Journal of the History of Medicine and Allied Sciences*, 30 (January 1975), 3-22.

The Society for Investigating the Nature and Cure of Cancer, a London group of English and Scottish physicians, was formed in 1801. In 1802 the society produced a series of questions about cancer and distributed them to as many other physicians as possible. The leading members of the society were John Abernathy, Sir Everard Home, John Pearson, Matthew Baillie, Thomas Denman, James Sims, and Robert Willan. The questions they posed involved finding the diagnostic signs of cancer, determining if cancer was contagious or hereditary, whether other diseases can turn into cancer, whether it always spreads, whether climate or nutrition can prevent or cure cancer, whether animals contract cancer, whether lymphatic glands could be affected primarily by cancer, whether certain types of people are immune, and whether there are any natural cures. These questions are still relevant today in the crusade against cancer, and many of them remain unanswered.

Serebrov, A. I., and N. P. Napalkov. "Osnovnye vekhi na puti razvitiia nauchno-prakitcheskogo onkologicheskogo instituta, osnovannogo N. N. Petrovym." *Voprosy Onkologii*, 22 (1976), 106-12.

(See Chapter 30: *Sorok let deyatelnosti Leningradskovo Instituta Onkologii*).

"75 let moskovskomu nauchno-issledovatel'skomu onkologicheskomu institutu im. P. A. Gertsen MZ RSFSR." *Voprosy Onkologii*, 24 (1978), 3-4.

(See Chapter 30: Kapatsinksii).

Shimkin, Michael B. "As Memory Serves—An Informal History of the National Cancer Institute, 1937-1957." *Journal of the National Cancer Institute*, 59 (August 1977), 559-600.

In 1937 Congress passed the National Cancer Act to begin a concerted effort at controlling the disease and seeking an ultimate cure. Funding, however, was limited to $400,000 the first year, and the outbreak of World War II in 1940 did little to increase interest in the scientific campaign. In fact, World War II redirected scientific research in other directions. After the war, however, Vannevar Bush, head of the Office of Scientific Research and Development, transferred his agency's funds to the Public Health Service, and the National Cancer Institute received a boost from the funding. Between 1945 and 1947 NCI research grants increased from $180,000 annually to $4 million. During the 1950s the support of congressmen like Claude Pepper, Lister Hill, and Frank Keefe, as well as the initial successes in the new field of chemotherapy, led to greatly increased funding for the National Cancer Institute. By 1952 NCI funding had reached $12 million a year and in 1957 it was up to more than $80 million. The National Cancer Institute had become one of the most influential sources of scientific research funding in the world.

Shimkin, Michael B. "A View from the Outside: 1963-1977—Historical Note." *Journal of the National Cancer Institute*, 63 (July 1979), 223-39.

The major focus of cancer research over the decades has steadily built on accumulated knowledge. German pathologists, beginning with Johannes Muller in 1838, established that cancer was a cellular aberration. Experimental research began in 1903 with Carl Jensen's work on transplantable tumors in rodents and Peyton Rous's discovery of the chicken sarcoma virus. The carcinogenic phase of cancer research began with Yamagiwa and Ichikawa's work on coal tar and Kennaway's discovery of hydrocarbons. The 1950s was the decade of chemotherapy. In the 1960s the thrust of research was viral oncology, although it failed to establish viruses as the cause of human cancer. In the 1970s research efforts again focused on carcinogens.

Shimkin, Michael B. "Committee on Growth, 1945-1956: Another Noble Experiment." *Cancer Research*, 39 (January 1979), 262-68.

In 1945 the National Research Council formed the Committee on Growth, a body of respected scientists and oncologists, to serve as an advisory body on research to the American Cancer Society. During its 11-year existence, the Committee on Growth recommended $19 million in grants for 2,700 projects. By the 1950s, however, the American Cancer Society and the National Cancer Institute became convinced that a more direct, targeted approach to research had to replace the existing arrangement. The Committee on Growth was discontinued in 1956 as the American Cancer Society began to work more closely with the National Cancer Institute in distributing its research funds.

Shimkin, Michael B. "Epizootiology of Cancer: The Contribution of George W. McCoy and the Abortive Federal Cancer Program of 1910." *Journal of the National Cancer Institute*, 58 (February 1977), 457-59.

George W. McCoy, a leading authority on leprosy and plague, served as director of the Hygienic Laboratory (the forerunner of the National Institutes of Health) between 1915 and 1937. He received his M. D. from the University of Pennsylvania and specialized in public health. While at the Plague Laboratory in San Francisco between 1908 and 1914, McCoy collected data on the occurrence of neoplasms in rats and squirrels in the area. In 1910 McCoy proposed a cancer research program for the Hygienic Laboratory, but the Public Health Service refused to extend a grant of $25,000. Not until 1922 was laboratory research on cancer initiated by the federal government, and not until the creation of the National Cancer Institute in 1937 did it begin in a systematic way.

Shimkin, Michael B. "Eponymic Cancer Institutes in the United States." *Cancer Research*, 39 (June 1979), 2211-14.

1. Monroe Dunaway Anderson (1873-1953): Anderson was a cotton merchant from Tennessee who moved to Houston in 1907. In 1938 he created the M. D. Anderson Foundation, and in 1942 a large philanthropic gift from the foundation to the University of Texas established the M. D. Anderson Hospital and Tumor Institute in Houston, Texas.

2. George D. Barnard (1846-1915): Barnard was a stationary manufacturer who had moved from Massachusetts to St. Louis, Missouri, in 1868. In 1906 he endowed the Barnard Free Skin and Cancer Hospital in St. Louis, which later became part of the Washington University School of Medicine.

3. Eugene C. Eppley (1884-1958): Eppley was a hotel magnate who established the Eppley Foundation in 1948. The Eppley Institute for Research in Cancer was established in 1967 and eventually became part of the University of Nebraska School of Medicine in Omaha.

4. Sidney Farber (1903-1973): Sidney Farber was born in Buffalo, New York, and became a renowned pathologist, pediatric oncologist, and chemotherapist. In 1931 he founded the Children's Cancer Research Foundation in Boston, Massachusetts, and shortly before his death it was renamed the Sidney Farber Cancer Center.

5. Samuel S. Fels (1860-1950): Fels was born in North Carolina and became a prominent soap manufacturer. From his charitable foundation, the Fels Fund, he endowed the Fels Research Institute at Temple University in Philadelphia, Pennsylvania, in 1947.

6. Ellis Fischel (1883-1938): Fischel, a prominent faculty member and cancer specialist at the University of Missouri, died in an automobile accident in 1938, and in honor of his memory the state legislature renamed the state cancer hospital in Columbia after him.

7. Leo Goodwin (1886-1971): Leo Goodwin was born in Missouri and founded the Government Employee Insurance Company. He contributed to the expansion of the Germfree Life Research Center (GLRC) at Tampa, Florida, and in 1972 the GLRC changed its name to the Leo Goodwin Institute for Cancer Research.

8. Hubert H. Humphrey (1911-1978): Humphrey was a prominent liberal Democrat from Minnesota who had served as a United States Senator and Vice-President of the United States. He died of bladder cancer in 1978, and shortly thereafter the Cancer Research Center of Boston University was renamed after him.

9. Fred Hutchinson (1919-1964): Hutchinson was a prominent professional baseball player from Seattle, Washington, who died of lung cancer in 1964. In 1965 the cancer division of the Pacific Northwest Research Foundation was named the Fred Hutchinson Cancer Center.

10. Roscoe Bradbury Jackson (1879-1929): Jackson was born in Michigan and founded the Hudson Motor Company. The Jackson Memorial Laboratory, a cancer genetics center in Bar Harbor, was named after him in 1929 by its founder C. C. Little.

11. J. Erik Jonsson (1901-): Jonsson was born in New York City and became head of Texas Instruments Company in 1951. A founder of the Jonsson Family Foundation, he made generous grants to the University of California at Los Angeles. In 1976 the UCLA Jonsson Comprehensive Cancer Center was so named.

12. Vincent T. Lombardi (1913-1970): Vince Lombardi, the prominent football coach of the Green Bay Packers and the Washington Redskins, died of colon cancer in 1970. The Georgetown Cancer Research Center in Washington, D. C., was named for him in 1974.

13. Ben May (1889-1972): May, a shipping magnate from Mobile, Alabama, endowed the Ben May Laboratory for Cancer Research at the University of Chicago in 1944.

14. Michael W. McArdle (1874-1935): McArdle, a prominent industrialist from Wisconsin, died of cancer in 1935, and his will helped endow the McArdle Memorial Laboratory for Cancer Research at the University of Wisconsin.

15. Samuel Roberts Noble (1853-1917): Noble was a railroad leader and merchant in Ardmore, Oklahoma, and in 1945 his son established the Samuel Roberts Noble Foundation as a memorial to his father. Its biomedical division has specialized in grants for cancer research.

16. Georges Nicholas Papanicolaou (1883-1962): Georges Papanicolaou was an immigrant from Greece who spent his medical career at the Cornell Medical College in New York City where he developed the cytological technique for early diagnosis of cervical cancer. In 1961 he moved to Miami, Florida, to head the newly founded Papanicolaou Cancer Research Center.

17. Roswell Park (1852-1914): Park was a prominent surgeon at the University of Buffalo and founder of its cancer institute. In 1946 the New York State Institute for the Study of Malignant Disease was renamed the Roswell Park Memorial Institute.

18. Claire Zellerbach Saroni (1896-1962): Zellerbach and her husband, lumber and paper magnates, both died of cancer, and in their wills they endowed the Claire Zellerbach Saroni Tumor Institute of Mount Zion Hospital and Medical Center in San Francisco, California.

19. Alfred P. Sloan, Jr. (1875-1966) and Charles F. Kettering (1876-1958): Sloan and Kettering were prominent figures in the development of the General Motors Corporation. With personal grants in 1945, they founded the Sloan-Kettering Institute for Cancer Research, which is now the research branch of the Memorial Sloan-Kettering Cancer Center in New York City.

20. John Keener Wadley (1877-1973): Wadley was a lumber magnate from Arkansas who endowed the Wadley Research Institute and Blood Bank in Dallas, Texas, in 1951. It was later renamed the Wadley Institutes of Molecular Medicine.

21. Earl Whedon (1872-1958): A prominent physician and businessmen, Whedon endowed the Whedon Cancer Foundation in Sheridan, Wyoming, in 1954.

Shimkin, Michael B. "In the Middle: 1954-63—Historical Note." *Journal of the National Cancer Institute*, 62 (May 1979), 1295-1317.

The major accomplishment of the National Cancer Institute between 1954 and 1963 was the irrefutable proof that tobacco smoking causes lung cancer, the creation of the national clinical cancer data collection system, the developmnent of mammography, the establishment of the Cancer Chemotherapy National Service Center, and the role of the American Cancer Society as the political spearhead for the NCI.

Shimkin, Michael B. "Lost Colony: Laboratory of Experimental Oncology, San Francisco, 1947-1954." *Journal of the National Cancer Institute*, 60 (February 1978), 479-88.

The Laboratory of Experimental Oncology was a collaboration effort between the National Cancer Institute and the University of California Medical School at San Francisco. It was founded in 1947 as a fifteen-bed hospital and concentrated on experimental chemotherapy. Eventually the facility admitted 500 patients, all with advanced, disseminated neoplasms. It closed because of budget cuts in 1954.

Shimkin, Michael B. "Thirteen Questions: Some Historical Outlines for Cancer Research." *Journal of the National Cancer Institute*, 19 (1957), 295-328.

(See Chapter 30: Schoenberg).

Skowronski, S. "Komunikat informacyjny, dotyczacy powstania i rozwóju wojewódzkiego ośrodka onkologicnego w Poznaniu." *Nowotwory*, 21 (October-December 1971), 329-30.

The article provides a brief history of the Provincial Oncological Center in Poznan.

Sorok let deyatelnosti Leningradskovo Instituta Onkologii, 1926-1966. 1966.

The Leningrad Institute of Oncology was founded in 1926 by Nikolai Petrov. Between 1926 and 1965 the Institute treated 55,000 patients and conducted a wide variety of basic and applied research.

Stephenson, George W. "The Commission on Cancer: An Historical Review." *Bulletin of the American College of Surgeons*, 64 (September 1979), 7-13.

In 1912 the American Gynecological Society and the American College of Surgeons organized the Commission on Cancer. On behalf of the Commission Dr. Thomas Cullen began writing popular articles in women's magazines about the importance of early detection of cancer. In the 1920s the Commission dedicated its efforts to classifying bone sarcomas. The Commission worked on establishing accreditation criteria for cancer hospitals in the 1930s, and in the 1940s it worked on improving end-result reporting of cancer cases.

Stolk, A. "Antoni Van Leeuwenkoek-Huis." *Acta Unio Internationalis Contra Cancrum*, 8 (1952), 194.

(See Chapter 30: "The Netherlands Cancer Institute").

Supady, J. "Działalność wileńskiego komitetu do zwalczania raka w latach 1931-1936." *Nowotwory*, 29 (May-June 1979), 151-56.

The article provides a brief history of the activities of the Committee for Combating Cancer in Poland between 1931 and 1936.

Supady, J. "Powstanie i działalność stowarzyszenia 'polski instytu przeciwrakowy we lwowie (1929-1939)." *Wiadomosci Lekarskie*, 35 (November 1, 1982), 1301-03.

The article provides a brief history of the establishment of the Polish Anti-Cancer Society in 1929 and its educational and fund-raising activities to 1939.

Taylor, Howard C. "Thirty Years of Cancer Control." *Quarterly Review of the American Society for the Control of Cancer*, 8 (1943), 39-41.

(See Chapter 30: Triolo and Shimkin).

Talbot, T. R., Jr. *History of the Institute for Cancer Research*, 1927-1976. 1977.

Dr. Stanley Reimann, a pathologist in Philadelphia, got department store baron Rodman Wanamaker to donate funds for a research laboratory in 1927. In 1945 it became known as the Institute for Cancer Research. In 1974 the Institute was incorporated as the Fox-Chase Cancer Center in Philadelphia.

"10 let zhurnalu 'Voprosy onkologii'." *Voprosy Onkologii*, 11 (1965), 3-5.

The premier journal of Soviet oncology, *Voprosy Onkologii*, was founded in 1955 and published by the Leningrad Institute of Oncology.

"30 años de actividad do Instituto Nacional de Cancer." *Hospital (Rio de Janeiro)*, 74 (November 1968), 1417-21.

The National Cancer Institute of Brazil was founded in 1938 in Rio de Janeiro and has evolved into a major treatment and research center.

Thurzo, Vladimir. "Cancer Research Institute in Bratislava 1951-1971." *Neoplasma*, 18 (1971), 549-50.

It took Czechoslovakia many years to recover from the ravages of World War II and the political instabilities which led to the Communist Revolution in 1947. In 1951 the Oncological Research Institute was established in Brataslava, and by 1971 it had evolved into one of the two major cancer treatment and research centers in the Czechoslovakia.

Triolo, V. A. "The Institution for Investigating the Nature and Cure of Cancer." *Medical History*, 13 (January 1969), 11-28.

(See Chapter 30: Schoenberg).

Triolo, V. A. and M. B. Shimkin. "The American Cancer Society and Cancer Research. Origins and Organization: 1913-1943." *Cancer Research*, 29 (1969), 1615-40.

In 1913 a group of physicians and non-professional volunteers established the American Society for the Control of Cancer. The American Medical Association and the American College of Surgeons had earlier advocated a public education campaign to inform people about the warning signs of cancer, and in 1913 Frederick L. Hoffman delivered a paper before the American Gynecological Society in which he argued that the incidence of cancer was rising and that a national society should be established to fight the disease. The founding members of the American Society for the Control of Cancer were Edward A. Woods, J. Leonard Levy, Curtis E. Lakeman, Frederick L. Hoffman, Mrs. Robert Mead, Edward Reynolds, and John A. Brashear. Its main purpose was public education. During the 1930s the Society campaigned for an anti-cancer program at the federal level, and in 1937 Congress passed the National Cancer Act. In 1944 the American Society for the Control of Cancer was reorganized and became the American Cancer Society.

Triolo, V. A., and I. L. Riegel. "The American Association for Cancer Research, 1907-1940." *Cancer Research*, 21 (1961), 137-67.

(See Chapter 30: Creech).

Vikol, Jakob. "Twenty-Five Years of Cancer Control in Hungary." In Jakob Vikol and C. R. Sellei. *Orszagos Onkologiai Ontezet. Twenty-five Years in the Fight Against Cancer. Reports of the State Oncological Institute.* 1966. Pp. 9-25.

The State Oncological Institute of Hungary was established in 1941, but because of World War II, its development as a research and clinical cancer center did not really begin until 1947. Since then the State Oncological Institute has evolved into a clinical and research center with branch offices around the country, in addition to the center in Budapest.

Voldman, D. "Guerir du cancer et mourir de vieillesse: Histoire de l'Hospice Paul-Brousse de 1905 a 1975." *Asclepio*, 35 (1983), 317-26.

The Paul-Brousse Hospice was established in Paris in 1905 to treat terminally ill patients and assist them in making their deaths as pain-free as possible. It was one of the earliest hospices established in the world and set the stage for the "quality-of-death" ideas which would become so powerful later in the twentieth century.

Wada, T. "History of Clinical Oncology in Hokkaido in the Last 50 Years." *Hokkaido Journal of Medical Science*, 49 (January 1974), 1-4.

The article describes the development of clinical oncology services, cancer control efforts, and public health education campaigns in Hokkaido, the northernmost of the Japanese islands, since the 1920s.

Weisburger, Elizabeth K. "History of the Bioassay Program of the National Cancer Institute." *Progress in Experimental Tumor Research*, 26 (1983), 187-201.

(See Chapter 7: Weisburger).

Weisburger, Elizabeth K. "History of the Journal of the National Cancer Institute." *Journal of the National Cancer Institute*, 59 (August 1977), 2 Suppl., 601-04.

Between its first issue in August 1940 and the present, the journal has grown from an in-house organ of the National Cancer Institute to an internationally renowned scientific journal.

Yarmechuk, William A. *The Movement to Establish the National Cancer Institute*. Bethesda, Maryland: 1977.

(See Chapter 30: Yarmechuk).

Yarmechuk, William A. "The Origins of the National Cancer Institute." *Journal of the National Cancer Institute*, 59 (August 1977), 551-58.

In 1927 Senator Matthew Neely of West Virginia introduced legislation for a federal reward of $5 million to the individual or group that developed a cure for cancer. In the economy-minded era of the 1920s the proposal did not succeed, nor did his 1928 proposal for a government-funded study by the National Academy of Sciences to develop a scientific crusade against cancer. Little was done about the matter until 1937. By that time the federal government had assumed new social responsibilities and a powerful movement for anti-cancer action by the federal government was being driven by the General Federation of Women's Clubs and the American Society for the Control of Cancer. In 1937 Senator Royal Copeland of New York introduced legislation creating the National Cancer Institute and the bill passed.

Author Index

— G —

— X —

— Y —

Subject Index

— I —

— J —

About the Compiler

JAMES S. OLSON is Professor of History at Sam Houston University, Huntsville, Texas. His earlier works include *Dictionary of the Vietnam War*, *Historical Dictionary of the New Deal: From Inauguration to Preparation for War* (Greenwood Press, 1988, 1985), *Herbert Hoover and the Reconstruction Finance Corporation, 1931-1933*, *The Ethnic Dimension in American History*, *Native Americans in the Twentieth Century*, and numerous articles.